SYSTEMS ANALYSIS
IN HEALTH CARE

SYSTEMS ANALYSIS IN HEALTH CARE

edited by
Vijay Mahajan and
C. Carl Pegels

PRAEGER PUBLISHERS
Praeger Special Studies

New York • London • Sydney • Toronto

Library of Congress Cataloging in Publication Data

Main entry under title:

Systems analysis in health care.

    1. Health services administration--Statistical methods. 2. Health facilities--Administration--Statistical methods. 3. System analysis. I. Mahajan, Vijay. II. Pegels, C. Carl. [DNLM: 1. Delivery of health care. 2. Health of welfare planning. 3. Systems analysis. W84.1 S993]
RA394.S94   658.4'032   78-11193

PRAEGER PUBLISHERS
PRAEGER SPECIAL STUDIES
383 Madison Avenue, New York, N.Y. 10017, U.S.A.

Published in the United States of America in 1979
by Praeger Publishers,
A Division of Holt, Rinehart and Winston, CBS, Inc.

9   038   987654321

© 1979 by Praeger Publishers

All rights reserved

Printed in the United States of America

PREFACE

The health care industry is complex and pervasive in our economy. Because it is comprised of mostly smaller institutions such as hospitals, physician practices, health care centers, nursing homes, laboratories, and state and municipal health departments, it is not always perceived as being as large as it is. However, in 1977, the health care industry consumed about 9 percent of the GNP, had a cost inflation rate higher than the overall economy, and was beset by numerous problems including unaffordable malpractice insurance for some medical specialties, hospitals near bankruptcy, nursing home fraud and poor treatment, medicaid and medicare fraud and overutilization, and numerous other "ills." Although we clearly cannot address all of these areas, we feel we have provided reasonably comprehensive coverage of the health care complex.

The major objectives of this book are (1) to supplement library reading lists with a collection of articles from different periodicals; (2) to provide a course in health care systems analysis with a viable primary text; and, (3) to provide practitioners in the health care field with a reference book on the application of systems analysis in the health care field. By providing an introductory set of readings applicable to the health care field in general, this book can also be used in an introductory course on systems analysis.

In the process of selecting published papers we have placed more emphasis on the quality of the work than on how recently it was published. As a result some of the studies may have been published several years ago. However, the material used is not time-dependent and as a result, this book should be useful and up-to-date for a considerable period of time.

This book has several distinguishing features. It provides an introduction to health care issues in general. The selected systems analysis articles provide a background in multivariate statistics and quantitative methods. Various areas of health care are covered and each selected article discusses an important aspect of health care and shows an application of a specific technique.

Chapter 1 provides an introduction to systems analysis especially as it relates to the health care field and a detailed summarization by chapter of the other 20 chapters. The 20 chapters are divided into three parts: multivariate analysis, management science/operations research, and other systems analysis techniques.

Each chapter contains at least one study on the application of the technique discussed in the chapter. A total of 23 application studies are used in the book.

A brief abstract of the application study or studies forms the introduction to each chapter. This is followed by an introduction and summary of the technique used in the application study. The summary of the technique is then followed by a list of references for further reading.

Chapter 3 deals with physician-related planning activities. It provides an analysis of medical care based on an extensive collection of medical records.

Chapters 5 and 7 are based on hospital and dental utilization. Hospital utilization as a function of average age and average income is discussed in Chapter 5, and dental utilization is discussed in Chapter 7.

In Chapters 2, 6 and 8, hospital classification is discussed. Chapter 2 presents a study of the case mix of 65 hospitals. Urban vs. rural location was determined to be an important determinant. Chapter 6 discusses classification of hospitals on the basis of several variables, while Chapter 8 presents a study of how patients select a hospital.

Chapters 9, 10 and 16 deal with hospital operations planning. Chapter 9 consists of two studies. The first work is a study on bed limitations imposed by a regional planning agency while the second work discusses the development of a severity index for burn patients. Chapter 10 presents a technique for determining surgical unit capacity in a hospital, while Chapter 16 discusses a model for deriving hospital service areas.

Hospital manpower planning is treated in Chapters 11 and 12. In Chapter 11, staff planning in a psychiatric hospital is presented while Chapter 12 is a study of staff planning in a messenger unit in a hospital.

Chapter 13 discusses the problems associated with the planning process of crossmatching blood in a hospital blood bank. Two different crossmatch policies are evaluated.

Chapters 14 and 15 are concerned with regional health planning. Chapter 14 deals with imbalances in the distribution of hospitals in a region and Chapter 15 discusses a technique for assessing community health needs.

The two studies in Chapter 17 are based on public health screening for diseases. The first study deals with the cost effectiveness of pap smear screening, while the second paper discusses a PKU screening program.

Chapters 4 and 18 deal with computers in medicine. Utilization of computers in non-Federal hospitals is discussed in Chapter 4 while Chapter 18 provides a comprehensive survey of computers in health care.

Finally, in Chapters 19, 20 and 21, the budgeting and forecasting process is discussed. A short-term blood inventory forecast model is presented in Chapter 19. Chapter 20 presents a technique for budgeting in hospitals, and forecasting patient tray demand in a hospital food service is discussed in Chapter 21.

We have provided you with a brief survey of the health care application areas covered in the book. Unfortunately the book cannot be totally comprehensive because it would become too lengthy. We have taken the more important areas and selected works that provide a reasonable coverage of the important application areas and also of relevant systems analysis techniques.

In conclusion, we want to thank the authors and publishers of the articles we have used, for their permission to include the respective contributions.

CONTENTS

	Page
PREFACE	v
LIST OF TABLES	xii
LIST OF FIGURES	xix

PART I: MULTIVARIATE ANALYSIS

Chapter

1	INTRODUCTION TO SYSTEMS ANALYSIS	3
2	MULTIPLE REGRESSION	16
	The Extent of Role Differentiation Among Hospitals Judith R. Lave and Lester B. Lave	18
3	FACTOR ANALYSIS	52
	Quality of Medical Care: A Factor Analysis Approach Using Medical Records Carl E. Hopkins, Robert W. Hetherington, and Eleanor M. Parsons	54
4	DISCRIMINANT ANALYSIS	69
	A Discriminant Analysis of Users and Nonusers of Computers in the Hospital Industry Vijay Mahajan and Milton E. F. Schoeman	70
5	CANONICAL CORRELATION ANALYSIS	93
	Hospital Utilization by Characteristic of Industry in Southwestern Ohio Howard Randall Garland	95
	Simple, Multiple, and Canonical Correlations P. Joseph Phillip and Stephen Gibson	115

Chapter		Page
6	CLUSTERING ANALYSIS	124
	Classification of Community Hospitals P. Joseph Phillip and Ramani N. Iyer	126
7	AUTOMATIC INTERACTION DETECTOR ANALYSIS (AIDS)	152
	Prediction of Dental Service Utilization: A Multivariate Approach Thomas T. H. Wan and Ann Stromberg Yates	154
8	CONJOINT MEASUREMENTS	179
	Analytical Approach To Marketing Decisions in Health Care Organizations Yoram Wind and Lawrence K. Spitz	181

PART II: MANAGEMENT SCIENCE/OPERATIONS RESEARCH

9	DECISION THEORY	207
	Use of Decision Theory in Regional Planning Richard M. Grimes, Catherine L. Allen, Ted R. Sparling, and Gerald Weiss	209
	A Decision Theory Approach to Measuring Severity in Illness David H. Gustafson and Donald C. Holloway	217
10	LINEAR PROGRAMMING	232
	The Application of Linear Programming to Decision-Making in Hospitals William L. Dowling	234
11	INTEGER PROGRAMMING	244
	A Staff Allocation Model for Mental Health Facilities Joseph P. Lyons and John P. Young	245

Chapter		Page
12	QUEUEING THEORY	268
	Hospital Manpower Planning by Use of Queueing Theory Ishwar Gupta, Juan Zoreda, and Nathan Kramer	270
13	MARKOV CHAIN APPLICATION	281
	A Comparison of Two Blood Bank Crossmatch Policies C. Carl Pegels and Andrew E. Jelmert	282
14	SIMULATION	296
	Locational Efficiency of Chicago Hospitals: An Experimental Model Richard L. Morrill and Robert Earickson	298

PART III: OTHER SYSTEMS ANALYSIS TECHNIQUES

15	DELPHI METHOD	321
	Delphi Forecasting of Health Care Organization David B. Starkweather, Louis Gelwicks, and Robert Newcomer	322
16	GRAVITY MODEL	340
	A Mathematical Model for Deriving Hospital Service Areas James Meade	342
17	COST EFFECTIVENESS AND COST-BENEFIT ANALYSIS	358
	Cost Effectiveness of Early Detection of Disease Stuart O. Schweitzer	360
	Application of Cost-Benefit Analysis to a PKU Screening Program Kenneth C. Steiner and Harry A. Smith	375

Chapter		Page
18	COMPUTER APPLICATIONS	388
	Overview of Computer Applications in a Variety of Health Care Areas Marion J. Ball and Gary L. Hammon	389
19	INVENTORY CONTROL	422
	Management Control of Blood Through a Short-Term Supply-Demand Forecast System George M. Frankfurter, Kenneth E. Kendall, and C. Carl Pegels	424
20	INPUT-OUTPUT ANALYSIS	438
	Input-Output Analysis and the Hospital Budgeting Process William O. Cleverley	439
21	TIME SERIES ANALYSIS	458
	Forecasting Patient Tray Census for Hospital Food Service Ronald J. Harris and Everett E. Adam, Jr.	460
APPENDIX—Health Care Journals		474
BIBLIOGRAPHY OF ARTICLES		478
ABOUT THE AUTHORS		481

LIST OF TABLES

Table		Page
1.1	System Types, Goals, and Behavior	5
1.2	Summary of Articles, Application Areas, and Techniques	8
2.1	Distribution of Diagnoses: 65 Hospitals, July-December 1968	23
2.2	Incidence of Surgery: 65 Hospitals, July-December 1968	24
2.3	Distribution of Surgical Procedures: 65 Hospitals, July-December 1968	25
2.4	Common Diagnoses: 65 Hospitals, July-December 1968	26
2.5	Common Surgical Procedures: 65 Hospitals, July-December 1968	30
2.6	The Extent of Commonality: 65 Hospitals, July-December 1968	33
2.7	Indexes of Surgical Complexity: 65 Hospitals, July-December 1968	34
2.8	Distribution of Primary Surgical Procedures by Complexity	35
2.9	Coefficients of Variation between Hospitals and within Hospitals	38
2.10	Coefficients of Variation for Selected Variables by Hospital Location	40
2.11	Regressions Explaining Variation in Some Case-Mix Measures	42
3.1	Hypothesized Dimensions and Selected Indicators of Quality of Medical Care Services	56
3.2	Factor Analysis of Content of 11,000 Medical Care Bits	58

Table		Page
3.3	Mean Factor Score, by Plan	62
3.4	Transformed Factor Score Means and Ranks, by Plan	63
4.1	Dictionary of Variables	74
4.2	Simple Correlation between Predictor Variables and Adoption	81
4.3	Intercorrelation Matrix between Predictor Variables which Have Simple Correlation Greater Than .40	81
4.4	Adopters-Nonadopters Discriminant Function Tests	83
4.5	Factor Interactions	83
4.6	Adopters-Nonadopters Discriminant Analysis Results	84
4.7	Adopters-Nonadopters Classification Matrices	86
4.8	Tests on Predictive Power of Discriminant Function	88
5.1	Age, Annual Income, and Use Rates per 1,000 Members, 1965	99
5.2	Simple Regression and Correlation Analyses	117
5.3	Multiple Regression and Correlation Analyses	118
6.1	Variables Initially Selected	133
6.2	Stratification of Hospitals by Number of Beds	134
6.3	Excerpt from Factor Structure Matrix: Stratum I	135
6.4	Subsets of Variables Selected for Cluster Analysis	136
6.5	Means and Coefficients of Variation of 21 Characteristics, by Stratum	137
6.6	Number of Hospitals in Each Cluster and Number of Nonclusterable Isolates, by Stratum	139
6.7	Nonclusterable Isolates in Stratum I	140

Table		Page
6.8	Profiles of Five Selected Nonclusterable Isolates	141
6.9	Generalized Mahalanobis Distances	142
6.10	Coefficients of Variation: First Cluster in Each Stratum vs. Randomly Selected Group of Same Size within Same Stratum	143
6.11	Classification Matrix for Stratum I	145
6.12	Performance of Discriminant Functions	146
7.1	Annual Average Number of Dental Visits per Person per Household ($\bar{Y}$) for Seven Independent Variables in Automatic Interaction Detector (AID) Analysis	163
7.2	Relative Importance of Seven Social and Demographic Variables in Predicting Dental Visits of 2,168 Households: AID Analysis	165
7.3	Multiple Classification Analysis of Dental Services Utilization for 2,168 Households	166
7.4	Multiple Regression Analysis of Dental Services Utilization for Total and Subgroups	170
7.5	Significant Predictors of Dental Services Utilization in the Total Sample and in Subgroups, Identified by Multiple Regression Analysis	173
8.1	Sample Composition	185
8.2	Stimulus Set	186
8.3	Fractional Factorial Design for 3^6 Stimulus Set	187
8.4	Illustrative Stimulus Card	188
8.5	Summary of Multivariate Analysis of Variance	192
8.6	Characteristics (and Their Associated Utilities) of "Best" Hospital for Two Respondents Groups	195

Table		Page
8.7	Comparison of Actual Evaluation of New Hypothetical Hospitals with Predicted Evaluation Based on Additive Conjoint Measurement Results	196
8.8	Illustrative Set of Multi-attribute Decision Problems of Various Health-Care Organizations	198
9.1	Sample Decision Matrix	210
9.2	Decision Matrix for Houston Service Area under Four Decision Alternatives	212
9.3	Expected Values for Various Decision Alternatives Using Bayes' Procedure	214
9.4	Expected Values for Various Decision Alternatives Using Unequal Probabilities	215
9.5	Criteria Used to Measure Burn Severity	222
9.6	Sample Calculation of Burn Severity	224
9.7	Comparison of Severity Index Model to Probit Analysis Model Using Selected Patients	226
9.8	Relationship between Survival Rates and Severity Index Ratings	228
11.1	Normalized Appropriateness Indexes, by Personnel Type and Therapeutic Activity	250
11.2	Analysis of Variance Comparing Raters, Therapists, and Therapies	251
11.3	Distribution of Time Spent in Noninterchangeable Activities, by Personnel Type	255
11.4	Total Number of Hours of Planned Therapeutic Activities per Month	256
11.5	Average Monthly Salary, by Personnel Type	257

Table		Page
11.6	Allocation of Planned Therapeutic Activities among Personnel Types on the Basis of 1974 Personnel Mix and Total Hours of Planned Therapeutic Activities Listed in Table 11.4	258
11.7	Allocation of Planned Therapeutic Activities among Personnel Types on the Basis of Modified Staff Mix and Total Hours of Planned Therapeutic Activities Listed in Table 11.4	260
11.8	Allocation of Planned Therapeutic Activities among Personnel Types in Expanded Tricounty Unit on the Basis of Available Staff	262
11.9	Allocation of Planned Therapeutic Activities among Personnel Types in Expanded Tricounty Unit on the Basis of "Ideal" Staff Mix	263
12.1	Distribution of Calls Grouped by Service Time Required	272
12.2	Observed and Theoretical Frequency Distributions of Calls per Mean Service Time	274
12.3	Expected Queue Length with Various Numbers of Messengers	277
12.4	Hourly Cost of Various Staffing Levels at Two Different Ratios of Waiting Cost (C_2) to Service Cost (C_1)	277
13.1	Input Probability Matrix—Common Policy	287
13.2	Output Matrix—Common Policy	287
13.3	A Typical Blood Demand Schedule	289
13.4	Input Probability Matrix—Modified Policy	290
13.5	Output Matrix—Modified Policy	291
13.6	Comparison of the Two Policies	292
13.7	Transfusion as a Function of Outdating before First Assignment	292

Table		Page
13.8	Probability of Outdating as a Function of Demand Distribution and the Ability of Blood Bank Managers to Estimate the Probability of Transfusion	293
13.9	Sensitivity of Reduction in Outdating of Modified Policy over Common Policy in Percentage Points	294
13.10	Percentage Outdating as a Function of the Mean Value of s	294
15.1	Predominating Health Service Organization Patterns	329
15.2	Predominating Methods of Medical Care Reimbursement	330
15.3	Predominating Methods of Consumer Medical Care Financing	333
15.4	Medical Service Organizational Patterns and Their Effect on Hospitals	334
16.1	Percentage of Patient Flow from Hospital to Nonhospital Areas	344
16.2	Selected Hospital Service Areas and Population	348
17.1	Age and Sex Distribution of Mentally Retarded Patients in Mississippi Mental Institutions in 1967	379
17.2	Summary of Direct Costs for Institutionalized Mentally Retarded Patients	380
17.3	Adjusted Present Value of Lifetime Earnings for Males: Amount Discounted at 4 Percent, Adjusted to 1967 Dollars and for Mississippi, by Age	381
17.4	Adjusted Present Value of Lifetime Earnings for Females: Amount Discounted at 4 Percent, Adjusted to 1967 Dollars and for Mississippi, by Age	382
17.5	Total Costs for Institutionalized PKU Patients in 1967	383
17.6	Retrospective Analysis of Program Costs	383

Table		Page
17.7	Program Costs for Live Birth Data	385
19.1	Collections Forecast	428
19.2	Partial Output of the Forecast Model	430
19.3	Comparison of Forecasted and Resultant Inventory Levels	434
20.1	Output Measures for Hospital Departments	442
20.2	Projected Dollar Cost per Unit	447
20.3	Charge/Cost Ratios for Selected Departments	448
20.4	Differences between Hospital Budget and I-O Budget in Cost per Unit	450
20.5	Comparison of Labor Budget Accuracy	453
20.6	Association of Labor Budget Variances	455
21.1	Daily Patient Tray Census, March 1971	466
21.2	Daily Patient Tray Census, June 12, 1972 to August 13, 1972	466
21.3	Error Measure Values Resulting from Selected Model Parameters	468
21.4	Error Measure Values over 31 Daily Forecasts by Five Computer Models	469
21.5	Error Measure Values over 61 Daily Forecasts by Four Computer Models and the Manual Estimate	469
A.1	Health Care Journals	474

LIST OF FIGURES

Figure		Page
1.1	Relationships among Systems	6
4.1	Factor Interactions	79
5.1	Age and Total Inpatient Incident Rate	101
5.2	Age and Surgical Incident Rate	101
5.3	Age and Medical Incident Rate	102
5.4	Age and Maternity Incident Rate	102
5.5	Income and Total Inpatient Incident Rate	106
5.6	Income and Surgical Incident Rate	106
5.7	Income and Medical Incident Rate	107
5.8	Income and Maternity Incident Rate	107
5.9	Income and Outpatient Incident Rate	108
7.1	A Schematic Model of Dental Services Utilization with Examples of Operational Specifications	156
7.2	Predictor Tree for Analysis of Dental Visits	164
8.1	Utility Scores for the Six Hospital Characteristics under the Two Scenarios: Total Sample	190
8.2	Utility Scores for the Six Hospital Characteristics under Scenario 1: Hospitalized vs. Nonhospitalized Group	193
9.1	Relative Contribution of Size of Burn to Severity of Full-Thickness Burn, As Independently Conceptualized by Four Physicians	220
9.2	Relative Contribution of Size of Burn to Severity of Partial-Thickness Burn, As Independent Conceptualized by Four Physicians	220

Figure		Page
9.3	Relative Contribution of Age to Severity of Burn, As Independently Conceptualized by Four Physicians	220
9.4	Relationship between Severity Index Scores and Percent Chance of Death According to Probit Analysis Model	225
12.1	The Queueing System: One Line, Multiple Servers in Parallel	271
12.2	Distribution of Service Times	273
12.3	Probability of Waiting Times Longer than t at Different Staffing Levels	276
14.1	Flow Chart of Model Process	303
14.2	Changes in Cluster Size and Patient Travel Resulting from Shifting Physicians	307
14.3	Changes in Patient Load and Patient Travel Resulting from Shifting Demand on Physicians	308
14.4	Changes in Bed Complement of Selected Chicago Area Hospitals Resulting from Shifting Capacity to Charity, Negro, and Other Patients	310
14.5	Changes in Charity, Negro, and Other Patient Travel in Selected Chicago Areas Resulting from Shifting Hospital Capacity	311
14.6	Changes in Patient Travel with Existing Distribution of Hospital Capacity when Race and Income Barriers are Removed	312
16.1	Location of Hospitals and Patient Supply Centers in Southwest Idaho, 1973	345
16.2	Hospital Service Areas in Idaho As Derived from Raw Data of an Idaho Hospital Association Patient-Origin Survey	347

Figure		Page
16.3	Hospital Service Areas in Idaho As Derived from Results of a Gravity Model	354
16.4	Comparison of Hospital Service Areas in Idaho	355
16.5	Service Area Nonalignment	356
17.1	Simple Decision Tree	363
17.2	Decision Tree with Test Errors	364
17.3	Decision Tree for Cervical Cancer Diagnosis Strategy	368
21.1	Observed Daily Patient Tray Count (▲), Adaptive Exponential-Smoothing Forecast (●), and Moving-Average Regression Forecast (■): 31 Days	470
21.2	Observed Daily Patient Tray Count (▲), Adaptive Exponential-Smoothing Forecast (●), and "Manual" Intuitive Forecast (■): 61 Days	470

PART I

MULTIVARIATE ANALYSIS

1

INTRODUCTION TO SYSTEMS ANALYSIS

INTRODUCTION

Systems analysis in health care is by its most simple definition an organized approach to analyze and study health care delivery services. Simple definitions do not always clarify completely what one intends to convey. Therefore, we shall discuss in some detail "systems," "systems analysis," "systems approach," "systems study," and "organizational and cybernetic systems."

Although numerous systems analysis studies in the health care field have been published in professional journals, as many or more systems analysis studies that are performed by practitioners never get published. However, published operations research studies, which usually are conceived by someone's desire to apply a technique to a hypothetical problem, appear much more frequently in print. Because of the above, the casual observer may feel that operations research is the technique to use in the health care field. The contrary is true. Most health services problems lend themselves much more to the systems study approach. In the next section we shall attempt to show how systems analysis is a most useful approach to study health care delivery services.

Systems

The word "systems" is an overused word that can be applied to a variety of situations. Since we use it in this chapter we shall attempt to define it. The word "systems" has been defined by a variety of authors, each for his own purposes and each with a slightly different meaning. The differences are, however, slight, and a common definition that can be developed is, "a system is a set of common related elements." The term "elements" tends to be used interchangeably with variables, objects, functions, activities, parts and subsystems but the central concept of relationship is always present.

To differentiate a system from an aggregation, one can define a set of common related elements as a system and the set of just the elements as an aggregation. Hence, we can also define a system as an organized aggregation. Systems and aggregations are also analogous to permutations and combinations. A system is more like a permutation whereas an aggregation is more like a combination.

A system can best be illustrated by a mechanical parallel with an internal combustion engine. Unless all parts (or elements) are assembled (or arranged) properly the engine (system) will not function at all or will not function satisfactorily.

In summary then, a system is a set of elements arranged in a certain way so that a desired function can be performed.

Organizational Systems

As was pointed out before, the word "systems" is overused but it also applies to many areas. There are at least three types of systems: engineered, organismic, and organizational. The engineered systems are products of technology and are of the electrical-electronic-mechanical variety. The internal combustion engine was one example. Other examples are computers, radios, refrigerators, etc. Organismic or biological systems are products of nature. Man is just one example of them. Organizational systems are the ones of concern in this book. See Table 1.1 for a variation of an analysis of systems as proposed by Cumming [1976, p. 139].

Of the three types of systems the engineered systems are clearly the most rigidly programmed. An engineered system performs the function for which it is designed and must function within those constraints. A biological system is also quite rigidly programmed but variations in input do not necessarily immobilize it. It is quite adaptive to changes in input and will adjust itself to continue to provide the desired output. For instance, an animal can be put on half rations and will continue to function for a long time. On the other hand cutting the voltage to an electrical device such as an electric motor by 20 percent will certainly immobilize it and may actually destroy it. This does not imply that engineered systems cannot be designed to be more adaptive. They can. However, seldom can an engineered system be as adaptive as a biological system.

Organizational systems can take the same or different inputs and by the same or rearranged process elements, may produce the same or different outputs depending on system objectives. Hence, organizational systems are the most adaptive and can continue to

TABLE 1.1

System Types, Goals, and Behavior

	System Type		
	Engineered	Organismic	Organizational
Inputs	Programmed	Given/Variable	Variable
Process (means)	Fixed	Program varied	Inventive
Output	Fixed	Fixed	Variable
Goal level choice	None	None	Ideal
Behavior	Deterministic	Purposive	Stochastic/ Purposeful
Environment	Closed	Open	Open

function, albeit sometimes less than optimally, under severely adverse conditions. Organizational systems can also be viewed as supersystems in the sense that they have as main ingredients organismic systems, humans, but also engineered systems such as computers, hospital beds, automobiles, etc., as components of the system.

Before leaving the discussion of systems we want to show graphically how systems relate to each other. Figure 1.1 shows that relationship. Note that we have added the parents or ancestors of the organismic system to complete the picture.

Systems Study Terminology

The most logical term to give to the study of a system is "systems study." This term is used but more common terms are "systems analysis" and "systems approach." All three terms can be viewed as synonymous.

Quade defined systems analysis as, [1970, p. 4] ". . . an inquiry to aid a decision maker choose a course of action by systematically investigating his proper objectives, comparing quantitatively where possible the costs, effectiveness, and risks associated with the alternative policies or strategies for achieving them, and formulating additional alternatives if those examined are found wanting."

FIGURE 1.1

Relationships among Systems

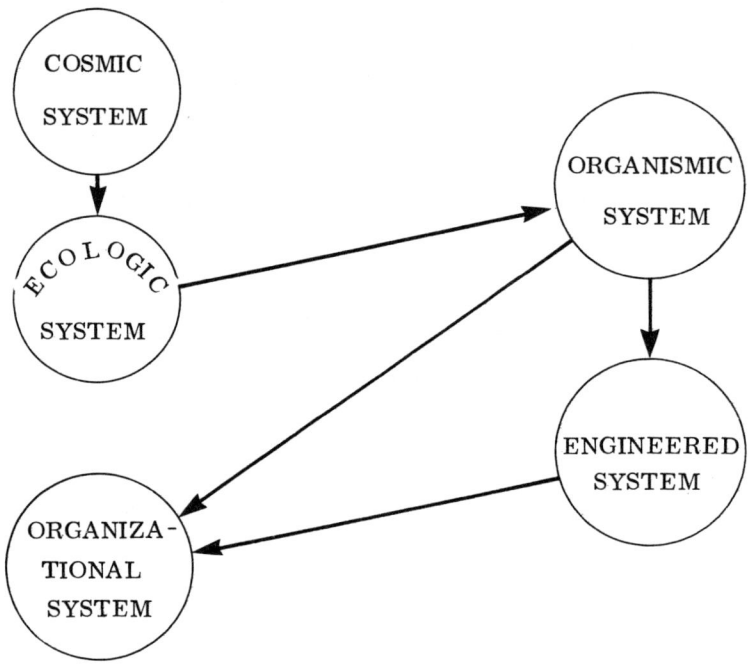

Ackoff (1973, p. 661), an authority on systems, prefers the term "systems approach." He also draws a fundamental distinction between analytic and systems modes of thought. He points out that analytic thinking involves reductionism, taking apart what is to be explained (the whole) and then explaining the whole in terms of its parts. By contrast, the study of systems problems requires the synthetic mode of thought, that is, to view what is to be explained (the part or element) in terms of its role or function in the larger system.

A relationship between systems analysis and operations research exists but needs explanation. Quade, [1970, p. 7] explains it not so briefly as, ". . . systems analysis is associated with that class of problems where the difficulty lies in deciding what ought to be done—not simply how to do it—and honors go to people who have the ability or good fortune simply to find out what the problem is. The total analysis is thus likely to be a more complex and a less neat and tidy procedure, one seldom suitable for quantitative optimization. In fact the process is to a large extent synthesis: The environment will have to be forecast, the alternatives designed, and the operational laws invented. Thus, with systems analysis, one associates 'broad,' 'long range,' 'high level,' 'choice of objectives' problems, and 'choice of strategy,' 'judgment,' 'qualitative,' and 'assistance to logical thinking.' In contrast with operations research one associates 'lower level,' 'overall maximization,' 'mensuration,' 'quantitative,' 'means to an end,' and the 'optimal solution.'"

Health Services System as a Cybernetic System

Navarro [1969, p. 179] has attempted to explain how the word "system" applied to health services should be viewed. He points out that the term system gives the impression of referring to a tight set of relationships that are fully deterministic, predictable or controllable. The above definition implies the existence of an organized, coordinated, planned undertaking which surely is not true of health services as a cybernetic system consisting of many components, being subject to many random uncontrollable influences. The models of a cybernetic system are mainly probabilistic rather than deterministic and they not only deal with probabilities but also with "black boxes" which indicate areas of ignorance and assumptions.

The deterministic view of a system emanates largely from the engineered system and the probabilistic or cybernetic system is analogous to the organizational system discussed before.

When thinking in terms of systems analysis in the health field, be aware that at all times you are working on a subsystem of the whole. Organizational systems, as opposed to engineered systems, have boundaries that are difficult to define and that part of the system must be identified or delineated, in order to be analyzed.

Systems Analysis Techniques in Health Care

Although we have argued in the previous pages that there is a difference between systems analysis and operations research, the

TABLE 1.2

Summary of Articles, Application Areas, and Techniques

Chapter	Article Title(s)	Setting or Application Area	Technique or Model	Major Analysis
		Part I: Multivariate Analysis		
2	The Extent of Role Differentiation Among Hospitals	Hospitals	Multiple Regressions	The case-mix variation defined by five measures based on diagnosis and surgical procedures is analyzed in terms of institutional, demographic, and locational variables.
3	Quality of Medical Care: A Factor Analysis Approach Using Medical Records	Medical Records	Factor Analysis	Analysis of medical records yields four important factors named prevention, rationality, verification, and continuity of medical care.

4	A Discriminant Analysis of Users and Nonusers of Computers in the Hospital Industry	Nonfederal Hospitals	Discriminant Analysis	Profiles of users and non-users of computers are developed in terms of hospital, hospital environment, and hospital administrator's characteristics.
5 a.	Hospital Utilization by Characteristics of Industry in Southwestern Ohio	Hospitals	Canonical, Correlation/ Regression Analysis	Demand for surgical, maternity, and outpatient services across ten employee groups is analyzed in terms of their average age and average income.
b.	Simple, Multiple and Canonical Correlations			
6	Classification of Community Hospitals	Community Hospitals	Clustering Analysis	A classification of hospitals is developed in terms of the hospital and its environmental characteristics.
7	Prediction of Dental Service Utilization: A Multivariate Approach	Dental care delivery planning	Automatic Interaction Detector Analysis	The utilization of dental services is analyzed in terms of three dimensions: Need for care, predisposing factors (social, demographic, and

(continued)

Table 1.2 (continued)

Chapter	Article Title(s)	Setting or Application Area	Technique or Model	Major Analysis
				psychological factors), and enabling factors (family or individual resources, characteristics of the dental care system).
8	Analytical Approach to Marketing Decisions in Health Care Organizations	Hospital Selection Process	Conjoint Measurement	Conjoint measurement is used for the analysis of hospital selection by patients. Six basic factors were selected as important predictors in the selection decision.

Part II: Management Science/Operations Research

Chapter	Article Title(s)	Setting or Application Area	Technique or Model	Major Analysis
9 a.	Use of Decision Theory in Regional Planning	Health care planning	Decision analysis	The impact of basing the bed limitation in a planning area is analyzed in terms of four extrapolations of bed usage rates.

10

b.	A Decision Theory Approach to Measure Severity in Illness	Burn Care units	Multi-attribute utility model	An index for illness severity in a burn care unit is developed by using multi-attribute utility model.
10	The Application of Linear Programming to Decision Making in Hospitals	Hospitals	Linear Programming (L.P.)	L.P. is used to determine the maximum number of surgical patients that can be admitted and treated in a hospital given fixed capacities of resources to produce the services.
11	A Staff Allocation Model for Mental Health Facilities	Mental hospital	Integer programming	A model which could provide an optimal mix of personnel to be employed in a psychiatric hospital is described.
12	Hospital Manpower Planning by Use of Queueing Theory	Messenger unit in a hospital	Waiting line Model	A model is developed and applied to determine the size of a staff in a hospital messenger unit.
13	A comparison of two Blood Bank Crossmatch policies	Blood Bank Management	Markov Chains	The absorbing Markov Chain Model is used to evaluate two blood crossmatch policies.

(continued)

Table 1.2 (continued)

Chapter	Article Title(s)	Setting or Application Area	Technique or Model	Major Analysis
14	Locational Efficiency of Chicago Hospitals: An Experimental Model	Regional Planning	Simulation	An experimental simulation model is described by which imbalances in the distribution of hospitals may be evaluated.

Part III: Other Systems Analysis Techniques

Chapter	Article Title(s)	Setting or Application Area	Technique or Model	Major Analysis
15	Delphi Forecasting of Health Care Organization	Health Planning Area	Delphi Method	Assessment of community health needs by using Delphi Method.
16	A Mathematical Model for Deriving Hospital Service Areas	Spatial Distribution of Patients	Gravity Model	A model is developed and applied to replicate patient flow around medical centers.
17 a.	Cost effectiveness of early detection of disease	Preventive Health Care Planning	Decision Trees	A methodological framework for the cost-effectiveness evaluation of diagnostic tests (Pap test) for mass screening is developed and applied.

b.	Application of Cost Benefit Analysis to PKU Screening Program	Preventive Health Care Planning	Cost Benefit Approach	Cost benefit approach is used to determine the parameters of a screening program.
18	Overview of Computer Applications in a Variety of Health Care Areas	Health Care Management Information Systems	Computer Application	Clinical and communication applications of computers in medicine, with a detailed state-of-the-art description on radiology systems as well as the entire area of finance and management are presented.
19	Management Control of Blood through a short-term supply-demand forecast system	Blood inventory control	Management Control	Design, development, implementation and operation of a short-term blood inventory system are described.
20	Input-output Analysis and Hospital Budgeting Process	Hospital	Input-output analysis	Input-output model is used for budgeting in hospitals.
21	Forecasting Patient Tray Census for Hospital Food Service	Hospital Food Service	Time Series Analysis	Five computer-based time series models that forecast patient tray demand in a medical center food service are compared.

foundations of systems analysis lie in the techniques that are used in systems analysis and many of these techniques are operations research oriented. However, systems analysis uses many other techniques that have an orientation toward multivariate analysis, decision analysis, cost analysis, planning, control, management information systems and other computer-based methods.

In the balance of this book we shall discuss, and illustrate with published reference articles, how systems analysis techniques are applied to study health care delivery systems.

The published references are organized into three sections. The first section deals with the application of multivariate analysis techniques; the second section contains articles describing the use of management science/operations research in various health situations, and the last section provides examples of other techniques which have been used to analyze health systems.

Table 1.2 contains a listing of all the references by title only. For each reference we have shown the setting/application area, technique/model and the major analysis conducted. Although the references have been organized by techniques, the reader may want to follow the references by setting or by the major analysis conducted in the articles. It may be emphasized at this point that the selection of these articles is by no means comprehensive and each article has been selected to merely illustrate an application of a specific systems analysis technique in a specific health care situation.

The first part, Multivariate Analysis, contains eight articles. These articles show applications of multiple regression, factor analysis, discriminant analysis, canonical correlation analysis, clustering analysis, automatic interaction detector program (AIDS), and conjoint measurements. The settings or application areas are hospitals, primary care physicians, medical records, hospital administrators and planners, regional health planning, and dental care needs of a planning area.

The second part, Management Science/Operations Research, contains seven readings on the application of management science/operations research. Included are applications of decision analysis and multiattribute utility models, linear programming, integer programming, queueing models, Markov Chains and simulation. The settings or application areas are health care planning, burn care unit, community hospital, mental hospital, blood bank and regional planning.

The final part, Other Systems Analysis Techniques, contains eight articles. The techniques used include the Delphi method, gravity model, cost-benefit models, decision trees, computer applications, management control, input-output analysis and time series model. The settings or application areas include health planning, patients, hospitals, preventive health care, blood services, and health care organizations.

Conclusions

In this introductory chapter we have attempted to provide a brief overview of systems and systems analysis which was followed by a description of the approach to be used in the remainder of the book.

We have used articles from health care and other journals which are systems analysis oriented. There are, however, many other health care journals in print and we urge the reader to familiarize himself or herself with these journals. In the Appendix we have provided a listing of these journals including the publishing organization, the main target audience, and a description of the contents.

REFERENCES

Ackoff, R. L., "Science in the Systems Age: Beyond IE, OR and MS." Operations Research 21 (May-June 1973):661-71.

Cumming, P. D., National Blood Policy and the American Blood Commission: A Systems Study, Ph.D. Dissertation, State University of New York at Buffalo, 1976.

Quade, E. S., Analysis for Military Decisions. Amsterdam: North Holland, 1970.

Navarro, V., "Systems Analysis in the Health Field," Socio-Economic Planning Sciences 3 (October 1969):179-89.

2

MULTIPLE REGRESSION

INTRODUCTION

Various statistical techniques are employed to measure case-mix of a group of 65 hospitals in the geographic area, as a step toward defining a measure of hospital output. Patients from the hospitals were aggregated into 17 diagnostic groupings. Based on the incidence of surgery, of secondary diagnosis, and of the estimates of the extent of common diagnostic and surgical procedures, an index of surgical complexity was derived. The mean, coefficient of variation and range of the surgical complexity indices were calculated. The results show that there is a considerable amount of variation among hospitals in the type of patients they treat. The coefficients of variation of the complexity indices were then compared across hospitals at a point in time as well as with 19 hospitals over a period of three years. The results show that the case mix within a particular hospital over a short period of time is relatively stable, whereas there is a much greater variation in case mix across hospitals. A similar methodology was employed to compare urban with rural hospitals. Finally, a series of regressions were performed to relate case mix to various institutional characteristics. The results reveal that such characteristics explained only about 25 to 45 percent of the variation in the case-mix measure.

Introduction to Technique

Multiple regression is concerned with the derivation of a model with which to relate quantitatively, the variation of a dependent variable Y with the variations of various independent variables (X_1, X_2, ..., X_k) as in:

$$Y = f(X_1, X_2, ..., X_k)$$

The functional linear form can be expressed as,

$$\hat{Y}_t = a_0 + a_1 X_{1t} + a_2 X_{2t} + \cdots + a_k X_{kt} + U_t$$

where $\hat{Y}_t$ is the dependent variable,

X_{it} are the independent variables, for all i,

a_i are the regression coefficients

and U_t is the disturbance or error term.

The regression coefficients, a_i, can be estimated by the Ordinary Least Squares Method, which states that the sum of the squares of the distances from the points to the line or plane should be minimized. That is, if

$$\sum (Y_t - \hat{Y}_t)^2 = f(a_0, a_1, \ldots, a_k)$$

where $\hat{Y}_t$ is the estimator for Y_t, and if we set

$$\frac{\partial f(a_0, a_1, \ldots, a_k)}{\partial a_i} = 0$$

for i = 0, 1, 2, ..., k, then we have k + 1 equations with k + 1 unknowns, and hence the coefficients can be determined.

The coefficient of determination, R^2, indicates the variance in the dependent variable explained by the regression. The significance of the regression coefficients can be tested by appropriate tests such as F-test.

REFERENCES

Cooley, W. W., and P. R. Lohnes, Multivariate Data Analysis. New York: Macmillan, 1971.

Draper, N. R., and H. Smith, Applied Regression Analysis. New York: Wiley, 1966.

Huang, D., Regression and Econometric Methods. New York: Wiley, 1970.

Nie, N., C. Hull, J. Jenkins, B. D. Steinbrenner, and J. Kim, SPSS: A Statistical Package for the Social Sciences. New York: McGraw-Hill, 1975.

Anderson, J. G., "A Social Systems Model of Hospital Utilization," Health Services Research 11 (Fall 1976):271-87.

Ernst, Richard, "Ancillary Production and the Size of Physician's Practice," Inquiry 13 (December 1976): 371-81.

Kaplan, S., "Analysis and Control of Nurse Staffing," Health Service Research 10 (Fall 1975): 278-85.

Lorant, J. H., and L. J. Kimbell, "Determinants of Output in Group and Solo Medical Practice," Health Services Research 2 (Spring 1976):6-20.

Worthington, P. N., "Prospective Reimbursement of Hospital to Promote Efficiency," Inquiry 13 (September 1976): 300-08.

Van Der Gaag, J., F. F. Rutten, and B. M. Van Praag, "Determinants of Hospital Utilization in the Netherlands," Health Services Research 10 (Fall 1975): 264-67.

THE EXTENT OF ROLE DIFFERENTIATION AMONG HOSPITALS

Judith R. Lave
and
Lester B. Lave

The case mix of 65 western Pennsylvania hospitals is studied from Hospital Utilization Project data comprising

---

Supported by PHS Grant No. R01 HS 00069 HSR from the National Center for Health Services Research and Development. Reprinted with permission from Health Services Research 6, No. 1, Spring 1971. Copyright 1971 by the Hospital Research and Educational Trust, 840 North Lakeshore Drive, Chicago, Illinois 60611.

The authors wish to thank Blue Cross of Western Pennsylvania and the Hospital Utilization Project for their data and cooperation. Robert Sigmond originally raised the question studied here: How a quarter of a million patient records, and five measures are constructed to describe the inpatient population on the basis of diagnoses and surgical procedures. The case-mix variation defined by these measures is then analyzed in a series of regressions on selected institutional characteristics and on demographic and locational variables, revealing urban vs. rural location to be an important determinant. While size, number of facilities and services, and teaching status of a hospital are shown to be correlated with case mix, they are found to explain too small a portion of the variation to be satisfactory surrogates for case mix.

It is commonly assumed that the case mix of hospitals reflects the wide diversity they reveal in size, control, facilities, and programs, so that the case mix of, for example, a teaching hospital will represent a much more serious and complex set of medical problems than, say, that of a small rural hospital. The quantitative aspects of the difference, however—how much the case mix varies across different types of hospitals—has not been investigated, and it is to this question, and an analysis of the factors in the variation, that the present article is addressed.

Using a number of measures constructed to describe the inpatient population in terms of the presenting diseases, the article attempts to answer the following questions:

1. For what reasons are people hospitalized?
2. How much specialization is there among hospitals in the types of patients they treat?
3. Is a hospital's case mix stable over short periods of time?
4. Is there more specialization among urban than among rural hospitals, in accordance with the economic principle that specialization is limited by the extent of the market?
5. Does the specialization follow differences in facilities and teaching programs—that is, do hospitals with expensive specialized facilities and large teaching programs handle a more complicated, less common set of medical problems than other hospitals?

---

different is the inpatient population in different hospitals? Thomas Fitzpatrick, Joseph Newhouse, and Lester Silverman offered comments and criticisms on an earlier draft of the article; and Lester Silverman, Eugene Seskin, and Howard Magid gave programming assistance.

Measures of case mix are a first step toward defining a measure of hospital output [1, 2]—an essential basis for statistical cost analysis and other types of analysis; and these measures are prerequisite to the design of effective cost-reimbursement procedures, since hospital costs are clearly affected by the types of patients treated. (Thus a hospital treating only patients requiring open heart surgery would have quite different costs from an obstetrical hospital [3].) In addition, the answers to the questions posed above have important implications for hospital administrators, in providing a basis for evaluating the performance of the individual hospital. Finally, they are important to health planning agencies, since coordinated planning is possible only when detailed information on the current situation is available.

DATA BASE AND METHODOLOGY

The study area in western Pennsylvania may conveniently be divided into Allegheny County (essentially the Pittsburgh metropolitan area) and a more rural portion outside Allegheny County. Most of the hospitals in the study are described as community hospitals, but data from one children's hospital and one eye and ear hospital are also included. The Allegheny County Hospital Planning Association has encouraged role differentiation by recognizing, in each of its five planning areas, a "lead" hospital, with more specialized facilities and personnel, for the care of patients the other hospitals are not equipped to treat. These "lead" hospitals, in turn, are linked to health center hospitals—the teaching hospitals of the University of Pittsburgh Medical School.

Patient data for this study were obtained from the Hospital Utilization Project (HUP), started in 1963. The study data extend from 1965, when HUP had 19 member hospitals, through 1968, at which time there were 65 participating hospitals. The HUP data are similar to those collected by PAS, although less complete. Participating hospitals report data on each discharged patient. HUP then codes (by ICDA, rev. ed.) and tabulates data on primary discharge diagnosis and up to eight secondary diagnoses; primary surgical procedure (if any) and up to five secondary surgical procedures; discharge status (dead or alive); age, sex, and marital status; hospital accommodation (private, semiprivate, ward); and method of payment (self-pay, Blue Cross, Medicaid, etc.). The HUP member hospitals are, of course, not a random selection of all hospitals in the area. They constitute, however, a large sample believed to be reasonably representative; in the greater Pittsburgh area, for example, all but 3 of the 27 short-term hospitals in the county planning association are HUP members.

A total of 249,696 patient records (133,017 of them surgical patients) were analyzed, representing 2,415,732 patient days (1,202,254 of them surgical patient days). These data covered all discharges from the 65 HUP hospitals for the second half of 1968, and additionally, for 19 member hospitals, the discharges for the preceding six half-year periods (that is, from the second half of 1965 through the first half of 1968).

One problem in using the HUP data is the likelihood of inconsistencies in the way primary and secondary diagnoses and surgical procedures are reported: it appears probable that some hospitals (e.g., teaching hospitals) may report finer diagnostic breakdowns and more secondary diagnoses. An effort was made to eliminate this source of bias by aggregating diagnoses and surgical procedures, as described below.

It should be mentioned that data on the newborn, except for abnormal conditions, were excluded from the analyses, since complete obstetrical information makes such data redundant. In a hospital handling 50 obstetrical cases, for example, no additional information is gained by tabulating, say, 50 newborn infants and 25 circumcisions.

On the basis of the HUP data, various measures were constructed to describe the inpatient population. For the first measure, patients were aggregated into 17 broad ICDA groupings, and the percentages of patients and of patient days in each grouping were determined. This imperfect measure of case mix was supplemented with measures of the incidence of surgery and of secondary diagnoses, estimates of the extent of "common" diagnoses and surgical procedures, and an index of surgical complexity. For each of these measures, the mean percent, the coefficient of variation, and the range were computed. The findings from this phase of the study provided answers to the first two questions raised at the beginning of this article.

In the second phase of the study, the variations in these measures across hospitals were analyzed and some hypotheses were tested in an effort to provide answers to the remaining questions. The coefficients of variation were compared across hospitals at a point in time, as well as within 19 hospitals over the time period 1965-68, to determine stability of case mix; a similar comparison was made between the urban (Allegheny County) and nonurban hospitals; and a series of regressions were performed to relate the variations to various institutional characteristics, including those listed in the Guide Issue of <u>Hospitals</u>, <u>J.A.H.A.</u>, and to demographic and locational variables.

EMPIRICAL MEASURES OF THE INPATIENT POPULATION

One basic approach to classifying patients—since the thousands of categories of medical diagnoses and surgical procedures found in manuals of classification are impractical as a basis for defining case mix—is to define groups by the amount and types of resources necessary to treat them. This categorization would start with the principal diagnoses, and the case mix would be defined in terms of the proportion of patients in each isoresource category [4]. A second approach is to aggregate patients by hospital service (pediatrics, obstetrics, male surgery, etc.) and to define case mix in terms of the proportion of patients in each service [3]. A third would aggregate patients into diagnostic groupings such as the 17 broad ICDA groupings (neoplasms, diseases of the circulatory system, diseases of the respiratory system, etc.) and define case mix in terms of the percentage of patients in each grouping.

The first classification would involve a major research effort requiring the judgment of both medical and nonmedical professionals. The second and third approaches are believed to be first approximations to a classification by isoresource categories. The third approach was chosen, focusing on the broad ICDA groupings, as the better approximation to an isoresource classification and more likely to be consistent across hospitals: the statement that a hospital treated 50 neoplasm cases appeared to offer more useful information than the statement that it treated 50 male medical cases, and there was, in fact, no uniformity in the way the study hospitals reported their service data.

The Crude Case-mix Measure

For each study hospital the percentage of patients and of patient days in each of the broad ICDA categories was first determined, as well as the mean percentages for the 65 sample hospitals for the second half of 1968 and, for patient days, the coefficient of variation and the range. These data, shown in Table 2.1, lead to two major conclusions. First, there is considerable variation in the case mix of the various hospitals. (Since the data base includes two specialized hospitals, as already noted, the results suggest somewhat more variation than if only general short-term hospitals had been included.) Second, the description of the hospitalized population is dependent on whether one focuses on number of patients or on patient days, because the average length of stay varies significantly across categories. For example, neoplasms represent, on average, 7 percent of discharges, but almost 10 percent of patient days; whereas deliveries and compli-

TABLE 2.1

Distribution of Diagnoses: 65 Hospitals, July–December 1968

ICDA Diagnostic Category	Patients, Mean Percent*	Patient Days Mean Percent*	Patient Days Coefficient of Variation	Patient Days Range
Infective and parasitic diseases	1.03	1.06	59.0	0.15– 3.34
Neoplasms	7.09	9.80	29.7	4.72–22.37
Allergic, endocrine, metabolic, and nutritional diseases	3.15	4.01	33.0	0.27– 7.07
Diseases of blood and blood-forming organs	0.58	0.72	50.7	0.04– 1.88
Mental, psychoneurotic, and personality disorders	2.06	2.43	162.1	0–29.67
Diseases of nervous system and sense organs	5.60	7.34	100.8	2.27–64.23
Diseases of circulatory system	11.12	16.77	24.5	0.24–26.70
Diseases of respiratory system	10.51	7.17	37.0	3.51–15.72
Diseases of digestive system	15.98	14.88	18.9	3.31–20.23
Diseases of genitourinary system	9.33	7.93	24.9	0–13.30
Deliveries and complications of pregnancy	13.08	6.62	41.1	0–13.18
Diseases of skin and subcutaneous tissue	1.51	1.48	37.0	0.25– 3.23
Diseases of bones and organs of movement	4.15	4.92	75.9	0.37–27.87
Congenital malformations	0.84	0.78	299.1	0.01–19.21
Diseases of early infancy	0.11	0.14	301.5	0– 3.24
Symptoms, senility, and ill-defined conditions	2.63	2.22	40.7	0.68– 5.57
Injuries and adverse effects of external cause	11.24	11.75	25.9	2.99–19.41

*These are simple, not weighted, mean percentages, determined by summing across hospitals the percentages in each category and dividing by 65.

cations of pregnancy represent, on average, 13 percent of discharges but only 7 percent of patient days.

Surgery and Multiple Diagnoses

The extent of surgery performed in a hospital depends partly on its diagnostically defined case mix. Even a perfect case-mix measure, however, will not completely determine the incidence of surgery, since many illnesses, such as ulcers, can be treated either medically or surgically. Since the broad case-mix measure does not take into account the different demands on hospital resources for the patient who undergoes surgery, the percentage of patients on whom at least one surgical procedure was performed and the average number of surgical procedures per surgical case were determined.

As shown in Table 2.2, surgery was performed on approximately 51 percent of all patients; the variation in this percentage across hospitals was not substantial. The hospital length of stay was, on average, shorter for patients who underwent surgery than for the general inpatient population. The mean number of surgical procedures per surgical case was 1.37, with little variation across hospitals.

The data on the distribution of surgical procedures (Table 2.3) show that there is more variation in the kinds of surgery than in the amount of surgery performed. As with nonsurgical diagnoses, the profile is dependent on whether patients or patient days are used as the base measure. The average length of stay for patients who had

TABLE 2.2

Incidence of Surgery: 65 Hospitals, July-December 1968

Measure	Mean	Coefficient of Variation	Range
Surgical patients, % of total patients	51.4	19.7	29.5-89.6
Surgical patient days, % of total patient days	46.8	21.4	25.9-86.5
Number of surgical procedures per surgical patient	1.37	7.2	1.07-1.60

TABLE 2.3

Distribution of Surgical Procedures: 65 Hospitals, July–December 1968

ICDA Category of Surgical Procedures	Patients, Mean Percent*	Mean Percent*	Patient Days Coefficient of Variation	Range
Nervous system	1.68	3.06	115.0	0–22.05
Endocrine system	0.50	0.50	79.4	0– 1.91
Eye	2.84	2.72	243.2	0–52.92
Ear, nose, throat	2.33	1.66	217.2	0–29.36
Buccal cavity and esophagus	15.22	5.09	42.2	1.00–15.10
Heart and intrathoracic vessels	0.49	0.71	275.5	0–10.45
Bronchi, lung, etc.	0.63	1.28	84.0	0– 4.87
Breast	2.43	1.97	42.0	0– 5.01
Gastrointestinal tract	17.40	25.42	22.4	0–42.64
Urinary and male genital systems	5.14	7.78	47.2	0–16.31
Female genital system, nonobstetrical	10.82	10.15	37.0	0–21.37
Obstetrical	19.28	11.37	46.3	0–30.23
Musculoskeletal system	12.91	19.27	36.3	0.75–43.58
Peripheral blood vessels and lymphatics	1.60	2.09	48.0	0.45– 5.19
Skin and subcutaneous tissue	6.70	6.93	42.1	0.19–16.96

*These are simple, not weighted, mean percentages.

TABLE 2.4

Common Diagnoses: 65 Hospitals, July–December 1968

ICDA Code	Description	Percent of Patients	Percent of Patient Days
660	Delivery without mention of complications	7.014	3.664
420	Arteriosclerotic heart disease, incl. coronary disease	4.611	7.488
510	Hypertrophy of tonsils and adenoids (incl. chronic tonsillitis)	4.262	0.844
560	Hernia of abdominal cavity without mention of obstruction	2.746	2.467
670	Complications of delivery	1.961	1.205
533	Disorders of occlusion, eruption, and tooth development	1.928	*
260	Diabetes mellitus	1.653	2.469
584	Cholelithiasis	1.483	2.276
634	Disorders of menstruation	1.300	0.688
385	Cataract	1.274	1.152
541	Ulcer of duodenum	0.988	1.204
571	Gastroenteritis and colitis, exc. ulcerative	0.960	0.642
461	Hemorrhoids	0.951	0.858
650	Abortion	0.936	*
735	Displacement of intervertebral disc	0.904	1.411
852	Concussion	0.891	*
648	Other complications arising from pregnancy	0.885	*
602	Calculi of kidney and ureter	0.871	0.684

550	Acute appendicitis	0.863	0.722
532	Other inflammatory disorders of supporting structures of teeth	0.817	*
391	Otitis media	0.796	*
530	Dental caries	0.749	*
572	Chronic enteritis and ulcerative colitis	0.749	1.086
630	Infective diseases of uterus, vagina, and vulva	0.724	*
741	Synovitis, bursitis, and tenosynovitis	0.722	*
434	Other and unspecified diseases of heart	0.720	1.107
610	Hyperplasia of prostate	0.714	1.198
723	Osteoarthritis (arthrosis) and allied conditions	0.711	*
620	Chronic cystic disease of breast	0.707	*
631	Uterovaginal prolapse	0.682	0.896
460	Varicose veins of lower extremities	0.674	0.762
214	Uterine fibromyoma	0.635	0.721
813	Fracture of radius and ulna (either or both)	0.634	*
324	Psychoneurotic disorder	0.629	0.792
331	Cerebral hemorrhage, nontraumatic	0.583	1.076
543	Gastritis and duodenitis	0.581	*
492	Primary atypical pneumonia	0.568	0.585
820	Fracture of neck of femur	0.565	1.666
332	Cerebral embolism and thrombosis	0.560	1.371
384	Strabismus	0.558	*
241	Asthma	0.553	*
450	General arteriosclerosis	0.544	1.168
500	Acute or subacute bronchitis	0.537	*

(continued)

27

Table 2.4 (continued)

ICDA Code	Description	Percent of Patients	Percent of Patient Days
527	Other diseases of lung and pleural cavity	0.527	0.731
578	Other diseases of intestines and peritoneum	0.522	0.640
447	Other hypertensive diseases	0.520	0.558
170	Malignant neoplasm of breast	0.518	0.879
491	Bronchopneumonia	0.506	0.555
153	Malignant neoplasm of large intestine	*	0.848
722	Rheumatic arthritis and allied conditions (or polyarthritis)	*	0.848
199	Malignant neoplasm of primary site or other and unspecified secondary sites	*	0.837
334	Other and ill-defined vascular lesions affecting central nervous system	*	0.740
162	Malignant neoplasm of bronchus and trachea and of lung specified as primary	*	0.701
540	Ulcer of stomach	*	0.645
581	Cirrhosis of liver	*	0.633
600	Infections of kidney	*	0.510
493	Pneumonia and thrombophlebitis	*	0.507
463	Phlebitis and thrombophlebitis	*	0.502
821	Fracture of other and unspecified parts of femur	*	0.501
		54.786	50.837

*Less than 0.5 percent.

operations on the buccal cavity and esophagus, for instance, was short; these patients (the majority of whom had tonsillectomies or tooth extractions) represented, on average, 15 percent of surgical cases but only 5 percent of surgical patient days—that is, their length of stay was only one-third of the average surgical stay. Patients who had operations on either the gastrointestinal tract or the musculoskeletal system had a long stay relative to the average, hence they represent a much higher proportion of patient days than of patients.

Another important dimension ignored in the crude case-mix measure is the coexistence of multiple diagnoses—which may indicate sicker patients, a more "complicated" case mix, or a higher proportion of geriatric patients. The average number of diagnoses per case was therefore determined for each hospital. (This measure is admittedly suspect, since the number of diagnoses reported may depend more on the characteristics of the attending physician than on the patient's state of health, with some physicians reporting only the main reason for hospitalization and others reporting everything wrong with the patient.) The mean number of diagnoses per case was found to be approximately 2, with little variation across hospitals (coefficient of variation, 15.8; range, 1.06-3.04).

The Extent of Commonality

Another approach to describing patient mix is to focus on the extent of what is here called the "commonality" of disease. If every known disease had an equal chance of occurring, no single disease would make up a significant part of a hospital's case mix. But some diseases do, of course, occur more often than others: a case of tonsillitis is more likely to turn up in a HUP hospital than one of malaria. Two questions were raised: (1) Are there certain diseases that make up a large part of the hospital case load? (2) Do some hospitals tend to treat more of these common diseases?

Four basic measures of commonality were constructed, two depending on the diagnosis and two on the surgical procedures performed. A common disease or condition was defined, for the purposes of the study, as one that accounted for at least 0.5 percent of all patients in the sample. Since length of stay for the more common diagnoses may be shorter than the average, those diagnoses which accounted for at least 0.5 percent of total patient days were also determined. Diagnoses were tabulated by the three-digit rather than the four-digit ICDA code (because not all physicians make the fine distinctions represented by the four-digit codes); and all uncomplicated deliveries (660-669) were grouped together as ICDA 660 and all complicated deliveries (670-689) as ICDA 670.

TABLE 2.5

Common Surgical Procedures: 65 Hospitals, July–December 1968

ICDA Code	Description	Percent of Procedures	Percent of Patient Days	Relative Value‡
76.0	Operations assisting delivery	12.323	3.670	22
27.2	Tonsillectomy with adenoidectomy	5.929	0.641	14
24.2	Surgical removal of tooth	4.775	0.846	5
89.1	Excision and destruction of skin lesion	3.608	1.616	16
40.0	Repair of inguinal hernia exc. recurrent	3.464	1.680	37
72.8	Dilation and curettage of uterus	2.672	0.781	14
77.0	Operations after delivery or abortion	2.549	0.575	37
53.5	Cholecystectomy	2.390	2.200	59
17.4	Extraction of lens, extracapsular	2.073	1.104	61
72.4	Hysterectomy, complete	1.902	1.370	60
45.1	Appendectomy	1.885	0.904	36
24.1	Simple tooth extraction	1.883	*	3
38.1	Partial mastectomy	1.721	0.541	15
49.3	Hemorrhoidectomy	1.705	0.918	16
82.3	Closed reduction of fracture of extremity (long bone)	1.452	0.650	†
27.1	Tonsillectomy with adenoidectomy	1.362	*	10
73.1	Local excision and destruction of lesion of cervix	1.302	*	4
20.4	Operations on tympanum	1.274	*	38
88.4	Excision and ligation of varicose veins	1.055	0.585	17

66.2	Prostatectomy	1.012	1.020	62
72.6	Hysterectomy, partial	0.967	0.720	60
82.5	Open reduction of fracture of extremity (long bone)	0.927	1.320	†
89.0	Incision of skin	0.891	*	3
83.4	Excision of intervertebral cartilage	0.788	0.854	†
89.4	Suture	0.773	*	10
64.5	Dilation of urethra	0.773	*	2
41.1	Incision of abdominal wall and umbilicus	0.773	0.975	36
78.0	Caesarian section	0.770	*	45
03.3	Spinal puncture	0.720	0.677	37
11.3	Advancement or recession of eye muscle	0.715	*	44
81.8	Traction or fixation without reduction	0.683	*	†
80.2	Partial excision of bone	0.670	*	†
83.5	Excision of semilunar cartilage of knee joint	0.634	*	†
21.4	Rhinoplasty	0.569	*	17
80.6	Sternal puncture for biopsy of bone marrow	0.532	0.601	†
85.2	Excision of muscle lesion	0.508	*	†
44.2	Partial gastrectomy	*	0.534	67
89.6	Skin graft	*	0.547	7
		68.029	25.329	

*Less than 0.5 percent.
†No relative value available.
‡Relates to index of surgical complexity; see following section.

The 48 conditions that by this definition are common as weighted by number of patients and the 43 conditions that are common as weighted by patient days are listed in Table 2.4. The former constitute approximately 55 percent of all discharges and the latter approximately 51 percent of all hospital days; 32 diagnoses appear in both listings.* In answer to the first question above, a small subset of diagnoses is found to account for a high proportion of all inpatient cases.

A similar procedure was followed to determine common surgical procedures, with similar adjustments of data. Table 2.5 lists 36 surgical procedures that made up 68 percent of all surgical procedures and 24 procedures that accounted for 25 percent of all surgical patient days; 22 procedures appear in both lists.† As with the medical diagnoses, a small subset of surgical procedures is found to account for a large proportion of all surgery performed.

The percent of discharges represented by the 48 common diagnoses, the percent of patient days represented by the 43 common diagnoses, the percent of the surgical case load made up of the 36 common surgical procedures, and the percent of the surgical patient days made up of the 24 common surgical procedures were then calculated for each hospital. Table 2.6 shows the mean percentages, coefficients of variation, and ranges for these measures.

Approximately 57 percent of the patients in the average hospital had one of the common diagnoses; but these diagnoses constituted as little as 27 percent of all total discharges in one hospital and as much as 66 percent in another, although variation in the fraction of the case load made up of common cases is, on average, only 11 percent. The distribution of common diagnoses by patient days is similar. In the average hospital common surgical procedures made up 72.5 percent of all primary surgical procedures. The range in the ratio of common surgical procedures to total surgical procedures is wider than that of common diagnoses to total diagnoses, but on average, the relative variation is similar. There is somewhat more variation in the ratio of

---

*The 44 diagnoses found to be the most frequent in the data of Blue Cross of Massachusetts are all included in the Table 2.4 list. A PAS list of the 50 most common reasons for admission (by four-digit ICDA code) contains seven diagnoses not included in Table 2.4; 13 of the Table 2.4 diagnoses—with dental disorders important among them—do not appear on the PAS list.

†The PAS list of the most frequently performed operations contains 11 not included in Table 2.5, and seven surgical procedures in Table 2.5 are not on the PAS list.

TABLE 2.6

The Extent of Commonality: 65 Hospitals, July-December 1968

Measure	Mean Percent*	Coefficient of Variation	Range
Common diagnoses (patients)	56.96	11.2	27.10-66.23
Common diagnoses (patient days)	56.46	14.0	12.93-66.25
Common surgery (patients)	72.50	11.8	38.34-84.26
Common surgery (patient days)	25.00	21.2	7.87-37.01

*These are simple, not weighted, percentages and hence differ from those of Tables 2.4 and 2.5, which are weighted percentages.

common surgery by patient days to total surgery by patient days. In answer to the second question above, it can thus be stated that some hospitals do treat proportionally more "common" cases than others.

Index of Surgical Complexity

One final way to describe the patient mix of a hospital is to focus on the degree of "complexity" presented by a case. Difficulty and complexity are surely related to, among other things, the rarity of the condition, the skill of the physician, and the supporting personnel and equipment needed to treat the condition. On the rather reasonable assumption that a hospital that receives the more complex surgical cases is also likely to receive the more complex medical cases, a measure of surgical complexity can be used as a surrogate for case-mix complexity.

In 1964 Blue Shield constructed a national index of relative values for surgical procedures, on the basis of charges for the procedures. The present study makes the assumption that these relative values (in effect, a relative fee schedule) are good approximations of the level of difficulty of a surgical procedure. If these procedures are priced at all rationally, the fee charged should be a function of the skill demanded of the surgeon, the amount of his time required, and the difficulty of the procedure. The study assumption is supported, moreover, by comparison of the Blue Shield relative values with a set of relative values constructed in Connecticut in 1953 on the basis of direct measurements of the complexity of certain surgical procedures. When the two relative value scales are standardized so that the value of an appendectomy is 1, they are found to be quite similar: the correlation between the two for 11 surgical procedures is .974 and the rank order correlation is .95.

The prime difficulty in using the Blue Shield relative values to construct an index of surgical complexity is the fact that they are associated with the Blue Shield Professional Index (BSPI) codes rather than the ICDA codes used for the study data. In some instances more than one BSPI surgical procedure is associated with a particular ICDA procedure (thus lobotomy, ICDA 01.0, covers leucotomy, lobectomy, and pallidectomy, BSPI 5133, 5164, and 5172); the BSPI relative values associated with an ICDA procedure may vary widely (in the lobotomy instance cited above, the BSPI values are 60.9, 97, and 58, respectively); and for some ICDA codes there are no corresponding BSPI relative values. These problems were met by averaging the relative values for those ICDA codes with more than one value; by excluding all orthopedic surgical cases, for which the range in values per ICDA code was extremely large; and by eliminating from the determination of the surgical complexity index those ICDA surgical procedures with no corresponding BSPI relative values. The relative value for each of the common surgical procedures has been shown earlier, in Table 2.5.

TABLE 2.7

Indexes of Surgical Complexity: 65 Hospitals, July-December 1968

Measure	Mean Complexity Index	Coefficient of Variation	Range
Based on number of surgical patients	26.82	10.4	19.58-34.44
Based on surgical patient days	35.22	9.7	22.52-44.75

TABLE 2.8

Distribution of Primary Surgical Procedures by Complexity

Relative Value	Mean Percent of Patients	Coefficient of Variation	Range
1- 10	20.93	25.9	11.2-36.9
11- 20	25.08	15.9	15.0-32.7
21- 30	14.77	30.6	12.9-25.7
31- 40	19.74	19.5	12.8-31.3
41- 50	4.94	44.3	1.8-16.1
51- 60	8.45	26.7	2.8-15.5
61- 70	4.44	61.8	0-13.5
71- 80	0.90	73.2	0- 2.8
81- 90	0.60	115.7	0- 4.1
91-100	0.14	337.7	0- 2.7

For each hospital two weighted complexity indexes were constructed, one based on the number of surgical patients and the other on the number of surgical patient days, as follows:

$$\text{Complexity index} = \sum_i C_{ij} W_i \left(\sum_i C_{ij} \right)^{-1}$$

where C_{ij} is the number of surgical patients (or of patient days) for ICDA procedure i in the jth hospital and W_i is the average relative value given to that procedure.

The mean percentage of a hospital's surgical cases included in the construction of the surgical indexes is 85.9 percent; of the 14.1 percent remaining approximately 13 percent were operations on the musculoskeletal system and 1 percent were other surgical procedures for which no relative value was available. Table 2.7 presents the mean complexity indexes across hospitals and the relevant information on the variation of the means. Table 2.8 gives more detailed information on the distribution of surgical procedures by weights (relative values).

The mean complexity index found across hospitals was 26.82, with a low of 19.58 and a high of 34.44. Obviously, then, some hospitals treat more complex cases than others, although the average variation in the index across hospitals is less than would perhaps be expected: 10.4 percent. The index based on surgical patient days is significantly higher than that based on surgical procedures, as might be expected, since surely the stay is longer for the more complicated surgical procedures.*

ANALYSIS OF CASE-MIX VARIATIONS

The case-mix measures discussed in the previous section showed substantial variation across hospitals; the inpatient populations of the various hospitals ranged widely in the proportion of "common" diagnoses and surgical procedures and in the type and complexity of surgery performed. In this section the variations in case mix are studied in an effort to determine some of the factors that explain such variation.

Stability of Case Mix within Hospitals

The case mix of all hospitals may be expected to change over time with the development of medical knowledge and technology and changes in the socioeconomic characteristics of the population. Thus some diseases, such as diphtheria, have been almost eradicated and others are treated differently: tonsillitis is less likely now to be treated by surgery than by drugs. Certain diseases (e.g., tuberculosis) are associated with poorer populations. Changing methods of financing medical and hospital care such as Medicare and Medicaid will also affect the types of cases found in hospitals. It was hypothesized that there would be little change in hospital case mix, however, over short periods of time, since the stability of the staff, the physical plant and equipment, and the time required to introduce changes ought to ensure relative stability.

This hypothesis was tested by comparing the coefficients of variation for the various output measures in the second half of 1968

---

*Roemer et al. [5] derived a surrogate case-severity index by focusing on the occupancy-corrected length of stay. The correlations between a similar index computed for the HUP hospitals and the surgical complexity indexes constructed here were only .39 (for the complexity index based on number of patients) and .38 (complexity index based on patient days). Thus the Roemer index is not a good surrogate for this direct measure of complexity.

with the mean coefficients of variation over time for the 19 hospitals
for which HUP data were available for seven six-month time periods
1965-68. The 1965-68 period might be expected to be one of great
change within individual hospitals, since it begins before Medicare
and Medicaid, covers the transition, and extends through the time
when both programs were fully implemented. The individual indexes,
then, should show more than the "normal" variation.

Table 2.9 shows, for selected output measures, the results of
this analysis; the same pattern emerged for all the output variables.
For all the variables the extent of variation within hospitals over time
is less than that between hospitals at a given period of time, and for
some measures the lack of variation over time is most striking.

A formal test for the hypothesis was constructed, under the
assumption that the case-mix category for a hospital is subject to a
binomial distribution over 6-month periods. This assumption is equivalent to saying that the arrival rate of patients of a given category
follows a Poisson distribution, since the mean probabilities are large
enough to make the binomial approximation to the Poisson distribution
quite good. For each of the categories in Table 2.9 a confidence interval of two standard deviations about the mean was established, and
the number of times an observation fell outside the confidence interval,
both within a hospital over time and across hospitals at a point in
time, was examined. The observations within hospitals over time
rarely fell outside the confidence interval—that is, case mix was
stable in a hospital over time. In looking at hospitals at a point in
time, many of the observations fell outside the confidence interval,
which is to say that case mix was quite different across hospitals.

The conclusion that the case mix of a hospital is stable over short
periods of time is an important one, since it means that results based
on a cross-sectional analysis of case mix need not be revised every year.

Effect of Urban Location

It was hypothesized that the hospitals of the Pittsburgh metropolitan area (Allegheny County) would display more role variation
than those of more rural areas not only because, as already mentioned,
the county hospital planning agency has deliberately encouraged and
structured such variation by its system of "lead" hospitals and health
center hospitals, but also because highly specialized equipment and
personnel (always in limited supply) can be expected to be concentrated
in areas with a large enough population base to support them, and the
practicing physicians in such areas are more likely to have ready
access to these specialized resources for referral. Distance may
also be a factor: because it imposes extra costs on the patient—both
financial and emotional—fewer patients may be referred by the physician associated with a small rural hospital. It seemed reasonable to

TABLE 2.9

Coefficients of Variation between Hospitals and within Hospitals

Output Measure	Variation between Hospitals: 65 Hospitals, 2d half of 1968	Variation between Hospitals: 19 Hospitals, 2d half of 1968	Variation within Hospitals: 19 Hospitals, 1965-68 (mean)
Distribution of diagnoses:			
Infective and parasitic disease	59.9	54.1	21.8
Neoplasms	31.3	27.8	6.9
Allergic, endocrine, metabolic, and nutr. dis.	34.8	47.0	11.5
Dis. of blood and blood-forming organs	50.1	69.5	25.9
Mental, psychoneurotic and personality dis.	124.1	76.5	23.3
Dis. of nerv. system and sense organs	114.0	151.0	9.8
Dis. of circulatory system	24.6	38.0	8.1
Dis. of respiratory system	31.4	45.4	11.4
Dis. of digestive system	18.4	21.1	6.0
Dis. of genitourinary system	25.1	33.1	13.3
Deliveries and complications of pregnancy	39.1	49.4	22.6
Dis. of skin and subcutaneous tissue	36.9	38.2	18.4

Dis. of bones and organs of movement	62.4	72.5	13.4
Congenital malformations	249.5	230.3	22.3
Dis. of early infancy	224.9	263.7	79.4
Symptoms, senility, etc.	32.2	30.1	12.9
Injuries and adverse effects of ext. cause	26.9	32.4	7.3
Index of surgical complexity:			
Based on no. surg. patients	10.4	11.4	3.3
Based on patient days	9.7	8.9	4.5
Measures of commonality:			
Common diseases (patients)	11.2	16.9	2.2
Common diseases (patient days)	14.0	23.6	6.1
Common surgery (patients)	11.8	17.7	2.8
Proportion of surgery	19.7	15.7	3.0
Diagnoses/case	15.8	8.9	3.4
Surg. proc./surgical patient	7.2	4.9	2.0

TABLE 2.10

Coefficients of Variation for Selected Variables
by Hospital Location

Variable	In Allegheny County	Outside Allegheny County
Proportion of common diagnoses	15.8	7.4
Proportion of common surgery	16.6	7.0
Average surgical complexity index	10.6	9.9
Proportion of complex surgery	86.8	71.5
Proportion of simple surgery	26.3	25.9
Percent of patients with surgical procedure	13.4	19.3

expect, then, that a 100-bed hospital in a rural area would be quite different in its case mix from a 100-bed hospital in Allegheny County.

To test this hypothesis, the coefficients of variation for the Allegheny County hospitals were compared with those for the hospitals outside the county on each of the 52 measures for which coefficients of variation were reported in the previous section. The coefficients of variation were found to be larger for Allegheny County hospitals than for noncounty hospitals on 38 of the 52 measures. (On a random basis the county-hospital coefficients would have been larger 26.5 times out of 52; there is less than 1 chance in 100 of their being found larger 38 times out of 52.) Table 2.10 shows the two coefficients for a selection of these measures. The results of the test support the hypothesis and affirm the important effect of urban vs. rural location on role variation.

Effect of Institutional Characteristics

It is reasonable to expect that a hospital's case mix will be related to its institutional characteristics. The more complex and uncommon cases should flow to the advanced teaching hospitals or to large hospitals with many services, since these cases, because they involve extensive diagnostic or surgical skills (supported by laboratories, technicians, and surgical teams), are more likely to require treatment by highly specialized physicians or to require expensive

equipment such as radiation apparatus or hyperbaric chambers—
skilled manpower and specialized equipment that tend to be concentrated in these types of hospitals. Correlatively, fewer common cases
should be found in the large teaching hospitals.

To test this hypothesis, and to determine the relative importance
of size, number of services, teaching status, and other variables in
explaining case-mix variation, regressions were estimated for
various measures of the variation in common diagnoses and common
surgery, in surgical complexity, and in the proportion of surgery.
As shown in Table 2.11, four regressions were estimated for each
measure. Regression 1 makes use of selected data on institutional
characteristics from the Guide Issue of <u>Hospitals</u>, <u>J.A.H.A.</u> [6] and
may be expressed as

$$CM_i = a_0 + a_1 B_i + a_2 S_i + a_3 AT_i + a_4 T_i + e_i$$

where CM_i is some measure of case mix in hospital i; B = the hospital's bed capacity; S = number of advanced services (intensive care
unit, premature nursery, outpatient department, postoperative recovery room, renal dialysis unit, X-ray therapy department, and physical therapy, occupational therapy, or rehabilitation unit);[*] AT is a
dummy variable indicating whether the hospital is an advanced teaching hospital; T is a dummy variable indicating whether it is a teaching hospital;[†] and e is an error term. Under general assumptions,
the a_i will be best linear unbiased estimates of the relation between
case mix and each of the hospital characteristics entered into the
regression.[‡]

---

[*]The technological adequacy index constructed by Roemer et al.
[5] could have been used instead of number of advanced services, but
preliminary investigation indicated that the latter was a slightly better
measure.

[†]The approvals listed in the Guide Issue as indicators of teaching
status were amplified from Blue Cross data on the basis of the Blue
Cross definitions: an advanced teaching hospital is one with medical
school affiliation and with three or more approved residency programs;
and a teaching hospital is one with an approved nursing school or
internship program or with at least one residency program.

[‡]The basic assumptions needed are that the model be linear and
that the distribution of the errors have an expected value of zero,
have finite variance, have a constant distribution over the various
observations, and be independent. In addition, no explanatory variable
may be omitted that correlates with included variables. In order to

TABLE 2.11

Regressions Explaining Variation in Some Case-Mix Measures
(Figures in parentheses are t statistics)

Independent Variables	Dependent variables: Regression number: R^2:	Proportion Common Diagnoses				Proportion Common Surgery				Average Surgical Complexity Index			
		1-1	1-2	1-3	1-4	2-1	2-2	2-3	2-4	3-1	3-2	3-3	3-4
		.264	.510	.555	.549	.447	.786	.797	.797	.283	.563	.591	.591
Constant term		58.451	58.495	55.286	56.628	76.699	86.201	85.798	85.819	24.089	18.656	17.268	17.247
Bed capacity		-.660	-1.130	-1.013	-.771	-1.557	-1.526	-1.783	-1.773	.374	.309	.253	2.62
		(-.82)	(-1.44)	(-1.34)	(-1.18)	(-1.66)	(-2.20)	(-2.56)	(-2.67)	(1.08)	(.96)	(.78)	(.85)
Bed capacity × AC		—	—	—	—	—	—	—	—	—	—	—	—
Lead		—	-2.758	1.692	—	—	1.236	4.032	4.016	—	-.844	.115	—
			(-.89)	(.48)			(.45)	(1.28)	(1.29)		(-.66)	(.08)	
Number of services		.249	.183	.777	.674	-.271	-1.010	-.981	-.982	.240	.536	.552	.553
		(.37)	(.30)	(1.23)	(1.15)	(-.35)	(-1.90)	(-1.88)	(-1.90)	(.84)	(2.17)	(2.27)	(2.29)
No. of services × AC		—	—	-2.733	-2.538	—	—	—	—	—	—	—	—
				(-2.35)	(-2.78)								
Advanced teaching		-5.317	-1.264	-2.440	-3.030	-8.184	-5.052	-2.428	-2.476	2.014	2.043	3.180	3.163
		(-2.24)	(-.51)	(-1.01)	(-1.67)	(-2.97)	(-2.33)	(-.93)	(-1.02)	(1.97)	(2.02)	(2.59)	(2.64)
Adv. teaching × AC		—	—	—	—	—	—	-5.564	-5.568	—	—	-2.164	-2.103
								(-1.72)	(-1.74)			(-1.43)	(-1.64)
Teaching		1.754	1.707	.997	—	.554	.126	.071	—	.577	1.059	1.086	1.081
		(.97)	(1.05)	(.62)		(.26)	(.09)	(.05)		(.74)	(1.58)	(1.64)	(1.66)
Proportion Medicare		—	.054	.057	—	—	-.231	-.201	-.202	—	.231	.299	.300
			(.39)	(.43)			(-1.87)	(-1.64)	(-1.68)		(4.02)	(4.14)	(4.20)
Prop. Medicare × AC		—	—	—	—	—	—	—	—	—	—	-.150	-.150
												(-1.28)	(-1.30)
Proportion Medicaid		—	-.113	-.020	—	—	.255	.223	.224	—	-.092	-.112	-.112
			(-.80)	(-.14)			(2.04)	(1.80)	(1.85)		(-1.58)	(-1.92)	(-1.94)
Prop. Medicaid × AC		—	—	—	—	—	—	—	—	—	—	—	—
Allegheny County		—	2.156	14.492	14.028	—	1.294	2.472	2.490	—	-.730	2.663	2.670
			(1.38)	(2.65)	(3.19)		(.94)	(1.63)	(1.70)		(-1.14)	(1.11)	(1.12)
Health center		—	-14.114	-18.169	-17.370	—	-27.533	-27.644	-27.637	—	7.905	7.181	7.241
			(-3.48)	(-4.27)	(-5.77)		(-7.69)	(-7.86)	(-7.93)		(4.75)	(4.16)	(4.72)

Dependent variables:	Proportion Complex Surgery				Proportion Simple Surgery				Proportion Surgery			
Regression number:	4-1	4-2	4-3	4-4	5-1	5-2	5-3	5-4	6-1	6-2	6-3	6-4
R^2:	.399	.590	.620	.619	.062	.203	.240	.240	.242	.529	.570	.578
Constant term	.022	-1.618	-1.096	-1.096	24.401	27.117	27.581	27.564	46.093	56.466	57.734	56.786
Bed capacity	.339	.353	.349	.334	.579	.495	.791	.807	2.634	1.625	2.644	2.789
	(2.26)	(2.40)	(2.35)	(2.33)	(.75)	(.58)	(.93)	(1.00)	(2.02)	(1.33)	(1.90)	(3.17)
Bed capacity × AC											-4.533	-4.344
											(-1.90)	(-2.61)
Lead		-.142	-.988	-.866		-4.545	-7.767	-7.756		-6.694	3.006	
		(-.24)	(-1.35)	(-1.29)		(-1.36)	(-2.02)	(-2.03)		(-1.39)	(.42)	
Number of services	.132	.217	.123	.121	-.817	-.789	-.823	-.827	-.630	.013	-.037	
	(1.07)	(1.93)	(1.02)	(1.01)	(-1.28)	(-1.22)	(-1.29)	(-1.32)	(-.59)	(.01)	(-.04)	
No. of services × AC			.426	.445								
			(1.88)	(2.02)								
Advanced teaching	.608	.476	.517	.667	-2.952	-2.225	-5.248	-5.333	4.750	4.154	1.118	
	(1.38)	(1.03)	(.90)	(1.46)	(-1.30)	(-.84)	(-1.63)	(-1.87)	(1.24)	(1.09)	(.23)	
Adv. teaching × AC			.302				6.411	6.445			3.520	6.522
			(.43)				(1.62)	(1.66)			(.56)	(1.50)
Teaching	.013	.194	.308	.310	-1.240	-2.334	-2.271	-2.289	1.687	-.118	-.957	
	(.04)	(.64)	(1.01)	(1.02)	(-.72)	(-1.33)	(-1.31)	(-1.35)	(.58)	(-.05)	(-.38)	
Proportion Medicare		.069	.067	.069		-.149	-.184	-.185		-.467	-.629	-.642
		(2.65)	(2.59)	(2.70)		(-.98)	(-1.22)	(-1.26)		(-2.15)	(-2.31)	(-2.53)
Prop. Medicare × AC											.597	.583
											(1.35)	(1.38)
Proportion Medicaid		-.025	-.037	-.040		-.045	-.009			-.611	-.478	-.364
		(-.93)	(-1.36)	(-1.48)		(-.30)	(-.06)			(-2.78)	(-2.10)	(-1.77)
Prop. Medicaid × AC												-.611
												(-1.25)
Allegheny County		-.464	-2.453	-2.471		3.736	2.379	2.395		6.638	5.257	6.714
		(-1.59)	(-2.35)	(-2.39)		(2.22)	(1.28)	(1.31)		(2.74)	(.53)	(.70)
Health center		3.160	3.799	3.820		-4.486	-4.358	-4.380		9.650	5.419	7.726
		(4.16)	(4.66)	(4.73)		(-1.03)	(-1.01)	(-1.03)		(1.53)	(.74)	(1.37)

In the second regression for each measure, additional explanatory variables a_5 to a_9 were entered, so that the equation becomes

$$CM_i = a_0 + a_1 B_i + a_2 S_i + a_3 AT_i + a_4 T_i + a_5 AC_i + a_6 L_i$$
$$+ a_7 HC_i + a_8 MC_i + a_9 MA_i + e_1$$

where AC is a dummy variable indicating whether the hospital is located in Allegheny County; L is a dummy variable indicating whether it is a "lead" hospital; HC is a dummy variable indicating whether it is a University of Pittsburgh health center hospital; MC = proportion of Medicare patients (a surrogate for patients over 65); and MA = proportion of Medicaid patients.

In a preliminary investigation these two regressions were estimated separately for the subset of Allegheny County hospitals and the subset of noncounty hospitals, to allow for the possibility that the parameter estimates might differ between the two, and the Chou test [7] was used to determine whether any explanatory power was lost by pooling the data into a single set and estimating a single regression. In every case the F test indicated that there was not a significant loss of explanatory power. Since some coefficients did appear to differ between the two subsets, however, the coefficients for the two subsets were estimated separately where the t of the separate variable (a test of whether the coefficient is significantly different from zero) was greater than 1. These separate estimates are shown in Regression 3 for each measure.*

Any variable whose coefficient was less than its standard error (t < 1) was eliminated in Regression 4, unless there was an overriding reason for keeping it; in Regression 3-4 of Table 2.11, for example, explaining the variation in the average surgical complexity

---

perform significance tests, some assumption about the distribution of the error must be made; since the residuals were found consistent with a normal distribution, normality was assumed.

*What was actually done was to form an interaction variable, number of services multiplied by the Allegheny County dummy variable; this variable takes on, for hospitals located in the county, a value of the number of services; for those outside it is zero. The Allegheny County effect is then found by adding the coefficient of services to the coefficient of S(AC); the noncounty effect is found by looking at the coefficient of S. Thus in Regression 1-3, the coefficient of number of services for Allegheny County hospitals is -2.733 + .777, or -1.956; for noncounty hospitals it is .777.

index, bed capacity was retained despite its t value of only .85 because of its importance in the regressions for the other measures, even though it did not make a significant contribution here.

Common Diagnoses and Common Surgery

As shown in Regression 1-1 of Table 2.11, the institutional characteristics of the study hospital account for only one-fourth of the variation in the extent of common diagnoses ($R^2 = .264$). The only important explanatory variable is advanced teaching status; on average, advanced teaching hospitals have 5 percent fewer common diagnoses (-5.317). Regression 1-2, with other explanatory variables added, is much more successful, since more than half the variation is explained. The size of the hospital now becomes an important variable, with common diagnoses falling by 1 percent for every hundred beds. Advanced teaching status loses its importance, and its role is usurped by the Allegheny County variable and the health center variable. Allegheny County hospitals have 2 percent more common diagnoses, after accounting for teaching status, size, number of services, lead status, and health center status. Health center hospitals have 14 percent fewer common cases than do other hospitals. Note that all health center hospitals are lead hospitals (-2.8) offering advanced teaching programs (-1.3) and are located in the county. These hospitals thus have 16 percent fewer common cases than nonteaching hospitals outside the county.

In Regression 1-3, allowing for the possibility of different coefficients inside the county, the only important case is the effect of the number of advanced services offered: within the county, hospitals with many advanced services have many fewer common cases, while the opposite is true outside the county. When all unimportant variables are eliminated (Regression 1-4), as expected large hospitals have fewer common diagnoses, as do hospitals offering many advanced services (within the county). Advanced teaching hospitals have fewer common cases (3 percent), as do health center hospitals (17 percent). Finally, in-county hospitals have many more common cases than hospitals outside the county, after accounting for size, teaching status, and number of advanced services. This result seems reasonable: since there are many more beds per capita within the county, people tend to be hospitalized for less important reasons.

Analysis of the proportion of common surgical cases in each hospital gave similar results. The explanatory power of the regressions is higher (ranging from .447 to .797). Size is seen to be an important variable: within large hospitals proportionally less common surgery is performed than in small hospitals. (Oddly, lead hospitals perform slightly more common surgical procedures; apparently the system of role differentiation is not all it might be.) As with the common diagnoses, fewer common surgical procedures are performed in hospitals with many advanced services; advanced teaching hospitals have fewer such procedures both within and outside the county. Hospitals handling many Medicaid patients do more common surgery, while those with a high proportion of Medicare patients do less. In the health center hospitals many fewer common surgical procedures are performed. Ceteris paribus, much more common surgery is done in hospitals within Allegheny County. The greater explanatory power of the final regression for common surgery (.797 as compared to .549 for common diagnoses) is evidence that surgical cases are more rationally allocated, with common surgery showing greater concentration than common diagnoses in small nonteaching hospitals.

Surgical Complexity

Since the two indexes of average surgical complexity reported earlier have almost identical implications, the analysis focuses on the index based on number of patients. As shown in Regression 3-1, the hospital institutional characteristics explained just over one-fourth of the variation in the index. As expected, size and advanced teaching status are the important variables: hospitals with the capability of treating difficult cases tend to get them. When the five additional explanatory variables are entered into the regression (Regression 3-2), its explanatory power rises from .283 to .563. Number of services and advanced teaching status become important variables. Within the hospitals in Allegheny County, after accounting for size and teaching status, the surgery performed is much less complex. The results suggest that operations on Medicare patients are more complex than average, while those on Medicaid patients are less complex.

Regression 3-3 indicates that in advanced teaching hospitals outside the county the surgery performed is much more complex, whereas in those within the county it is only slightly more complex;[*] the difficult cases here flow to the health center hospitals. The surgery in hospitals outside Allegheny County with a high proportion of Medicare patients is much more complex, while that in hospitals within the county is only slightly more complex.

However, when interaction variables are inserted for advanced teaching status and for proportion of Medicare patients, the sign of the Allegheny County coefficient changes. From the results in Regression 3-3, the explanation of the change from Regression 3-2 would

---

[*]As explained earlier, the two coefficients are added to determine the effect for Allegheny County: thus the county effect is the sum of $-2.164 + 3.180$, or 1.016; the noncounty effect is 3.180.

appear to be that advanced teaching hospitals within the county are relatively less specialized than their counterparts outside the county and that Medicare patients within the county have surgery of less complexity than those outside; when size and some aspects of case mix are held constant, advanced teaching hospitals within the county do surgery of greater complexity than those outside the county, but location makes less difference for these hospitals than for teaching and nonteaching hospitals. After these two effects within the county are accounted for, hospitals within the county perform more complex surgery than those outside. When the insignificant variables are dropped (Regression 3-4), the major results are unchanged.

In addition to analyzing the variation in the average complexity index, the investigation studied the variation in the percentage of surgical cases consisting of very complex surgical procedures (here defined as those with a relative value greater than 70) as well as the variation in the percentage of quite simple surgical procedures (defined as those with a relative value under 20). Approximately 40 percent of the variation in the percent of complex surgery is explained by the hospital institutional characteristics (Regression 4-1), while only 6 percent of the variation in percent of simple surgery is explained (Regression 5-1). When only the important variables are included, 62 percent of the variation in complex surgery is explained. This complex surgery takes place in large hospitals, in hospitals with many advanced services (especially those within Allegheny County), in advanced teaching and teaching hospitals, and in health center hospitals. Fewer complex surgical procedures are done in Allegheny County hospitals (after accounting for other characteristics), in lead hospitals, and in hospitals with many Medicaid patients. (Those with many Medicare patients do more of the complex procedures.)

When only the important variables are included, 24 percent of the variation in the proportion of the "quite simple" category of surgical cases is explained. Proportionally more simple surgery is performed in the large hospitals and in hospitals located in Allegheny County; less is performed in the lead hospitals, in hospitals offering many services, in advanced teaching hospitals outside the county, in teaching hospitals, in health center hospitals, and in hospitals with many Medicare patients.

It will be recalled that musculoskeletal surgical procedures (approximately 13 percent of all surgery) and all other surgical procedures without a relative value were omitted in the construction of the indexes of surgical complexity. Would the information on these variables have affected the results of analysis of the variation in surgical complexity? An unsuccessful attempt was made to explain the variation in the proportion of all excluded surgery by focusing on hospital characteristics. The variation in the excluded nonmusculoskeletal surgery was then analyzed. These would be expected to be rare and complicated procedures, since all the common surgical procedures listed in Table 2.5 either had a relative value or were operations on the musculoskeletal system. These cases were found to be concentrated in large hospitals (especially within Allegheny County) and in health center hospitals. Within the county, they represented a smaller proportion of the surgical case load in hospitals with many services, in advanced teaching hospitals, and in teaching hospitals. These results, although somewhat inconclusive, do not seem inconsistent with the conclusion that the findings reported would not have been different if relative values had been available for these procedures.

Extent of Surgery

One of the ways in which inpatient populations were found to differ among hospitals was the extent to which patients undergo surgery. It was posited earlier in this article that the extent of surgery performed was partly a function of the diagnostically determined case mix; and analysis showed that, as expected, for all hospitals the 17 diagnostic categories accounted for 79 percent of the variation in the extent of surgery. The four regressions described above were then computed to see how much of this variation could be accounted for by the institutional characteristics.

As shown in Regression 6-1, just under one-fourth of the variation is explained by the institutional characteristics. In large hospitals and those with advanced teaching and teaching programs, proportionally more surgery is performed. In Regression 6-2, with the additional variables entered, the explanatory power rises to .529; in health center hospitals and in hospitals in Allegheny County, ceteris paribus, more surgery is performed. Medicare and Medicaid patients tend to have fewer operations. When the location variables are included (Regression 6-3), only the effect of size changes significantly: in large hospitals in Allegheny County proportionally less surgery is performed, whereas in large hospitals outside the county more is performed.

DISCUSSION

The analyses reported here, in general, support the conclusion that the variations in case mix across hospitals follow a rational pattern, in that uncommon and difficult cases tend to flow to those hospitals with the institutional capability for handling them. Reviews of the literature [8-10], however, cite many researchers who have used these characteristics as a surrogate for case mix, assuming that hospitals with similar services and facilities, or even with the same number of these, would produce a similar output. It should be pointed out that although the characteristics of size, number of advanced services, and teaching status selected as likely indicators of treatment capability did, indeed, show some correlation with case mix, they were found to explain only about one-fourth to something less than half of the variation in proportions of common surgery and common diagnoses, in surgical complexity, and in extent of surgery performed. On this basis, then, they cannot be considered good surrogates for case mix.

It is apparent, moreover, that not all the facilities and programs listed in the Guide Issue of <u>Hospitals</u> should be given equal weight. In an additional series of regressions (not reported in Table 2.11) to explain the variation in number of neoplasm cases, hospital size was found to be the only important variable; the effect of an approved cancer program in a hospital was to reduce its percentage of neoplasm cases (both benign and malignant; aggregation of the study data by broad ICDA categories did not permit separation of cancer cases). Although this variable never attained significance, the coefficients were negative in all regressions.

The importance of the location variable in the analyses lends further support to the thesis that the institutional characteristics alone cannot be used to define case-mix variation. The factor of urban vs. rural location was found to have two important effects. The hospitals in Allegheny County (the greater Pittsburgh metropolitan area) showed, as expected, a tendency to greater role variation than those outside the county; and they tended to have a greater concentration of common diagnoses and common surgery, to do more quite simple surgery and less very complex surgery, and to perform more surgery in general (although they also appeared, somewhat anomalously, to have a high average index of surgical complexity). The general tendency of small urban hospitals to produce medical care that is less complex than that of small rural hospitals may, it is speculated, be related to the fact that the ratio of hospital beds to population is much higher within the county than outside, so that people may be hospitalized for less serious illnesses.

The case-mix measures constructed in this study showed important differences in the distribution of broad categories of diagnoses and surgical procedures in a hospital population according to whether the distribution was measured by the percentage of patients or by the percentage of patient days, since the average length of stay varies significantly across categories. Thus neoplasms represented, on average, 7 percent of the discharges but almost 10 percent of patient days, while deliveries and complications of pregnancy represented

13 percent of discharges but only 7 percent of patient days; and operations on the buccal cavity and esophagus accounted for 15 percent of surgical patients but only 5 percent of surgical patient days, as compared with operations on the gastrointestinal tract or on the musculoskeletal system, which made up a much higher proportion of patient days than of patients. Such findings can serve as important input in future investigations of hospital cost functions.

The data required for this type of analysis are available for hospital systems in many areas, hence there is a high potential for replication of the study. Similar investigations elsewhere might help to refine the methodology and to test, extend, and generalize the findings; and unquestionably the results of such community or regional studies would be of real value to hospital administrators and hospital planning agencies.

CONCLUSIONS

The major conclusions of the study can best be summarized in the form of answers to the five questions posed at the beginning of the article.

1. A small subset of diagnoses and of surgical procedures was found to account for a large proportion of all cases in the 65 hospitals studied.

2. There is a considerable amount of variation among hospitals in the types of patients they treat. This variation is more apparent in the broad case mix of hospitals than in the extent to which they treat common diseases or uncommon and difficult diseases.

3. The case mix within a particular hospital over a short period of time is relatively stable—that is, there is much more variation in case mix across hospitals at a point in time than within hospitals over short periods of time. A cross-sectional analysis of case mix therefore need not be revised every year.

4. There is greater role specialization among hospitals in the metropolitan area. Small urban hospitals tend to have more of the common diagnoses and surgical procedures and fewer uncommon and difficult cases than small rural hospitals.

5. The amount of specialization in case mix shows a tendency to follow differences in hospital institutional characteristics. Common cases, both surgical and nonsurgical, tend to be concentrated in small nonteaching hospitals, and the complexity of surgery performed rises with the teaching capability of a hospital. The institutional characteristics of size, teaching status, and number of advanced services, however, explain only about 25 to 45 percent of the variation in the case-mix measures constructed, hence they cannot be considered good surrogates for case mix.

REFERENCES

1. Yett, D., and J. Mann, "The Analysis of Hospital Costs: A Review Article," J. of Bus. 41 (April 1968):191.

2. Lave, J., and L. Lave, "Hospital Cost Function," Amer. Econ. Rev. 60 (June 1970):379.

3. Feldstein, M., Economic Analysis for Health Service Efficiency. Amsterdam: North Holland, 1967; Chicago: Markham, 1968.

4. Gurfield, R., and J. Clayton, Jr., Analytic Hospital Planning: A Pilot Study of Resource Allocation Using Mathematical Programming in a Cardiac Unit. RM5893-RC. The Rand Corporation, Santa Monica, Calif., April 1969.

5. Roemer, M., A. Moustafa, and C. Hopkins, "A Proposed Hospital Quality Index: Hospital Death Rates Adjusted for Case Severity," Health Serv. Res. 3 (Summer 1968):96.

6. Hospitals, J.A.H.A. Guide Issue, August 1, 1968 and August 1, 1969.

7. Johnston, J., Econometric Methods. New York: McGraw-Hill, 1968.

8. Berry, R., "Returns to Scale in the Production of Hospital Services," Health Serv. Res. 2 (Summer 1967):123.

9. Carr, W., and P. Feldstein, "The Relationship of Cost to Hospital Size," Inquiry 4 (June 1967):45.

10. Hefty, T. R., "Returns to Scale in Hospitals: A Critical Review of Recent Research," Health Serv. Res. 4 (Winter 1969):267.

3

FACTOR ANALYSIS

INTRODUCTION

The authors use factor analysis to identify underlying dimensions presumed to measure quality of care for six health insurance plans. Over 11,000 medical care bits were coded from the medical records of the insured population, with 32 variables designated as potential indicators of quality of care. Twelve of these variables were dropped because of failure to load on any factor, thus leaving 20 variables which loaded on four factors.

Five dimensions with corresponding variables were initially hypothesized, but when factor analysis was undertaken only three of the initial dimensions resulted (along with a fourth unanticipated dimension) and many variables did not "load" as anticipated. Factor scores were calculated for each factor and then weighted by the amount of variance explained by each factor to obtain transformed score means. The mean scores for each plan were summed over the four factors to obtain an overall ranking of "quality of care" for each insurance plan.

Introduction to Technique

The primary purpose of factor analysis is to reduce a large number of variables in a data set to a smaller more meaningful set of underlying dimensions, called factors. The original variables are ordinarily considered "indicators," not important in and of themselves. What is important is the structure of underlying dimensions (factors) which explain the common variance of the variables. Four distinct steps are common: inter-item correlation, factor extraction, factor rotation, and factor scaling.

Inter-Item Correlation: A correlation matrix is constructed to display the correlations (normally product-moment) between all variables in the analysis. The matrix may contain a dimensional structure, but the researcher generally cannot see it. Factor extraction is the search for that structure.

Factor Extraction: Extraction (e.g., principal-component analysis) transforms the set of variables of the correlation matrix into a factor matrix. The factor matrix displays the "loading" of each variable on the underlying dimensions, called common factors. Loading defines the degree to which each variable is correlated with the underlying factor. The factor structure can be mapped on a two-dimensional coordinate space (for two factors at a time) with variable coordinates corresponding to factor loadings.

Factor Rotation: The initial factor structure is both arbitrary—there are an infinite number of equally good ones—and difficult to interpret. There is no way to overcome the first problem; there simply is no unique solution. The problem of interpretation is approachable by use of factor rotation. The purpose of rotation is to enable the researcher to simplfy the factor columns and to display a meaningful pattern. The "varimax" criterion forces rotation of the axes to line up factors in such a manner as to produce loadings that approximate, as close as possible, either 1 or 0. It allows the analyst to define the meaning of factors in terms of those variables which clearly load on them and those which clearly do not. The initial factor solution typically produces moderately high loadings of most variables on the first, i.e., most important, factor. The varimax solution strengthens the loading of the most important of those variables and diminishes the rest—which, in turn, load more highly on secondary factors. Inferences can then be made about the meaning of the underlying factors. Inferences are based on the judgment of the analyst, not on mathematical criteria.

Factor Scaling: If factor analysis is to be used as a measurement tool, scores on the underlying factor—a newly created variable—can then be generated for all original cases.

REFERENCES

Nie, N., C. Hull, J. Jenkins, K. Steinbrenner, D. Bent, and J. Kim, SPSS: A Statistical Package for the Social Sciences, Second Edition. New York: McGraw-Hill, 1975.

Green, P., and D. Tull, Research for Marketing Decisions. Englewood Cliffs, N.J.: Prentice-Hall, 1970, Chapter 12.

Harris, D. M., "Effect of Population and Health Care Environment on Hospital Utilization," Health Services Research 10 (Fall 1975): 229-43.

Kimbell, L. J., and J. H. Lorant, "Methods for Systematic and Efficient Classification of Medical Practices," Health Services Research 8 (Spring 1973):46-60.

QUALITY OF MEDICAL CARE: A FACTOR ANALYSIS
APPROACH USING MEDICAL RECORDS

Carl E. Hopkins
Robert W. Hetherington
Eleanor M. Parsons

A relatively inexpensive, reliable, and unobtrusive method is described for measuring the content of medical care. Factor analysis of the content of the records of more than 11,000 physician-patient encounters from six different health insurance plans extracted four main factors or dimensions that together explained 42 percent of the variance in record content. Appropriate names for these dimensions appear to be: "prevention," "rationality," "verification," and "continuity." The method is tested by scoring the six insurance plans on the four factors.

Based on a paper read at the 23rd annual conference of the American Institute of Industrial Engineers, Anaheim, Calif., June 1, 1972. Research supported by Public Health Service Grant No. HS-00274. Reprinted with permission from Health Services Research 10, No. 2 (Summer 1975). Copyright 1975 by the Hospital Research and Educational Trust, 840 North Lakeshore Drive, Chicago, Ill. 60611.
Immeasurable assistance from the (anonymous) reviewers is gratefully acknowledged. Any remaining shortcomings are the authors'.

Most professionals (physicians, dentists, etc.) are wary of defining quality explicitly but are sure they know it when they see it. They commonly believe only a professional can judge quality of medical care. Hence the popularity of peer review. Objective or mechanical audits—even those that strictly follow physician-developed algorithms—are generally distrusted. Case review, either through examination of medical records [1,2] or by direct observation of physicians at work [3,4] is the only method trusted by the professionals, and even this with reservations. Case review usually means an expert judging without use of explicit criteria, since physicians rarely agree on particular criteria.

Some basic themes are found throughout the rhetoric of quality of care [5-8]. They make it clear that "quality" of care is not a unitary dimension and may be captured only by some weighted combination of a number of measurable criteria.

The problem, then, is to find a set of salient procedures in the content of medical care that reflects the "quality" of that care and to find a set of weights for the procedures such that a single composite score for quality of medical care encounter may be obtained. For economy and unobtrusiveness of the method, the procedures to be measured should be those that commonly are recorded in the patient chart.

The approach taken in this work was to find 40 such common procedures, using the advice of especially knowledgeable physicians and health record specialists. Then, in the well-known procedure of content factor analysis, the data themselves sort out the variables into factors (or dimensions) and define relative weights for the formation of a composite score. If these clusters make medical sense or can be validated by comparison with direct medical appraisal, one has a relatively inexpensive, unobtrusive, objective measure of "quality."

ASPECTS OF QUALITY MEASURED

From the literature [2-6, 8-11] and from extended discussions with physician consultants, five major qualitative dimensions of medical care were hypothesized. These five dimensions and their associated indicators are exhibited in Table 3.1. The indicators were limited to those procedures and activities that could be determined reliably from the medical chart. The inclusion of some procedures, such as "pelvic examination," may seem arbitrary and debatable, but the empirical analysis to follow will test these hypothesized relations. Some items, such as "well-baby checkup" and "Papanicolaou

TABLE 3.1

Hypothesized Dimensions and Selected Indicators
of Quality of Medical Care Services

Dimension	Indicators	
Prevention	Checkup examination Chest X ray Papanicolaou smear Prenatal checkup Immunization Well-baby examination	Advice on avoidance of future problems Rectal examination Pelvic examination Serology

Comprehensiveness	Secondary condition
	  found during visit
	  for another condition
		Social factors

Continuity	Follow-up visit
	Follow-up visit
	  requested
	Continuity of
	  medical personnel
		Continuity of medical
		  record
		Progress notes
		Rehabilitation services

Coordination	Referral: specialist Referral: paramedic	Consultation services

Rationality	Chief complaint
	History
	Physical examination
	Diagnosis
	Laboratory work
	  ordered
	Laboratory results
	  recorded
	Physician seen
	Surgery (amount)
		Treatment: injection
		Treatment: prescription
		Treatment: other
		Complete blood count
		Urinalysis
		Other laboratory work
		  done (amount)
		Other radiology work
		  done (amount)

smear," are age or sex-limited, and suitable statistical adjustments were made to correct for this problem.

DEVELOPMENT OF THE METHOD

The Data

Subscriber lists for 1968-69 for six different Los Angeles health insurance plans [12] were sampled randomly by taking every nth name from a random starting point. The lists were 100-percent oversampled to allow for an expected 50-percent response to a mailed questionnaire. (A subsample of nonrespondents was tracked down and interviewed to estimate nonresponse bias; this was significant on only three variables, for which an appropriate adjustment was made in the data analysis.)

From the random sample, 805 families responded to mailed questionnaires and authorized release of their medical records to investigators; 570 families had had some kind of care during the study year. This group provided 1,215 complete medical records (including hospital records) covering a 12-month period in the lives of the family members.

The medical records were photocopied in physicians' offices and hospital libraries by a company that specializes in this activity. The aim was to score each record on quality and then compare means and distributions of quality under the six plans.

Coding

The medical records were cut up (literally) into discrete bits of service, a medical care bit (MCB) being defined as a single patient-physician encounter and its associated laboratory, radiology, and other ancillary services. The MCB is the smallest discrete unit of medical care with substantive meaning. Bits may be combined or added to form more aggregated units of study, such as a patient, a family, a physician, a hospital, or a health insurance plan. From the 1,215 records, 11,379 bits were coded on each of 40 items of information. Most of the procedures coded were dummy variables (simply occurring or not), but some, such as "physical examination," were coded on a Likert-type scale, i.e., from one for a scanty examination to three for a full and detailed examination not limited to presenting complaint. Subjective judgment of the appropriateness of procedures was not attempted.

With this concept a lengthy series of training sessions and testing were held. Two physicians and three advanced nursing students

TABLE 3.2

Factor Analysis of Content of 11,000 Medical Care Bits

Variable	Factor 1 (Prevention)		Factor 2 (Rationality)		Factor 3 (Verification)		Factor 4 (Continuity)	
	r[a]	weight[b]	r	weight	r	weight	r	weight
Papanicolaou smear	0.82*	0.386*	-0.04	-0.101	0.00	-0.018	-0.07	0.008
Pelvic examination	0.81*	0.367*	0.14	0.004	0.02	-0.117	0.02	0.059
Checkup examination	0.71*	0.308*	-0.10	-0.142	0.18	0.011	-0.17	-0.060
Rectal examination	0.49*	0.173*	0.14	0.006	0.31	0.081	0.00	0.020
Physical examination	0.49*	0.159*	0.50*	0.221*	0.18	-0.023	0.03	0.041
Chief complaint	-0.01	-0.008	0.68*	0.381*	0.04	-0.038	-0.16	0.091
History	0.23	0.022	0.64*	0.315*	0.26	0.039	0.19	0.117
Diagnosis	0.11	0.014	0.51*	0.274*	0.02	-0.061	0.18	0.107
Progress notes	-0.07	-0.052	0.43*	0.262*	-0.12	-0.097	0.15	0.084
Complete blood count	0.16	-0.037	0.07	-0.050	0.77*	0.374*	0.01	-0.003
Urinalysis	0.14	-0.039	0.06	-0.049	0.71*	0.347*	-0.01	-0.012
Serology	-0.04	-0.115	0.04	-0.034	0.66*	0.343*	0.03	0.001
Chest X ray	0.10	-0.042	-0.04	-0.040	0.57*	0.282*	-0.06	-0.043
Follow-up visit	-0.10	0.005	-0.06	-0.021	0.01	-0.021	0.86*	0.473*

Follow-up visit requested	-0.02	0.035	0.05	0.032	0.06	0.022	0.85*	0.473*
Continuity of medical personnel	-0.10	0.010	-0.30	-0.146	-0.12	0.023	0.25	0.137
Social factors	0.11	-0.012	0.32	0.150	0.22	-0.068	-0.08	-0.040
Laboratory, radiology results recorded	-0.08	0.047	0.24	0.160	-0.16	-0.094	-0.16	-0.088
Referral: specialist	-0.07	-0.078	0.22	0.124	0.08	0.037	-0.16	-0.097
Immunization	0.02	0.001	-0.07	-0.043	0.02	0.017	-0.26	-0.143
Total percentage of variance explained	17.5		9.5		7.9		7.5	

aFactor loading (correlation of the variable with the factor).
bContribution of variable to factor variance.
*The correlation coefficients that define the factors.

each coded the same 20 records, and the results were tested for agreement (percent of coder pairs in exact agreement), intercoder correlations (Goodman's and Kruskal's gamma statistic [13]), concordance (Kendall's coefficient [13]), and bias (consistent deviation from the group average). Most of the items, such as "urinalysis ordered," required no judgment, simply care and attention. Several, however, required judgment (e.g., "level of seriousness," "completeness of physical exam"), and on these items agreement and reliability were low and bias was high. After group discussions of these items, modification of their definitions and scaling, and reiteration of the coding procedures, satisfactory coding (from 62-percent to 95-percent agreement) was achieved on 32 of the 40 variables; the unreliable variables were discarded. The coding of the 32-item set was then adopted as a standard, and as new coders were added they were trained on each item until they reached 85-percent agreement with the group coding, with no signs of nonrandom error (bias). The coders were retested frequently. Of the 32 variables in the final set, 8 remained difficult to code and test because they were infrequent or because they required some element of judgment. These were "advice on future problems," "social factors," "referral: paramedic," "annual checkup," "rectal examination," "pelvic examination," and "serology." These eight items were assigned to a specially trained (and audited) coder who did no others.

Although imperfections in the method and resulting data may remain despite the rigorous precautions, it was felt that a significant step had been achieved in making possible objective statistical analysis of data obtainable from medical records.

Analysis of the Data

Empirical verification of the existence of underlying dimensions in the data was accomplished by application of factor analysis (varimax rotation). After two reiterations to clear out redundant or meaningless variables, the 20 "best" variables were retained for the final factor analysis: 15 that had highly significant loadings on at least one of the first four factors, plus five that, although low on correlation with the factors, seemed to have conceptual significance ("continuity of medical personnel," "social factors," "lab and radiology results recorded," "referral to specialist," and "immunizations").

Final Dimensions of Quality

Results of the factor analysis are shown in Table 3.2; the correlation coefficients that define the factors are marked by asterisks.

The five hypothesized dimensions (Table 3.1) did not emerge; instead, the data yielded four major factors. While no single factor explained a great deal of the variance, the four factors combined explained 42 percent—still not high, but sufficient to encourage further exploration of the method. Five variables ("Papanicolaou smear," "pelvic examination," "checkup examination," "rectal examination," and "physical examination") had significantly high correlations (0.49 to 0.82) with the first factor and (with the exception of "physical examination") no appreciable correlation with any other factor. This factor seemed clearly to be "prevention."

"Physical examination," "chief complaint," "history," "diagnosis," and "progress notes" comprised a second cluster that corresponded fairly closely to the dimension originally labeled "rationality."

Four other variables, "complete blood count," "urinalysis," "serology," and "chest X ray," formed a cluster obviously related to rationality, but apparently distinct; its content seemed to represent adequate work-up, so it was given the name "verification."

The fourth factor picked up "follow-up visit" and "follow-up visit requested," the two variables remaining under the heading of "continuity" after the factor analysis.

The remaining five variables ("continuity of medical personnel," "social factors," "laboratory and radiology results recorded," "referral: specialist," and "immunization"), which had been forced into the factor analysis because of presumed conceptual significance, turned out to have no significant relation to any of the four factors and failed to form a fifth factor. For all of the factors that did emerge, the sign of the correlation coefficient makes sense: i.e., more Pap smears are associated with "prevention," more histories are associated with "rationality," and so on.

The coefficient for each variable composing a factor indicates the relative importance (weight) of that variable in the factor. Thus a factor score for a given MCB is obtained by summing over all the variables the product of the observed value of each variable times that variable's weight in the factor.

APPLICATION OF THE METHOD

The four factors were tested for their ability to differentiate among the six health insurance plans, which represent quite different approaches to the provision of medical care. Two were closed-panel prepaid group practice plans of different sizes ("small" and "large"); another pair comprised a large and a small commercial indemnity insurance plan; and the third pair was two provider-sponsored "open" service plans operated respectively by a medical society and a hospital association. The general hypothesis was that the more centralized

TABLE 3.3

Mean Factor Score, by Plan

Plan	Factor			
	Prevention	Rationality	Verification	Continuity
All six plans	0.421 ± 0.119*	0.513 ± 0.120	0.138 ± 0.097	0.587 ± 0.101
Large group	0.455	0.531	0.148	0.589
Small group	0.435	0.506	0.153	0.567
Hospital sponsored	0.401	0.526	0.118	0.625
Physician sponsored	0.410	0.504	0.139	0.587
Small commercial	0.435	0.501	0.153	0.567
Large commercial	0.375	0.504	0.133	0.556

*Standard deviation of individual medical care bit.

TABLE 3.4

Transformed Factor Score Means and Ranks, by Plan
(1 = Highest Rank, 6 = Lowest)

Plan	Factor				Overall Score and Rank
	Prevention	Rationality	Verification	Continuity	
Large group	15.01 (1)	11.43 (1)	10.81 (2)	10.15 (3)	47.40 (1)
Small group	12.06 (2)	9.45 (3)	11.22 (1)	8.52 (5)	41.25 (2)
Hospital sponsored	7.06 (5)	11.03 (2)	8.37 (6)	12.82 (1)	39.28 (3)
Physician sponsored	8.39 (4)	9.29 (4.5)	10.08 (3)	10.00 (4)	37.76 (5)
Small commercial	8.67 (3)	9.05 (6)	9.02 (5)	11.18 (2)	37.92 (4)
Large commercial	3.23 (6)	9.29 (4.5)	9.59 (4)	7.69 (6)	29.80 (6)

and organized plans, i.e., the group practice plans, would rank superior on the four dimensions of quality developed through the factor analysis. To test this, the records were sorted by plan, factor scores were computed for each medical encounter, and average scores were calculated for each plan for each of the four factors.

Plan Performance

Table 3.3 presents the mean factor scores for the six plans. In order to compare mean scores across the factors it was necessary to put the four factors on the same scale. This was done with the transformation $\bar{x}' = (\bar{x} - X)/S$, where $\bar{x}$ is the mean score for a plan, $\bar{X}$ is the mean of the plan means, and S is the all-plan standard deviation for each dimension. To permit addition of the factors to get an overall plan score, an additional transformation was applied: $10 + w\bar{x}$, where w is the relative weight of the factor (actually the percentage of variance explained by the factor, namely 17.5, 9.5, 7.9, and 7.5 percent for the four factors, respectively). The constant 10 is added to make all transformed means positive. Table 3.4 presents the transformed means and ranks (1 = highest rank). In this table any differences greater than one are statistically significant because of the large ns. The numbers have no direct physical meaning.

By summing the transformed mean scores over the four factors it was possible to get an overall ranking of the plans. Although no plan was highest on all factors and none was in the same rank on all scores, there was some general consistency in the rankings, with the group practice plans having more high scores, the provider-sponsored plans falling generally in the middle, and the commercial plans scoring generally low.

Prevention. When all six plans were analyzed together the "prevention" factor accounted for 17.5 percent of the variance in medical services content (Table 3.2).

As shown in Table 3.4, the group practice plans ranked first and second on this dimension. Performance was highest in the small group practice plan on two of the five indicators ("checkup examination" and "pelvic examination"), and the large group practice plan was highest on the remaining three ("physical examination," "Papanicolaou smear," and "rectal examination"). The hospital association plan and the large commercial plan ranked lowest. This result agrees with expectation: one can infer that in the group plans the physician "manages" the consumer's health, and has incentives to maintain health and prevent disease, while in the other plans the consumer tends to manage his own health, making decisions on when and where to get care with no visible incentive to seek preventive care.

Rationality. This factor accounted for 9.5 percent of the variance in services recorded for all six plans (Table 3.2).

The large group practice plan ranked highest, with the hospital-sponsored plan second (Table 3.4). A previous study [14] has shown the large group plan's medical records to be more complete than those of the others, which may explain this finding. A physician attitude survey [12] showed an association between rationality score and the attitude that good medical records are necessary to high quality care, but physicians who believed in good medical records were spread evenly across the plans, so this potentially confounding variable does not explain the differences observed.

Another potentially confounding variable was the level of seriousness of the conditions treated, which could conceivably give rise to more MCBs in the form of progress notes connected with lengthy hospitalizations. However, the level of seriousness did not differ much among the plans and so could not explain the observed differences.

Of the individual variables comprising the rationality factor, rate and extent of "physical examination" and "history" were greatest for the two group practice plans. In addition, "diagnosis" and "chief complaint" were more frequently recorded in the group plans.

Data from the physician survey mentioned before [12] indicated that across all plans rationality scores were higher for specialists, younger physicians, and physicians who see fewer than four patients per hour.

Verification. This accounted for an additional 7.9 percent of the variance in services recorded for the six plans.

Again the two group practice plans ranked first and second. The small group plan was highest on use of all four of the tests (complete blood count, urinalysis, serology, and chest X ray).

A surprising side-finding was that although many laboratory and radiology tests were ordered, reports of the results were found in only 13 percent of the applicable medical care bits, with somewhat more test reports found in the records of the commercial and provider-sponsored plans.

Continuity. This accounted for an additional 7.5 percent of the variance in services recorded for the six plans.

On the continuity factor the hospital plan and the small commercial plan ranked highest, as might be expected, with the group practice plans low. This finding is explained by the structure of the group plans, in which a patient is less likely to see the same physician on every visit, and in which more paramedical personnel are used. The group plans generally try to assign each patient to a primary physician, but the patients are free to go to specialty clinics without referral and they often do.

DISCUSSION

These dimensions of the content of medical care could be used to compare the products of different physicians, hospitals, or health insurance plans.

The method has some obvious advantages. Once the development costs are sunk (for identification of variables, development of a coding manual, and collection and coding of a large sample of medical records) and the procedure has been established, (1) it is relatively inexpensive to repeat, (2) it is mechanical, reliable, and does not require expensive expert judgment, and (3) it is unobtrusive with respect to the activities being measured.

On the other hand, however, the method is limited by the completeness and legibility of the medical records, which vary enormously [1]. A separate study [14] indicated that it is possible to score medical records on their own quality; it might be worthwhile to use these two scoring systems to explore the relationship between quality of records and quality (content) of care. If there should be a substantial relationship between the two, it might then be worthwhile to include record quality as a variable in the factor analysis, or even to use record quality measures as a surrogate for quality of medical care.

The method could be validated by comparing medical record factor scores with quality scores assigned by a panel of physicians using the Delphi technique or the direct judgments of the peer review process. More direct validation would relate factor scores to various outcome measures such as subsequent morbidity, disability, and mortality. This would require quite large samples and probably would not be worth the cost on its own account; but grafted onto some other large-scale study, such as the current Rand Corporation health insurance study [15], it might be accomplished at a reasonable cost-to-benefit ratio.

However validated, and whether or not it measures "quality," the method appears to offer a feasible means of aggregating and assessing the content of medical care. Large-scale purchasers of medical care (governments, trade unions, professional societies, etc.) have a considerable interest in what they are getting for their money and in comparing the outputs of alternative plans. Such entities could well afford the investment required to find the relevant parameters (procedures) and their factor coefficients. Once this is accomplished they could monitor the content of care over time and across alternative plans with small periodic samples.

The plans themselves would appear to have a stake in maintaining and improving their output through similar surveillance. Analysis of which factors were substandard—and which variables (procedures) were included in such factors—would point fairly precisely to areas requiring remedial action. For example, in the present study, the large group practice plan is clearly above average in the first three factors, but could benefit from improvement of the "continuity" factor. Having identified this weakness of the system, the operations analysts could study the system of appointments, callbacks, and referrals to pinpoint the means of improving it.

Finally, individual hospitals and physicians could be similarly monitored as to their output.

Since large medical care purchasers are increasingly requiring more complete and uniform data systems of their provider sources [16], the quality of the data to be fed into this method should improve, making the quality of care scores more precise, more reliable, and less expensive to collect.

REFERENCES

1. Lembcke, P. A., "Evaluation of the Medical Audit," J. Am. Med. Assoc. 199 (February 20, 1967):543.

2. Daily, E. F., and M. A. Morehead, "A Method of Evaluating and Improving the Quality of Medical Care," Am. J. Public Health 46 (July 1956):848.

3. Peterson, O. L., "Medical Care: Its Social and Organizational Aspects—Evaluation of the Quality of Medical Care," New Engl. J. Med. 269 (December 5, 1963):1283.

4. Clute, K. F., The General Practitioner. Toronto: University of Toronto Press, 1963.

5. Lee, R. L., and L. W. Jones, The Fundamentals of Good Medical Care. Committee on the Costs of Medical Care, Publication No. 22. Chicago: University of Chicago Press, 1933.

6. Brook, R. H., "Quality of Care Assessment: Choosing a Method for Peer Review," New Engl. J. Med. 288 (June 21, 1973):1323.

7. DeGeyndt, W., "Five Approaches for Assessing the Quality of Care," Hosp. Adm. 15 (Winter 1970):21.

8. Williamson, J. W., "Evaluating Quality of Patient Care: A Strategy Relating Outcome and Process Assessment," J. Am. Med. Assoc. 218 (October 25, 1971):564.

9. North, R. C., O. R. Holsti, M. G. Zaninovich, and D. A. Zinnes, Content Analysis. Evanston, Ill.: Northwestern University Press, 1963.

10. Cochrane, A. L., Effectiveness and Efficiency: Random Reflections on Health Services. London: Nuffield Provincial Hospital Trust, 1972.

11. Donabedian, A., Medical Care Appraisal—Quality and Utilization: A Guide to Medical Care Administration, Vol. 2. New York: American Public Health Association, 1969.

12. Hetherington, R. W., C. W. Hopkins, and M. I. Roemer, Health Insurance Plans: Promise and Performance. New York: Wiley, 1975.

13. Kendall, M. G., and A. Stuart, The Advanced Theory of Statistics. New York: Hafner, 1967.

14. Horiuchi, H. T., "Evaluation of the Quality of Health Plan Patient Records." Unpublished thesis, University of California—Los Angeles, 1970.

15. Veney, J. E., "The Rand Health Insurance Study," Inquiry 11 (March 1974):3.

16. Kovner, A. R., and E. J. Lusk, "State Regulation of Health Care Costs," Med. Care 13 (August 1975):8.

4

DISCRIMINANT ANALYSIS

INTRODUCTION

The incorporation of computer and information management techniques has been considered by many to be a possible solution to some of the major management problems currently facing hospitals. Nevertheless, in 1970, only 40 percent of the nonfederal hospitals in the United States were using computers. It seems relevant to investigate the reasons that some hospitals have adopted computer use and others have not. Based on an open system conceptualization of a hospital, this paper presents a basis hypothesis on the factors that distinguish adopters from nonadopters. Data from the state of Texas are used to support the hypothesis. Moreover, through discriminant analysis, characteristic profiles of adopters and nonadopters are developed.

Introduction to Technique

Discriminant analysis is a technique to study group differences. The dependent variable, in discriminant analysis, is nominal scaled, whereas independent variables are (typically) interval scaled. The objectives of this technique are to: (a) test whether significant differences exist among the average 'score' profiles of two or more a priori defined groups, (b) determine which independent variables account most for such intergroup differences in average profile, (c) find linear combinations of the independent variables that best separate the group means, that is which maximize among group variance relative to within group variance, and (d) classify new subjects whose characteristics, but not group identity, are known and assumed to be from one of the a priori defined groups. In case of two groups, multiple regression techniques may be used to achieve the same objectives.

REFERENCES

Green, P. E., and D. S. Tull, Research for Marketing Decisions. Englewood Cliffs, N.J.: Prentice-Hall, 1970.

Tatsuoka, M. M., Discriminant Analysis: The Study of Group Differences. Champaign, Ill.: Institute for Personality and Ability Testing, 1970.

Wentz, B., Marketing Research Management and Methods. New York: Harper & Row, 1972.

A DISCRIMINANT ANALYSIS OF USERS AND NONUSERS OF COMPUTERS IN THE HOSPITAL INDUSTRY

Vijay Mahajan
and
Milton E. F. Schoeman

INTRODUCTION

Information binds together the many components of any modern organization; it is the key variable in the process of managing organizations. We are, in fact, living in an information society [30]. A modern hospital, perhaps more than any other social institution, is dependent upon rapid and accurate information flow. In the practice of modern medicine, correct information at the right time can be vital to save a life or prevent a catastrophe. A systems expert of the Lockheed Missile and Space Corporation says, "The real practice of medicine is an information handling art" [15].

Two of the many problems which concern experts in the health services are the rising cost of and the quality of health care. Lockheed studies estimate that approximately 30 percent of each hospital bill is attributable to nonproductive information handling [15]. Other independent estimates are somewhat more conservative, ranging from 20 to 25 percent, but the fact remains that these expenses represent a significant portion of total costs [10, 26]. Furthermore, it is estimated that professional personnel (the largest component of a hospital's budget is salaries) often spend over 30 percent of their time in information handling [7, 17]. According to the National Communicable Disease Center, 10 to 40 percent of bacteriological testing in clinical laboratories is unsatisfactory, along with 30 to 50 percent in simple chemistry tests, 40 to 80 percent in different blood counts, and 20 to 30 percent in assessments of serum electrolytes. Most of these errors belong in the 'paper and pencil' category; they are caused by transcription, arithmetic miscalculation, and inaccurate patient identification [4].

The above statistics suggest that computers may provide a means to reduce or at least stabilize the cost of health care and to improve the quality of care. In fact, "the introduction of the computer and information management techniques is considered by many informed health professionals and knowledgeable leaders in the medical computer field to be a solution to some of the major health management problems we are confronted with today" [3]. The above statement is supplemented by the results of a survey conducted by the Hospital Financial Management Association where 93 percent of responding hospitals reported that electronic data processing has enhanced the effectiveness of their information flow [22].

In 1970, the estimated installed computer value in the hospital industry was $0.24 billion, one percent of the total installed computer value in all industries [29]; this figure was expected to rise to $1.4 billion by 1975, 3 percent of the total installed computer value [29]. Indeed the hospital industry has the greatest computer-usage growth rate among all industries [29]. In recent years, the availability of small computers and mini-computers and service organizations, outside the hospital organization, which supply shared computer use to hospitals are all having a powerful effect on the rate and areas of diffusion of computer usage in hospitals.

Nevertheless, only about 40 percent of the hospitals in the United States were using computers in 1970 [31]. Why have only 40 percent of the hospitals adopted computers? What are the differences between the adopters and nonadopters? This paper analyzes the characteristics of the adopters and nonadopters of computers. To accomplish this purpose, a hospital is conceptualized as an open system. This conceptual framework is used to derive the hypothesis that the differences between the adopters and nonadopters can be attributed to (a) the characteristics of hospitals, (b) the environment in which a hospital operates, and (c) the characteristics of the hospital administrator.* Discriminant analysis of variables related to these three

---

*These three factors are also suggested in other research conducted on the diffusion of innovations in the health system dealing with programmatic services; see, for example, [27] or [28].

sets of factors is used to distinguish between adopters and nonadopters. The state of Texas, in which about 30 percent of the nonfederal hospitals[*] have adopted computers, is chosen as a specific study site. Of all states in the west south central census region, Texas has the highest number of hospitals and medical schools, including some which are known nationwide and worldwide for being on the forefront of medical research.

CONCEPTUAL FRAMEWORK AND MAJOR HYPOTHESIS

A Hospital as an Open System: A Conceptual Framework

A hospital, like any other organization, is a social system designed for attaining some specific goals and serving a certain purpose or purposes. In an open-system framework, the hospital is in constant interaction with its environment and there is an importation of energy from the external environment into the hospital [6]. Literally, the hospital is viewed as importing resources from the environment in terms of people, materials, capital, and so forth. It is expected to use these inputs to output a product (that is, healthy patients) or a service to its environment in exchange for new inputs. A hospital's survival, then, depends upon its ability to favorably exchange its outputs over time with the environment to get continued inputs. For example, today's hospitals are plagued by rapidly escalating workloads and cost, both of which suggest unfavorable exchange; such a situation, in turn, gives rise to alternative systems or organizations, such as Health Maintenance Organizations or neighborhood health centers, that may improve this exchange, and thereby attract environmental resources away from hospitals.

The history of the American hospital reflects its continued struggle to change its objectives and structure to cope with its changing environment [8, 11]. From almshouses and pesthouses, orphanages, and shelters for the aged, infirm, and insane, hospitals have developed into agencies of medical care, research, and education, directly and indirectly benefiting almost all members of the modern community. As Heydebrand [20] points out, the modern hospital is a "multipurpose institution" possessing some or all of the following functions: economic enterprise, medical care institution, social

---

[*]Federal hospitals are excluded from the analysis since they have an atypical set of resources which can be applied to the implementation of computer systems.

agency (which nevertheless is subject to the "test of financial solvency" like a business enterprise), educational enterprise (this role being "among the most diverse purposes of the hospital" and "much more than a sideline activity"), research enterprise, religious institution (especially when spiritual care is seen as an additional responsibility in church-affiliated hospitals), community enterprise, and public enterprises (because hospitals' costs are of public concern).

From the preceding discussion it may be hypothesized that the adoption, or nonadoption of computers may be attributed to the goals of a hospital and its own organizational structure created to attain these goals. Thus, the first factor in distinguishing adopters from nonadopters consists of hospital characteristics.

Clearly, a second factor arising from an open systems framework is the environment. The environment of an organization is important in two different ways. First, changes in the environment create a situation of stress or pressure to which the adoption unit must respond if it is to remain in a relationship of "dynamic equilibrium" with the environment. Thus, an adoption unit is more likely to innovate when its relevant environment is rapidly changing than when it is steady. Furthermore, for two adoption units operating under the same environment, depending upon their structural characteristics, different amounts of stress or pressure from the environment may be required to result in adoption of the innovation by them at different times. Second, if the response to the dynamic environment is an innovation, environmental norms may or may not favor the changes this innovation implies. Therefore, it is hypothesized that the environment in which a hospital operates or serves should contribute to the differences between the adopters and nonadopters. A hospital environment in this study is divided into three segments: (a) its physical location, (b) the health of the population it serves, and (c) the relevant economics.

Finally, in any organization, the ultimate decision to adopt and/or implement an innovation is the responsibility of the management. It is not an overstatement to say that the management of an organization provides the driving force to lead an organization in a dynamic environment. The management may represent the 'style' or the 'image' or the 'behavior' of an organization. In the case of hospitals, "there is no element of health manpower whose impact on hospital effectiveness is more important than the hospital administrator's" [34]. A number of studies and articles have emphasized the important role played by the hospital administrator in the process of adopting innovations or more specifically the use of computers [5, 12, 19, 21, 25, 41]. Therefore, it is hypothesized that the third factor which should distinguish between the adopters and nonadopters is the training and background of the hospital administrator.

TABLE 4.1

Dictionary of Variables

Variable	Variable Index	Definition
Computer activity	y	y = 1 if hospital uses computer activity = 0 otherwise
Hospital Characteristics		
Teaching designation	x_1	x_1 = 1 if hospital is a major unit of a teaching facility = 0 otherwise
Control	x_2	x_2 = 1 if hospital is governmental, nonfederal = 0 otherwise
	x_3	x_3 = 1 if hospital is nongovernmental, not-for-profit = 0 otherwise
If $x_2 = x_3 = 0$, then hospital is nongovernmental for profit		
Service	x_4	x_4 = 1 if hospital is general medical and surgical = 0 otherwise
Stay	x_5	x_5 = 1 if hospital is short-term = 0 otherwise
Bed size	x_6	x_6 = Number of beds
Census	x_7	x_7 = Average number of patients receiving care each day during a 12-month period; does not include newborn
Occupancy	x_8	x_8 = Ratio of average daily census to the average number of beds maintained during the 12-month period
Facilities	x_9	x_9 = Total number of facilities (AHA identifies 46 different facilities in a hospital, e.g.,

Variable	Variable Index	Definition
		Intensive care unit, Emergency department, Volunteer services department, etc.)
Advanced technological facilities	x_{10}	x_{10} = Number of advanced technological facilities. These are: open-heart surgery; diagnostic radioisotope; therapeutic radioisotope; organ bank; electroencephalography; inpatient renal dialysis; outpatient renal dialysis; burn care.
Total expenses/bed	x_{11}	x_{11} = Total expenses per bed in thousands of dollars for a 12-month period.
Payroll/employee	x_{12}	x_{12} = 12-month salary per full time employee in thousands of dollars. It does not include salaries paid to interns, residents, students, nurses and other trainees.
Personnel/bed	x_{13}	x_{13} = Number of full time personnels per bed. It does not include trainees, private nurses, and volunteers.

Hospital Environment

Location Characteristics:

Urban/Rural	x_{14}	x_{14} = 1 if county in which hospital is located is in a SMSA (standard metropolitan statistical area). There are 24 SMSAs in Texas. = 0 otherwise

(continued)

Table 4.1 (continued)

Variable	Variable Index	Definition
Density	x_{15}	x_{15} = county population per square mile.
Age	x_{16}	x_{16} = median age of county populace.
	x_{17}	x_{17} = percent of population below 14 years of age.
	x_{18}	x_{18} = percent of population above 65 years of age.
Income	x_{19}	x_{19} = median per capita income.
	x_{20}	x_{20} = percent of families with income below poverty level.
	x_{21}	x_{21} = percent of population earning greater than $10,000 per annum.
Health characteristics:		
	x_{22}	x_{22} = number of licensed hospitals in the county.
	x_{23}	x_{23} = number of medical schools in the county.
	x_{24}	x_{24} = hospital beds per 1000 population in the county.
	x_{25}	x_{25} = physicians per 1000 population in the county
Economic characteristics:		
	x_{26}	x_{26} = percent of administrators and managers in county population. Included are such occupations as public administrators, bank officers, buyers, inspectors, pilots, school administrators, etc.

Variable	Variable Index	Definition
	x_{27}	x_{27} = percent of professional, technical workers in county population. This group includes such occupations as lawyers, accountants, computer specialists, engineers, mathematical specialists, physicians, nurses, teachers, and scientific technicians.
	x_{28}	x_{28} = percent change in total bank deposits in county since 1959.

Hospital Administrators

Administrator's background and training:

	x_{29}	x_{29} = 1 if hospital administrator is a member of the American College of Hospital Administrators. = 0 otherwise
	x_{30}	x_{30} = 1 if hospital administrator is a physician. = 0 otherwise
	x_{31}	x_{31} = 1 if hospital administrator is a nurse. = 0 otherwise
	x_{32}	x_{32} = 1 if hospital administrator is church trained. = 0 otherwise.

If $x_{30} = x_{31} = x_{32} = 0$, then hospital administrator has training and/or college education in hospital administration.

To summarize, the overriding hypothesis of this study is that the differences between adopters and nonadopters can be attributed to (a) the characteristics of the hospitals, (b) the environment in which a hospital operates, and (c) the training and background of the hospital administrator.

Selection of Predictor Variables

Thirty-two predictor variables are selected to represent the above three factors; thirteen predictor variables represent the characteristics of the hospital; fifteen predictor variables represent the hospital environment segmented into locational, health, and economic environment; and four predictor variables represent the training and background of hospital administrator. The rationale for the selection of these variables is given in detail in [31]. Table 4.1 gives the listing and the definition of these variables. The variables listed represent a compromise between those characteristics that should be ideally measured and those characteristics on which data were available. In the case of hospital characteristics, the data were relatively straightforward to collect. In the cases of environmental and hospital administrator characteristics, however, most of the available data came from secondary sources with some overlap in categorizations. Even so, categories were structured as independently as possible. Where necessary correlation analyses were performed to permit accurate interpretation of the results.

DATA COLLECTION AND DATA ANALYSIS METHODOLOGIES

As of December 1973, of the 490 non-federal hospitals in the state of Texas, 142 hospitals were using computers, about 30 percent of the population. References 1, 2, 13, 14, 23, 24, 35, 36, 39, and 40 were used to compile data on the 32 predictor variables for the whole population. Data could be collected only for 367 hospitals (this includes 117 adopters and 250 nonadopters). This sample represents about 75 percent of the population. Furthermore, all the adopters in the state of Texas were short term hospitals (x_5). A chi-square analysis on the sample showed that the sample does not represent nongovernmental-for-profit hospitals which have bed capacity less than 50; such a shortcoming was not considered major since the overwhelming majority of hospitals in the population are not in this category.

The results are presented in terms of the four objectives of discriminant analysis [18], which are:

A. <u>Group differences</u>: Testing whether significant differences exist among the average 'score' profiles of two groups (adopters and

FIGURE 4.1

Factor Interactions

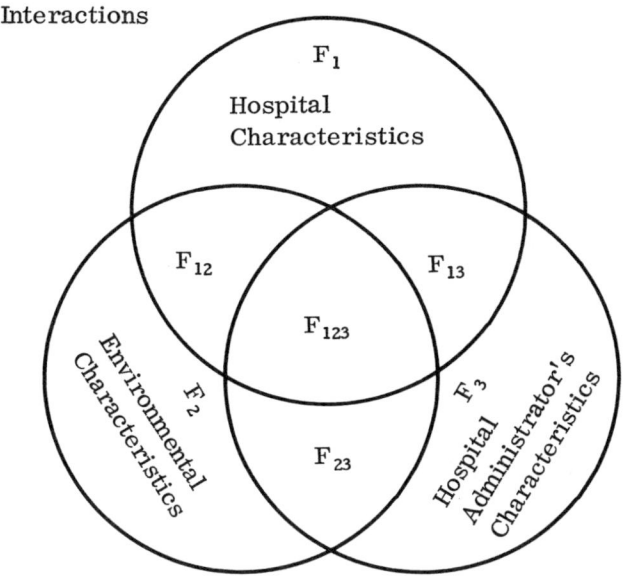

$$\hat{\omega}^2_{123} = F_1 + F_2 + F_3 + F_{13} + F_{12} + F_{23} + F_{123}$$
$$\hat{\omega}^2_{12} = F_1 + F_2 + F_{12} + F_{13} + F_{23} + F_{123}$$
$$\hat{\omega}^2_{13} = F_1 + F_3 + F_{12} + F_{13} + F_{23} + F_{123}$$
$$\hat{\omega}^2_{23} = F_2 + F_3 + F_{12} + F_{13} + F_{23} + F_{123}$$
$$\hat{\omega}^2_1 = F_1 + F_{12} + F_{13} + F_{123}$$
$$\hat{\omega}^2_2 = F_2 + F_{12} + F_{23} + F_{123}$$
$$\hat{\omega}^2_3 = F_3 + F_{13} + F_{23} + F_{123}$$

nonadopters) in terms of predictor variables, assuming group co-variation and dispersion are equal and the distributions are multinormal. Testing is done by Wilk's lambda test [9].

B. <u>Strength of discriminators</u>: Determining which variables account most for any intergroup differences in average profile; this is done by examining structural coefficients between the predictor variables and discriminant function, and with a univariate F-test on each predictor variable [9]. The total discriminatory power of the whole battery of predictor variables is measured by the index

$\hat{\omega}^2$ [37]. The total discriminatory power attributable to each factor (F_j) and their interactions ($F_{i,j}$) is determined by calculating $\hat{\omega}^2$ and performing discriminant analysis on each individual factor and their combinations.*

C. <u>Linear combination</u>: Finding linear combination of the predictor variables by maximizing among-group relative to within-group separation, measured by separation index λ.

D. <u>Classification</u>: Classifying new subjects whose characteristics, but not group identity, are known by using the linear combination of predictor variables. Confidence in the predictive power of the discriminant function is obtained by comparing the classification obtained by the discriminant function to the classifications obtained by three chance criteria [32, 16].

RESULTS

Simple Correlation Analysis

In our earlier discussion, it was pointed out that the predictor variables selected to represent different characteristics may be intercorrelated. Table 4.2 presents the simple correlation between predictor variables and the dependent variable (that is, computer adoption) for the entire population of 400 hospitals.

Examination of Table 4.2 indicates that there are only two predictor variables x_9, total number of facilities, and x_{11}, total expenses/bed, which have simple correlation greater than .50. There are only three predictor variables x_6, number of beds, x_7, census, and x_{10}, number of advanced technological facilities, which have simple correlation greater than .40 but less than .50. The correlations of other predictor variables with the adoption are not too strong. The intercorrelations among these five variables are presented in Table 4.3. Examination of these intercorrelations indicates that the five variables are highly intercorrelated. The large bed size hospitals tend to have high census, a greater number of total number of facilities, and advanced technological facilities. The correlation between x_{11}, total expenses/bed, with the other four predictor variables, though not very strong, is also high. These results suggest that adopters of computers have large bed size, serve more patients (that is, high census), have a greater number of total and advanced technological facilities and tend to have high expenses/bed.

An examination of simple correlations, though it gives some insight about the structure of the problem, does not directly take into

---

*See key below Figure 4.1.

TABLE 4.2

Simple Correlation between Predictor Variables
and Adoption

Predictor Variable	Correlation	Predictor Variable	Correlation
x_1	.23	x_{17}	.18
x_2	-.18	x_{18}	-.34
x_3	.12	x_{19}	.33
x_4	.09	x_{20}	-.26
x_5	.12	x_{21}	.34
x_6	.45	x_{22}	.32
x_7	.45	x_{23}	.30
x_8	.36	x_{24}	-.07
x_9	.51	x_{25}	.29
x_{10}	.46	x_{26}	.09
x_{11}	.52	x_{27}	.37
x_{12}	.23	x_{28}	.10
x_{13}	-.02	x_{29}	.37
x_{14}	.37	x_{30}	-.12
x_{15}	.32	x_{31}	-.05
x_{16}	-.04	x_{32}	.19

TABLE 4.3

Intercorrelation Matrix between Predictor Variables
which Have Simple Correlation Greater Than .40

Predictor Variable	6	7	9	10	11
6	1.0				
7	.99	1.0			
9	.81	.81	1.0		
10	.78	.79	.88	1.0	
11	.45	.49	.59	.53	1.0

consideration the interactions between the predictor variables. For this reason, discriminant analysis is performed next on the sample of 367 hospitals.

Group Differences

Are the two groups of adopters and nonadopters significantly different? If μ_1 and μ_2 are the centroids of the two groups (adopters and nonadopters) respectively, the null hypothesis is:

H0: $\mu_1 = \mu_2$

and alternate hypothesis is:

H1: $\mu_1 \neq \mu_2$

The following results are obtained for Wilk's lambda test for group means:

```
Wilk's lambda                       =  .547
F-ratio                             = 8.646
Degrees of freedom                  = 32 and 334
Probability of group differences
  due to chance                     =  .0000
```

Therefore, we reject the null hypothesis and conclude that, statistically, there are significant differences among the adopters and nonadopters in terms of the defined predictor variables.

Strength of Discriminators

Which variables account most for the differences between the two groups?

The variance between the two groups is explained along one discriminant axis. Table 4.4 presents these results. The separation index or the discriminant criterion value λ is .8284. Thus, the total discriminatory power of the battery of predictor variables, $\hat{\omega}^2$, is .4509. That is, about 45.09 percent of the total variability of the discriminant function is attributable to group differences. Or, 45.09 percent of the variability in the discriminant space is relevant to group differentiation; and 100 percent of the total discriminatory power of predictor variables is explained by one discriminant function.

Table 4.5 gives results for factor interactions. 30.30 percent of the total discriminatory power of the battery of predictor variables

TABLE 4.4

Adopters-Nonadopters Discriminant Function Tests

$$\text{Trace} = .8284$$
$$\lambda = .8284$$
$$\hat{\omega}_2 = .4509$$

	Axis 1
Percent of variance explained	100.0000
chi-square	211.9500
Degrees of freedom	32.0000
Probability of no difference	0.0000

TABLE 4.5

Factor Interactions*

Factors	$\hat{\omega}_2$	F	Percent of the Explained Variability
1	.4064	.1366	30.30
2	.2436	.0257	5.70
3	.1505	.0159	3.53
(1, 2)	.4350	.1381	30.63
(1, 3)	.4252	.0548	12.15
(2, 3)	.3143	.0029	0.64
(1, 2, 3)	.4509	.0769	17.05

*1. Hospital characteristics.
 2. Environmental characteristics.
 3. Hospital administrator's characteristics.

TABLE 4.6

Adopters-Nonadopters Discriminant Analysis Results

Variables	Correlation Axis 1	F-Ratio	P	Discriminant Function Weight 1
x_1	.3300	18.9467	.0001	-.6846
x_2	-.2730	12.7549	.0007	-.2647
x_3	.1796	5.4104	.0194	-.1976
x_4	.1285	2.7504	.0940	.2999
x_5	.1948	6.3827	.0115	.0685
x_6	.6689	92.8023	.0000	-.0002
x_7	.6901	100.4241	.0000	.0019
x_8	.5486	57.6258	.0000	-.0009
x_9	.7874	142.5907	.0000	.0339
x_{10}	.7063	106.6006	.0000	-.0755
x_{11}	.7545	126.8633	.0000	.0374
x_{12}	.3374	19.8498	.0001	-.0531
x_{13}	-.0432	.3093	.5855	-.0006
x_{14}	.5893	68.1503	.0000	.0556
x_{15}	.4852	43.5847	.0000	.0002
x_{16}	-.0732	.8893	.3485	.0090
x_{17}	.2550	11.0825	.0013	-.0214
x_{18}	-.5518	58.4042	.0000	-.0257
x_{19}	.5085	48.4355	.0000	.0001
x_{20}	-.4420	35.4456	.0000	.0126
x_{21}	.5541	58.9693	.0000	.0110
x_{22}	.4623	39.1259	.0000	-.0179
x_{23}	.4479	36.4834	.0000	.1442
x_{24}	-.0965	1.5478	.2116	.0112
x_{25}	.4960	45.7883	.0000	.0447
x_{26}	.1604	4.3069	.0363	.0355
x_{27}	.6210	77.2744	.0000	.0132
x_{28}	.1335	2.9691	.0818	.0002
x_{29}	.5436	56.4091	.0000	.1254
x_{30}	-.1659	4.6107	.0304	-.2339
x_{31}	-.0538	.4789	.4965	.3998
x_{32}	.2582	11.3696	.0012	.2387

is attributable to hospital characteristics, 30.63 percent to the interaction between hospital characteristics and environmental characteristics, 12.15 percent to the interaction between hospital and hospital administrator's characteristics, and 17.05 percent to the three-way interaction between hospital, environmental, and hospital administrator's characteristics. Individually, the environmental characteristics have 5.70 percent and the hospital administrator's characteristics have only 3.53 percent of the total discriminatory power of the predictor variables.

Table 4.6 gives the structural correlation between predictor variables and discriminant scores and univariate F-ratio test results. Examination of univariate F-ratios in Table 4.6 indicates that predictor variables, x_4, type of service, x_{13}, personnel per bed, x_{16}, median age of county populace, x_{24}, hospital beds per 100 population, x_{28}, percent change in total bank deposits in county since 1959, and x_{31}, hospital administrator is a nurse, do not, independently, separate the groups. All other predictor variables, independently, are likely to contribute significantly to the overall differences between groups. Predictor variables x_{26}, percent of administrators and managers in county population, and x_{30}, hospital administrator is a physician, are significant at the .03 level of significance and all others are significant at less than the .01 level of significance.

Examination of structural coefficients between predictor variables and discriminant axis shows that hospitals which have adopted computers are likely to have large bed size, higher census, higher percent occupancy, a greater number of total facilities and advanced technological facilities, and higher total expenses per bed. Such hospitals are likely to be located in counties which are in a SMSA, have a low percent of population above 65 years of age, a higher median per capita income, a higher percent of population earning greater than $10,000 per annum, a higher number of physicians per 1000 population, and a higher percent of professional, technical workers in county population. Such hospitals are more likely to have a hospital administrator who is a member of the American College of Hospital Administrators.

The above results show that the best discriminators in hospital characteristics are, in order of their importance: (a) x_9, total number of facilities, (b) x_{11}, total expenses per bed, (c) x_{10}, total number of advanced technological facilities, (d) x_7, census, and (e) x_6, bed size.

In the environmental characteristics, the best discriminators are, in order of their importance: (a) economic environment, (b) locational environment, and (c) health environment. The best discriminator in the hospital administrator's characteristics is membership in the American College of Hospital Administrators (ACHA).

TABLE 4.7

Adopters–Nonadopters Classification Matrices

A. Sample[a]

			Predicted Group		
			1	2	Total
Actual	1	Adopters	97	20	117
Group	2	Nonadopters	42	208	250

B. Subsample 1[b]

			Predicted Group		
			1	2	Total
Actual	1	Adopters	44	15	59
Group	2	Nonadopters	22	103	125

C. Subsample 2[c]

			Predicted Group		
			1	2	Total
Actual	1	Adopters	47	11	58
Group	2	Nonadopters	30	95	125

[a]Classification is obtained by using discriminant function weights of the whole sample.
[b]Classification is obtained by using discriminant function weights of subsample 2.
[c]Classification is obtained by using discriminant function weights of subsample 1.

Linear Combination or Discriminant Function

Table 4.6 gives the weights of the predictor variables in the discriminant function. The y_{crit} value is 1.7095; that is, if the score of a hospital is greater than 1.7095, it will be classified as an adopter and if less than 1.7095, a nonadopter.

Classification

To verify the discriminatory and predictive power of the predictor variables, discriminant analysis is performed on two subsamples of the original sample of 367 hospitals. Subsample 1 contains 184 hospitals, selected at random from the whole sample, and subsample 2 contains the remaining 183 hospitals. Separate discriminant function weights are calculated for each subsample. For crossvalidation, discriminant weights of subsample 1 are used to predict the group classification of hospitals in subsample 2, and vice versa. Table 4.7 gives (a) the classification matrix for the whole sample using the discriminant function weights of the whole sample, (b) the classification matrix for subsample 1, and (c) the classification matrix for subsample 2 using the discriminant function weights of subsample 1. Tests on the predictive power of the discriminant functions are summarized in Table 4.8.

As expected, the highest percent of correct classifications is obtained for the whole sample, 83 percent. The discriminant function of subsample 2 gives about 78 percent correct classifications for subsample 1 and the discriminant function of subsample 1 gives about 80 percent correct classifications for subsample 2. Results of t-test analysis show that these percentages are significantly better than the percent of correct classifications that can be obtained by any random classification criteria (that is, proportional chance criterion, maximum chance criterion, or pure chance criterion).

Summary

The two groups, adopters and nonadopters of the use of computers, are found to be significantly different in terms of the 32 predictor variables, measuring the characteristics of the hospital, the environment in which a hospital operates, and the hospital administrator. The total discriminatory power of the battery of 32 predictor variables is 45.09 percent; 30.30 percent of which is contributed by the characteristics of the hospital, 30.63 percent by the interaction between hospital and environmental characteristics, 12.15 percent

TABLE 4.8

Tests on Predictive Power of Discriminant Function

A. Random Classification Tests

	Percent of Correct Classifications		
	Sample	Subsample 1	Subsample 2
P, Correct classifications by discriminant function	83.11	77.60	79.89
Qp, Proportional chance criterion	56.56	56.70	56.42
Qm, maximum chance criterion	68.12	68.31	67.93
Qc, Pure chance criterion	50.00	50.00	50.00

B. t-test

Chance Criterion	Sample		Subsample 1		Subsample 2	
	t value	Level of Significance	t value	Level of Significance	t value	Level of Significance
Qp	10.2613	<.001	8.0807	<.001	9.0674	<.001
Qm	6.1624	<.001	3.8312	<.001	4.9089	<.001
Qc	12.6863	<.001	10.5751	<.001	11.4521	<.001

by hospital and hospital administrator's characteristics, and 17.05 percent by the interaction of all three of them. Individually, environmental characteristics contribute 5.70 percent and hospital administrator's characteristics 3.53 percent; while 0.64 percent is contributed by their interaction.

The best discriminators are, in order of their importance: x_9, total number of facilities; x_{11}, total expenses/bed; x_{10}, number of advanced technological facilities; x_7, census; x_6, number of beds; x_{27}, percent of professional, technical workers in county population; x_{14}, location in an SMSA; x_{21}, percent of population earning greater than \$10,000 per annum; x_{18}, percent of population above 65 years of age; x_8, percent occupancy; x_{29}, membership in ACHA; x_{19}, median per capita income; and x_{25}, physicians per 1000 population.

Hospitals that have adopted computers are likely to have large bed size, higher census, higher percentage occupancy, greater number of total facilities and advanced technological facilities, and higher total expenses/bed. Such hospitals are likely to be located in counties which are in an SMSA, have low percent of population above 65 years of age, higher median per capita income, higher percent of population earning greater than \$10,000 per annum, higher number of physicians per 1000 population, and higher percent of professional, technical workers in county population. Such hospitals are more likely to have a hospital administrator who is a member of the ACHA.

Confidence in the discriminatory power of the predictor variables and the predictive power of the discriminant function is obtained by sample validation and cross-validation. Sample validation yields 83.11 percent correct classifications and cross-validation on two subsamples yield 77.60 and 79.89 percent correct classifications, which is significantly better than any classification that can be obtained by any chance criterion.

Results of the study support the hypothesis that differences between the adopters and nonadopters can be explained by (a) the characteristics of the hospitals, (b) the characteristics of the environment in which a hospital operates, and (c) the training and background of the hospital administrator.

REFERENCES

1. American Medical Association, Distribution of Physicians in the United States. Chicago, 1974.

2. Atlas of Texas, Bureau of Business Research, The University of Texas at Austin, Fall 1973.

3. Ball, M. J., "The Need for a Hospital Information System," in *How to Select a Computerized Hospital Information System*, edited by M. J. Ball, p. 1. New York: S. Karger, 1973.

4. Ball, M. J., "An Aid to Diagnosis: The Use of Computers in Automated Clinical Pathology Laboratories," *J. Med.* 1 (1970):265.

5. Becker, M., "Sociometric Location and Innovativeness: Reformulation and Extension of the Diffusion Model," *American Sociological Review* 35 (April 1970):267.

6. vonBertalanffy, L., *General System Theory*. New York: George Braziller, 1968.

7. Budd, P. J., "ADP as Aid in Personnel Shortages Enables Better Use of Professionals," *Hospital Topics* XLVII (April 1969):49.

8. Burling, T., et al., *The Give and Take in Hospitals*. New York: Putnam, 1956.

9. Cooley, W. W., and P. R. Lohnes, *Multivariate Data Analysis*. New York: Wiley, 1971, p. 227.

10. Copeland, W. C., "A New Approach to Hospital Information System: The Design of Hospital Report Generators for Statistical Reports to Agencies Outside the Individual Hospital," *Inquiry* 4 (March 1967):37.

11. Corwin, E. H. L., *The American Hospital*. New York: Commonwealth Fund, 1946.

12. Danziger, E. M., F. Greenwood, and J. H. Steinert, "The Administrator's Role and Responsibility in Computer Mechanization," *Hospital Administration* 12 (Spring 1967).

13. *Directory of American College of Hospital Administrators*, 1973.

14. *Directory of Approved Internships and Residencies*, American Medical Association, 1973.

15. *Forbes*, "Medicine in Hot Water," pp. 34-38, March 15, 1968.

16. Frank, R. E., W. F. Massy, and D. G. Morrison, "Bias in Multiple Discriminant Analysis," *J. of Marketing Research* 2 (August 1965):252.

17. Goodard, J. L., "Reducing Hospital Costs Through EDP Application," The Hospital Forum, February 1969, p. 11.

18. Green, P. E., and D. S. Tull, Research for Marketing Decisions, 3rd ed., Chapters 12 and 13. Englewood Cliffs, N.J.: Prentice-Hall, 1975.

19. Hammon, G. L., "Planning and Involvement Are the Words to Remember for an In-House Computer System," Hospital Financial Management, February 1974.

20. Heydebrand, W., Hospital Bureaucracy. New York: Dunellen, 1973.

21. Hickey, W. J., "Management Requisites for Success in Data Processing," Hospital Progress 47 (July 1966).

22. Hospital Financial Management, The State of the Art of Information Processing in the Health Care Industry. Chicago, 1970.

23. Hospitals: Guide Issue. J. of the American Hospital Association, August 1974.

24. Hospitals and Related Institutions in Texas, 1973-1974. Texas Hospital Association, Austin, Texas, 1974.

25. Jacobus, G. C., "Sorting Sense from Nonsense in Hospital ADP Programs," Hospitals 41 (May 1967).

26. Jydstrup, R. A., and M. J. Gross, "Cost of Information Handling in Hospitals," Health Services Research 1 (Winter 1966).

27. Kaluzny, A. D., "Innovation in the Health System: A Selective Review of System Characteristics and Empirical Research," Health Services Research 9 (Summer 1974).

28. Kaluzny, A. D., and J. B. Sprague, "Innovation in Health and Welfare Organizations: A Review and Critique of Current Theory and Research," in Innovation in Health Care Organizations, edited by A. D. Kaluzny and J. T. Gentry. University of North Carolina, Chapel Hill, 1974.

29. Kanter, J., Management-Oriented Management Information Systems. Englewood Cliffs, N.J.: Prentice-Hall, 1972, p. 33.

30. Kozmetsky, G., T. W. Ruefli, and D. S. Morris, Information Technology, Initiatives for Today—Decisions That Cannot Wait. New York: The Conference Board, 1972, p. 31.

31. Mahajan, V., Computers in Hospitals: A Diffusion Study, Ph.D. dissertation, The University of Texas at Austin, May 1975.

32. Morrison, D. G., "On the Interpretation of Discriminant Analysis," J. of Marketing Research 6 (May 1969):153.

33. Rao, C. R., Advanced Statistical Methods in Biometric Research. New York: Wiley, 1952.

34. Rome, W. J., "What is Management Effectiveness in a Small Hospital?" Hospitals 43 (June 1, 1969):111.

35. Selected Demographic Characteristics from Census Data—Fourth Count. Office of the Governor, State of Texas, Office of Information Services. OIS-GRS, August 1972.

36. Selected Demographic and Health Care Characteristics, Texas Health Data Institute, Austin, Texas, February 1971.

37. Tatsuoka, M. M., Discriminant Analysis: The Study of Group Differences. Champaign, Ill.: Institute for Personality and Ability Testing, 1970.

38. Tatsuoka, M. M., Multivariate Analysis: Techniques for Educational and Psychological Research. New York: Wiley, 1971, p. 157.

39. Texas Almanac, Dallas Morning News, Dallas, Texas. 1974.

40. Utilization of Automated Data Processing, Final Report, Texas Hospital Information Systems Society, Austin, Texas, February 1974.

41. Wiechevs, J. E., "Planning Hospital Automation Programs," Inquiry 5 (September 1968).

5

CANONICAL CORRELATION ANALYSIS

INTRODUCTION

The first paper uses multiple regression analysis and also provides data to which canonical correlation analysis is applied by the authors of the paper described below. The author's purpose was to investigate and analyze hospital utilization or the demand for hospital services within various industries in southwest Ohio. He attempts to show a relationship between income and age as one set of variables and types of hospital care: medical, maternity, surgical, and outpatient as the other set of variables. The author believed before he conducted the study that an increase in age or increase in income should increase the demand for hospital services. His findings after his investigations indicated that age was a dominant factor in the demand for hospital services but the study did not show the significance that had been obtained in previous studies. He also showed that there is no relationship between income and demand for hospital services. He anticipated this result since all the populations he studied had hospital insurance coverage. Other results dealt with two factors, one objective and one subjective, which created the variance from the demand trend sustained by the medical services classification. The objective factor indicated that the more accessible hospital services are, the more they were demanded and utilized. The subjective factor indicated that mental awareness of physical conditions increases hospital utilization.

In the second paper, the authors take the data from Garland's article and analyze it, first using multiple regression analysis and then canonical correlation analysis. When the data are put through multiple regression, three sets of variables are shown to have a positive relationship: surgical incidence and average annual income; medical insurance and average age; and inpatient incidence and average age. When the combined influence of age and income on various utilization measures is determined, the size of the correlation coefficient increased, although none of them reached the significance level. The partial correlation coefficients indicate possible causal relationships between surgical incidence and average age. Particularly noteworthy is the fact that the effect of age on medical incidence seems to increase when income is held constant.

The final implication of the second article is that among the predictor variables, the major determinant of the relationship is average age. The effect of average annual income is relatively low. Among the criterion variables, inpatient incidence contributes about twice as much as outpatient incidence toward the relationship.

Introduction to Technique

Canonical analysis is used to test whether or not two sets of variables are independent. It can also be used to determine which variables in each of two sets contribute most to the association of the sets. If a researcher is able to separate the variables of interest into sets, he is then in a position to postulate flows of influences.

Canonical analysis answers the following questions.

1. What is the total relationship between the dependent and independent variable sets?

2. What are the relative contributions of each subset to the total amount of variation explained in the dependent set?

3. Which variable in the dependent and independent set(s) respectively contributed most to the total amount of variation shared between the sets? The rationale and the mathematical form of canonical correlation analysis are provided in Phillip and Gibson's paper.

REFERENCES

Alpert, M. I., and R. A. Peterson, "On the Interpretation of Canonical Analysis," Journal of Marketing Research 9 (May 1972): 187-92.

Green, P. E., and D. S. Tull, Research for Marketing Decisions, 3rd ed. Englewood Cliffs, N.J.: Prentice-Hall, 1975.

Green, P.E., M. H. Halbert, and P. J. Robinson, "Canonical Analysis: An Exposition and Illustrative Application," Journal of Marketing Research 3 (February 1966):32-39.

HOSPITAL UTILIZATION BY CHARACTERISTIC OF INDUSTRY IN SOUTHWESTERN OHIO

Howard Randall Garland

INTRODUCTION

Our nation's total health bill in 1966 came to $30.6 billion and represented 6 percent of our national disposable income [1], a significant increase of approximately 50 percent over the totals for 1950. These figures not only indicate the American public is being convinced that increasingly more money should be spent for health care, but that the public is demanding more and better care. The result is that the price for care is increasing faster than the balance of the items used in computing the Consumer Price Index. The Index shows an increase of 13.1 percent for all expenditures in 1966, over the base period 1957-59, while medical care increased 27.7 percent.

Health insurance coverage has been expanding even more rapidly than the cost of health care and has become the fourth necessity of life. Today, health benefits alone come to 4.2 percent of an employee's basic salary, and, since World War II, the burden of payment has shifted to the employer [2]. Employers, being more cost conscious, are now taking greater care in the selection of health coverage and "shopping" for the best buys. For the same reasons, the health care industry is also becoming more sophisticated in analyzing the utilization of health care.

Of the total medical dollars spent, the largest increase in recent years has been that portion represented by hospital payments. Hospital care per patient day increased 216.3 percent, from $18.35 in 1952 to $58.04 in 1967 [3]. In 1966, 158 million persons had some type of hospital bill coverage; of these, 42 percent, or over 66 million, had Blue Cross coverage [4].

Because of these recent changes and the increasing emphasis on health economics, this paper will investigate and analyze hospital utilization or the demand for hospital services within various industries in Southwestern Ohio.

Howard Randall Garland is Manager, Actuarial and Statistics, Blue Cross of Southwest Ohio, Cincinnati.

Reprinted with permission of the Blue Cross Association, from Inquiry 6, No. 1, pp. 60-71. Copyright 1969 by the Blue Cross Association. All rights reserved.

THE DATA

The main emphasis in this investigation will be placed on the demand for hospital services of various individual employee groups. The empirical information was compiled during the year 1965 by the local Blue Cross Plan in Cincinnati, which provides coverage of hospital services for approximately 60 percent of the population in the 15-county area of southwest Ohio. The source of the statistical information should be kept in mind at all times, since many prior studies indicate that increased hospitalization is incurred when individuals have some type of hospital service coverage. However, this should not have any effect on the relationship of variances in the amount of hospital services demanded by each individual industry.

Two general sets of conditions can be defined which affect the utilization of medical care facilities: 1) the socioeconomic characteristics of the population, and 2) the medical care organization of the area [5]. In essence, this indicates that both supply and demand affect the utilization of hospital services. While authorities agree that Say's Law, "supply creates its own demand," is present and applies to hospital facilities, the current analysis is based on the demand factors, both due to time limitation and to the relatively constant supply factor within the time period under study.

Two Socioeconomic Characteristics Analyzed

The current study analyzes two main socioeconomic characteristics in relation to demand: From previous studies, as well as general knowledge obtained by experience in the health field, several preconceptions were harbored regarding the results which would be achieved. It is almost a certainty that a strong correlation will exist between the age of the employees of a particular industry and the utilization of hospital services. Studies have differed in regard to the degree of correlation in respect to age, but almost without exception all agree that hospitalization increases with age.

It is also assumed that the income of the employees of a particular industry will have a positive correlation to the demand for hospitalization. The degree of correlation, however, has been reduced in recent years by new government programs that provide hospital benefits for the low income segment of the population, and by the increase in the proportion of the population covered under hospitalization insurance. The significance of income in this analysis is doubtful because the population under study has prepaid coverage for hospital benefits.

Age and Income Factors by Industry

As indicated previously, studies have been conducted correlating age and income to hospital utilization [6]. Past studies have also analyzed the degree of hospital utilization by particular industries [7]; however, this analysis will view the factors of age and income within particular industries. This type of analysis is, of course, extremely important to an organization such as Blue Cross, since it is through group enrollment, either employee groups, unions, or professional groups, that most members are enrolled.

METHODOLOGY

The hospital utilization patterns of the various employee groups were divided into ten categories. In order of total membership, these were: manufacturing, retail and wholesale, local government, education and schools, medical services, transportation and utilities, service organizations, farming, professional associations, and finance and insurance.

In considering the various classifications, the following limitations must be recognized. Education and school group employees are actively engaged in their profession. Retired employees of these groups have not been included in the experience outlined in this study since their membership after retirement is not maintained in or connected with their original group. This limitation also applies, in most cases, to local government groups.

Farming groups are maintained through local farming associations, and membership requirements are not limited. Therefore, the chance of adverse selection is present, and the retention of members no longer actively working is possible. The membership for professional associations is handled in a similar fashion, and the same limitations would apply.

The membership in the remaining categories is handled in the following manner: If the employee group has an established retiree group, this group's hospitalization statistics were included in the particular classification to which their parent group is assigned. The manufacturing classification has the highest percentage of retiree groups due, in most cases, to pressure from organized labor.

The statistics for the calendar year of 1965 were selected for analysis to secure the latest data and yet obtain the most complete information available. To avoid any erratic fluctuations which might be sustained in the analysis of small employee groups, only those with a minimum of 1,200 contract months (or an average of 100 contract holders per month) were selected for study. Information pertaining to utilization is based on claims incurred and paid during the period. To project these figures to the total incurred for the period, a completion factor of 14.4 percent was used for the dollar amounts and 8.1 percent for the claim totals. These factors were derived from separate studies which covered completion experience during prior periods.

Choice of Basic Hospital Coverages

The groups studied had a choice between two basic hospital coverages: 1) "Standard" which covers a ward room (five or more beds) in full, with an allowance toward better accommodations and full ancillary coverage, or 2) "Comprehensive," which covers a semi-private room (two or more beds) in full, with an allowance toward private accommodations and full ancillary coverage. Outpatient benefits under standard and comprehensive coverages are the same and provide full benefits for accident, surgical, and emergency care. Since the fees charged for each type of coverage are based on the benefits provided, the utilization percentage of total dollar amounts is compatible.

The type of hospital care received was divided into four basic categories: surgical, medical, maternity, and outpatient. Maternity care covers all admissions pertaining to pregnancy, including miscarriage, false labor, and so forth. Outpatient or nonbed care refers to admissions to the emergency room of the hospital where the patient is discharged the same day.

The number of admissions or individual incidence of demand in the various categories is indicated as incidence per 1,000 members. The number of members per family contract for calculation of these figures is 3.29. This factor was developed from a random sample of all family contracts prior to undertaking this study.

It should also be noted that the contracts in our analysis limit covered days to 70, 120 or 365, and the statistics regarding length of stay would not include any days in excess of these limits.

The statistics utilized are pure figures and are not adjusted in any respect to minor deviations in hospital coverage which is present in some cases. In relation to the total population in this analysis, these deviations play a minor role and will not cause any inflationary tendency to a measurable degree.

ANALYSIS OF UTILIZATION PATTERNS

Table 5.1 shows the average age, average income and the various use rates per 1,000 members for each of the 10 groups. After reviewing these data it was decided that the analysis of age and income in

TABLE 5.1

Age, Annual Income, and Use Rates per 1,000 Members, 1965

Classification	Average[a] Age	Average[b] Annual Income	Inpatient Incidents	Surgical Incidents	Medical Incidents	Maternity Incidents	Outpatient Incidents
Manufacturing	39.9	$ 7,296	139.6	57.5	60.2	21.9	129.8
Retail and wholesale	40.8	4,730	117.8	51.4	47.3	19.1	118.9
Local government	41.3	6,355	141.4	60.4	60.5	20.5	152.0
Education and schools	40.7	6,802	120.4	49.3	51.2	19.9	108.2
Medical services	34.3	4,124	150.8	59.8	73.1	17.9	175.3
Transportation and utilities	43.5	6,918	133.3	54.0	58.8	20.5	115.7
Service organizations	43.5	4,366	131.2	54.3	52.7	24.2	125.4
Farming	50.9	2,097	157.1	54.5	88.6	14.0	82.5
Professional associations	44.9	26,930	148.6	65.5	63.4	19.7	145.2
Finance and insurance	32.8	5,477	105.9	43.9	42.3	19.7	96.2

[a]"Age and Income by Industry," Characteristics of Population—Ohio 1960 Census, Vol. 37 (Columbus: State of Ohio, 1960), pp. 733-37.

[b]McCormick, Francis B., et al. Ohio 1965 Farm Income (Columbus: State of Ohio, 1966), pp. 12-13; Papier, William, et al. Employment, Payroll, and Earnings Under the Ohio Unemployment Compensation Law by County, 1943 through 1965 (Columbus: State of Ohio, 1966), pp. 1-69; and Characteristics of Population—Ohio 1960 Census, op. cit., pp. 733-37.

relation to hospital utilization could best be achieved through the use of regression analysis.

Simple regression, referring to the relationship between two variables, will be utilized; therefore, age and income are considered separately. If each pair of values (incident rate and age/incident rate and income) are plotted as a point, we obtain a scatter diagram. Assuming that a relationship exists between the variables, they are related to each other by the linear equation $y = a + bx$.

It is the purpose of regression analysis to predict the value of y for a given value of x; however, it will also give the best estimates of the unknown parameters in the equation a and b. The estimated values of the unknown parameters are computed by the method of least squares. The linear equation for the series is then $\hat{y} = \hat{a} + \hat{b}x$ (^ denotes estimated values).

$\hat{y}$ = incident rate
x = age (or income)
$\hat{a}$ = coefficient of determination
$\hat{b}$ = regression coefficient

It is necessary to determine the adequacy of the values derived since errors are expected in any such estimates. It was assumed in the analysis that the existing errors were random and independent. The standard error of the retression coefficient was computed for the equation derived for each series.

The hypotheses established in the analysis were subjected to a "test of significance," which is a probability test based on sampling theory, designed to determine whether the data in the analysis are reasonable. The level of significance, which can be set at various degrees, is used to decide whether we will accept or reject a hypothesis as true or false.

One important qualification to this analysis should be noted. While the regression analysis of rates and averages can show whether the rates or averages are related within specified population groups, such analysis, in general, is not applicable to individuals within the specific groups. This problem is not acute, however, as it is the groups, rather than individual members, which are the primary focus of analysis [8].

AGE AND INCIDENT RATES

Age and Total Inpatient Incident Rate

Immediate visual inspection of Figure 5.1 indicates verification of the preconceived idea that a positive correlation of the demand for

FIGURE 5.1

Age and Total Inpatient Incident Rate

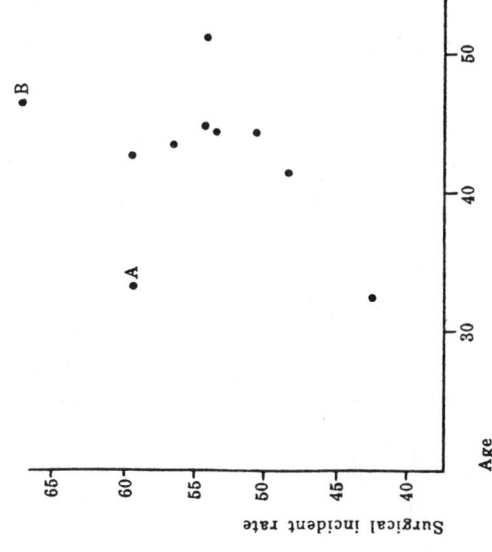

FIGURE 5.2

Age and Surgical Incident Rate

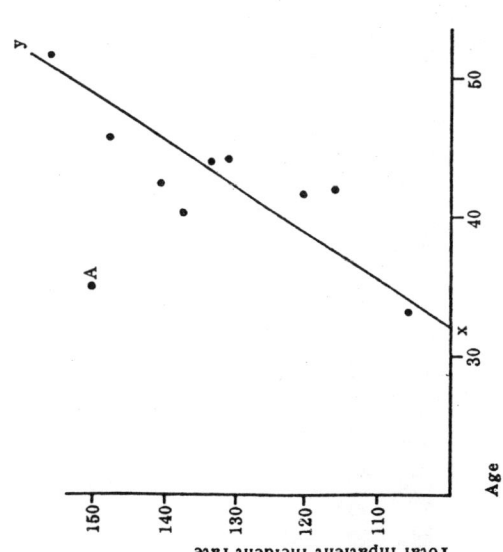

FIGURE 5.3

Age and Medical Incident Rate

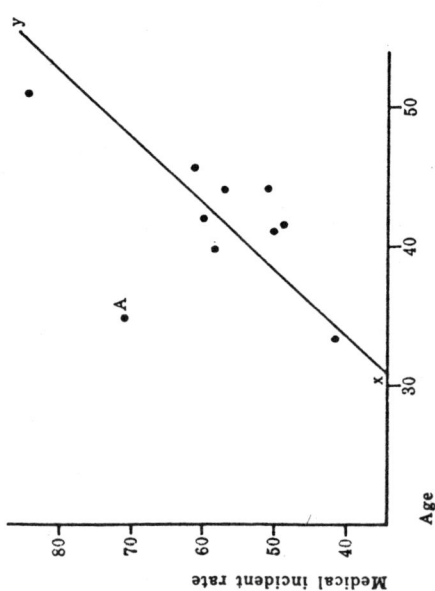

FIGURE 5.4

Age and Maternity Incident Rate

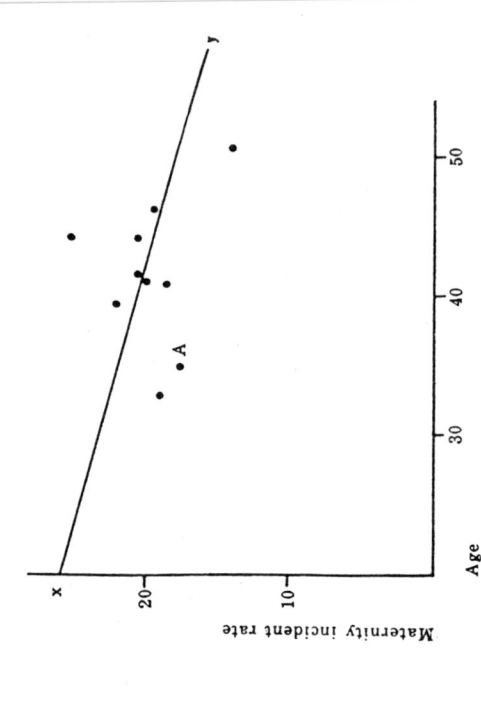

hospital services and age exist. The regression coefficient was calculated as +1.66 which, although not significant at the 5 percent level, was in excess of the standard deviation of error (.89).

To investigate the above factors in greater detail in an attempt to secure a higher correlation, the medical service category (point A) was omitted and the remaining statistics again subjected to regression analysis. The regression coefficient was then determined to be +2.82 which was significant at the 1 percent level (line xy). The coefficient of determination indicating the dependency of inpatient incidence on age was .714. The high degree of correlation achieved after omitting medical services is due to the fact that although this particular classification had the second lowest income in the study, its demand for hospitalization was second highest. Even more unusual is the fact that a high percent of the employees, although female, are single, thus eliminating the possibility of the high incident rate being caused by high maternity incidence.

The correlation outlined in the regression analysis between the total inpatient incident rate and age was more significant than any derived for the individual categories of service.

Age and Surgical Incident Rate

In considering the surgical incident rate the regression analysis offered no correlation. This result could be expected after reviewing Figure 5.2. Several notable characteristics exist, however, which were considered in analyzing the surgical incidents. If medical services (point A) and professional associations (point B) are excluded from the regression analysis, a positive correlation is derived, although significance was not obtainable at the 5 percent level. One reason for the low degree of correlation is the farming group which had the highest age level of any classification in the study, but only the fifth highest level of surgical incidence. The age factor in this classification, however, would have a tendency to reduce surgical incidence since many health conditions in higher age groups are treated on a medical basis due to the higher risk involved in surgery.

Age and Medical Incident Rate

The medical incident rate differs from surgical in that positive correlation was achieved considering all classifications, although significance was not present at the 5 percent level. Once again, medical services (point A) was omitted and the regression analysis recomputed. The results achieved in the second computation indicated a regression coefficient of +2.38 which was significant at the 1 percent level (line xy). The farming classification, although not contrary to this pattern, indicated a medical incident rate far in excess of the next closest classification thereby adding support to the assumption made in regard to surgical incidence for this age group.

Age and Maternity Incident Rate

Although the total inpatient incident rate and age indicate positive correlation, maternity as a category of inpatient service showed a negative correlation with respect to age. This result would obviously be expected since the higher the average age of a classification, the lower the number of members of child-bearing age. The regression coefficient derived from the factors presented in Figure 5.4 is -.135 which is significant at the 1 percent level (line xy). The coefficient of determination was extremely low, .065, indicating that the dependency of the incident rates on age is not great. This fact should be viewed in consideration of the population of the study which included, for the most part, employees still actively working.

The pattern of excluding medical services in previous computations for an in-depth view of the data was again followed. When the data were analyzed with this category (point A) omitted, a regression coefficient of -.253 was achieved. The most outstanding changes occurred in the coefficient of determination which increased to .188. The low maternity incidents in relation to age was to be expected due to the high percentage of single contracts in this classification.

Age and Outpatient Incident Rate

There was no correlation possible between age and outpatient incidence from the data secured. All classifications were fairly consistent, with three exceptions: medical services, finance and insurance, farming.

Although correlation could not be achieved, each of the classifications deviating from the central pattern was analyzed to see if any reasonable explanation for the deviation could be found. It has long been thought that outpatient incidents occur more frequently on family contracts since children are more prone to minor accidents and emergency cases. In reviewing the individual classifications in question, it was found that medical services and finance and insurance had the highest percentage of single contracts, which should indicate a low outpatient incident rate. This conclusion was verified by finance and insurance. However, for medical services, which should have had an even lower incident rate since it was the only classification where single contracts outnumbered family contracts, the complete reverse was true. The great variance could not be justified by any of the statistical data included in the study.

The contract mix of farming indicated a higher single content than the average but not enough to justify the low utilization sustained. There is another factor, however, to consider in the analysis of this category—the location of the membership. Most members in the farming classification live in rural areas where access to hospitals is limited. Therefore, if injuries of minor nature are sustained, they are either cared for in the home or treated by the local family doctor, since the time and expense involved in obtaining the services of a hospital is prohibitive.

The reverse of the above explanation, the availability of service, may be the cause for the high incident rate sustained by medical services. This reasoning in regard to utilization will be reviewed more fully later.

INCOME AND INCIDENT RATES

Income and Total Inpatient Incident Rate

Adequate correlation of income and inpatient incidents as illustrated in Figure 5.5 could not be achieved without noting and excluding two classifications, farming (point A) and medical services (point B). With the exclusion of these two categories a positive correlation is obtained with a regression coefficient of +.0011 (line xy). The coefficient of determination applying to this analysis was .341.

The exceptions made are unique in this pattern, since farming which had the lowest income also had the highest incident rate, and medical services which had the second lowest income had the second highest incident rate. The indication in regard to farming is that age is by far superior to income as a determining factor in the demand for hospitalization. However, once again we are faced with the fact that medical services, for no apparent reason thus far in the analysis, has an exceptionally high demand for hospital services.

Income and Surgical Incident Rate

A positive correlation can be obtained without exceptions between income and surgical incidence. The regression coefficient for the data illustrated in Figure 5.6 is +.0029 (line xy). The analysis is significant

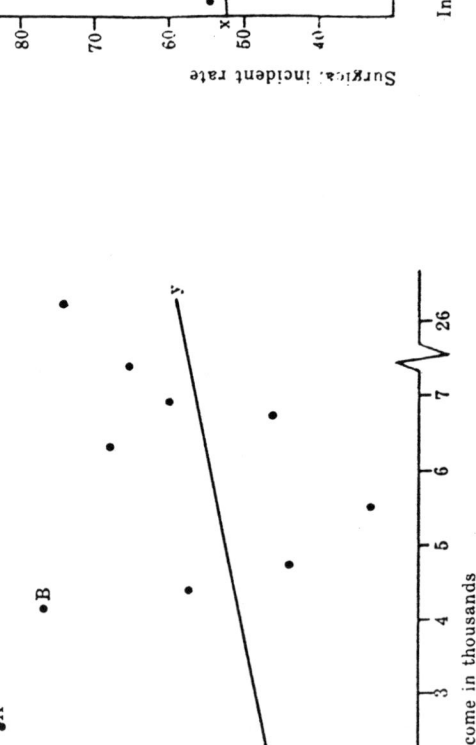

FIGURE 5.5

Income and Total Inpatient Incident Rate

FIGURE 5.6

Income and Surgical Incident Rate

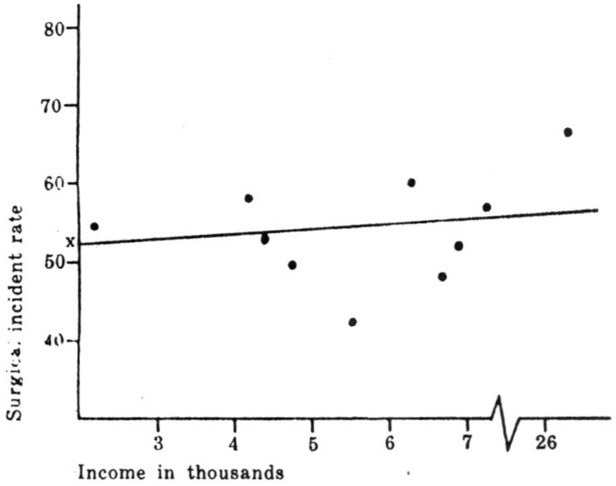

FIGURE 5.7

Income and Medical Incident Rate

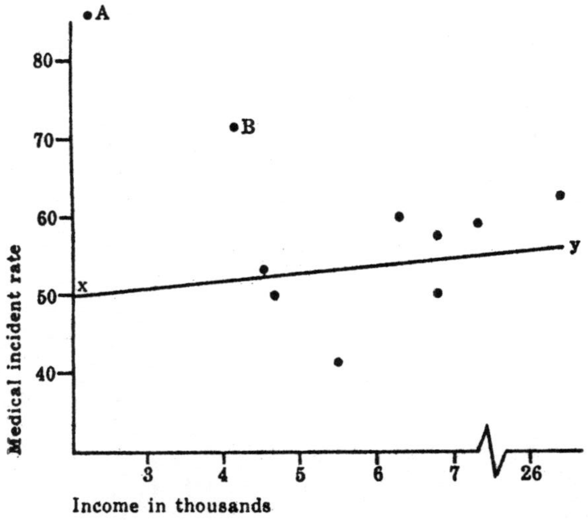

FIGURE 5.8

Income and Maternity Incident Rate

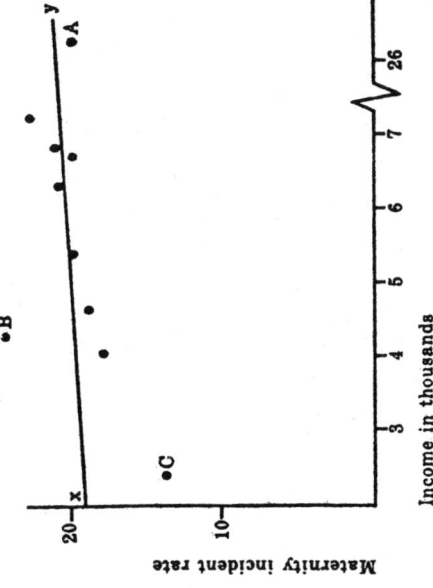

FIGURE 5.9

Income and Outpatient Incident Rate

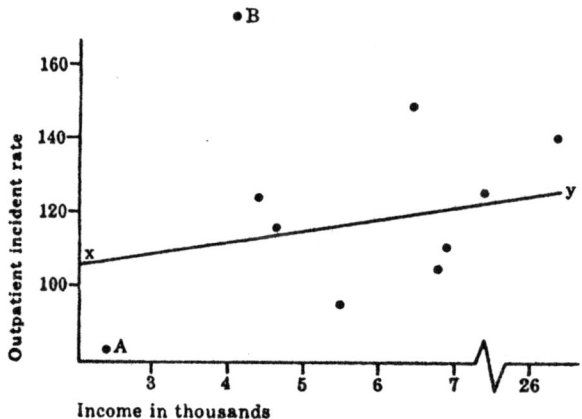

at the 1 percent level, but the coefficient of determination (.10) indicated little influence of income on incidence.

Income and Medical Incident Rate

In analyzing the medical incidence in relation to income, we are presented with the same two exceptions made in consideration of the total inpatient incident rate, those being farming (point A) and medical services (point B). Making these exclusions, the regression coefficient was computed as +.0005 and the coefficient of determination as .30 (line xy).

This computation, as well as the previous ones in regard to income, shows that the variance in demand for hospital services in relation to income is slight. This can easily be seen by reviewing Figures 5.5-5.9. One outstanding point, however, is that the patterns in Figures 5.5 and 5.7 are very similar. This is the same result found in comparison of Figures 5.1 and 5.3.

Income and Maternity Incident Rate

A positive correlation can be obtained between income and maternity incidence, but the dependency of the incident rate on income is practically zero, yielding a coefficient of determination of only +.015 (line xy). The hypothesis that the birth rate declines with an increased standard of living may be true since professional associations (point A) which had the highest annual income had a maternity incident rate of 19.7 compared to the average of 21.0. The information in this study, however, is inconclusive in respect to confirming any hypothesis of this nature.

The incident rate for service organizations (point B) and farming (point C) deviated more from the pattern than the other classifications. The deviation in farming was to be expected due to the age of the group rather than income. The movement from the pattern by service organizations was not justified to any degree by any of the variables included in this study.

Income and Outpatient Incident Rate

Positive correlation existed in relation to income and outpatient incidence; however, the dependency of incidence on income is slight. If we again exclude medical services (point B) in our regression analysis, the dependency of incidence on income, the coefficient of determination, increases from .088 to .292.

The farming classification (point A) conformed to the pattern of "low income—low utilization." However, this low demand, as explained previously, may be caused by availability of service and not low income.

FINDINGS OF EMPIRICAL INVESTIGATION

This investigation has produced several facts relating to the original factors of analysis, age and income, and also to various characteristics of several of the industries under study. The presentation of the findings will be made first in regard to our original factors of consideration, and second in regard to the dominant variations which were not explained by the control data.

Age

This study indicated that age is a dominant factor in the demand for hospital services. The degree of association between age and demand did not show the significance that has been obtained in prior studies; however, this study was not based on age alone but on the type of employment in which the study population was engaged. In this respect, the results were significant.

The analysis of the total inpatient incident rate showed immediate positive correlation of age and demand. After eliminating one category, medical services, significance was obtained at the 1 percent level. The inpatient incidence was analyzed not only in regard to the total but by the three individual types of service comprising the total to see if the association of age and demand was present in all categories.

The surgical incident rate did not offer any similarity to that of the total inpatient incidence. In fact, there was no correlation between age and demand for hospitalization considering all classifications. When the medical services and professional association classifications were excluded from our analysis, positive correlation was achieved. One oddity, mentioned previously, is that farming, which had the highest age, was surpassed in demand by several other classifications. This exception was created in all probability by the risk involved in surgery which increases with the age of the patient. The medical incidence differed from surgical in that the utilization conformed to the pattern established by the total inpatient incident rate. The degree of correlation for medical incidence was, however, higher than that achieved for the total. The maternity incident rate also showed a high correlation between age and demand for hospital service. The results were negative, however, instead of positive, which is a natural phenomenon to be expected.

A review and analysis of the outpatient incident rate offered no correlation of age and demand. Actually, the statistical data indicated a strong tendency toward an equalized demand level for the various industrial classifications with the exception of those categories outlined earlier: finance and insurance, medical services, and farming. The possible reasons for these exceptions were reviewed previously, and only the incident rate of the medical services classification remained alone as fully unexplained.

Income

This study indicated that income was not a determining factor in the demand for hospital utilization. This lack of association between income and demand was considered a possibility prior to this analysis since the population in the study all had hospital benefit coverage. If the population had been selected at random from the general population, different results might have been expected. However, in recent years the changing economy has undoubtedly reduced income as a significant factor in determining demand. This reduction of income as an influential factor in determining demand has been caused primarily for two reasons: 1) the increasing number of our population securing coverage for hospital benefits either on an individual basis or through employee groups, and 2) the increasing role of government health programs in providing benefits for the needy and elderly (principally those who cannot afford to purchase coverage themselves).

The total inpatient incident rate with respect to income did not offer any correlation. Correlation, however, was achieved after making several exceptions and eliminating from the regression analysis the following three categories: farming, medical services, and finance and insurance. The necessity for exclusion of farming and finance and insurance indicated that the effect of age as a factor of hospital demand was far superior to income. However, medical services once again stood alone in seeking an explanation of the high demand sustained.

The surgical incident rate in relation to income offered a significant level of correlation, but the regression coefficient once again indicated the influence of income is small. The medical incidence followed the same pattern as the total inpatient incident rate offering no correlation without exception. Significant correlation was obtained in regard to the maternity incident rate, but once again the dependency of the demand on income approached zero.

The analysis of the outpatient incident rate yielded results similar to those obtained for the inpatient incidence. The reliance of demand on income was negligible, and medical services was once again the exception to the general trend of the other industrial categories.

Factors Creating Unusual Deviations

All factors other than age and income were considered parameters in our analysis. However, while analyzing the data, an important fact was discovered regarding the deviations in the demand of hospital services for the medical services classification. In the analysis of utilization patterns this category was persistent in its deviation from the trend. In each regression computation, higher significance was achieved when the data pertaining to medical services were omitted. Considering the total inpatient incidence with regard to age, the regression coefficient was increased from +1.66 to +2.82 with the exclusion of medical services, and the coefficient of determination increased from .280 to .714. The results were similar for each category of hospital service with the degree of correlation being increased each time the data for this classification were omitted. The variance, however, was more predominant in the analysis of age rather than income.

The reason for the adverse effect of the data pertaining to medical services on correlation is that while this classification had the second lowest age and income in the study, its utilization rate was one of the highest. It is for these reasons that a detailed analysis was made of this particular industry.

The classification was composed primarily of hospital employees having, therefore, a high percentage of nurses (including student nurses) enrolled for benefits. The high concentration of nurses explains why this category was the only one in which the single contracts outnumbered the family. These facts—low age, low income, and high single contract mix—all would indicate a low utilization pattern. This conclusion was generated by the verified assumption that lower age groups, in general, demand less hospital service, and the predominance of single contracts dictates a lower maternity incident rate. The results in this particular case, however, are the reverse of our expectation.

Each employee group in this classification was reviewed to see if any particular characteristics were present which would generate the usual utilization sustained by this category. At this point in our analysis an outstanding discrepancy developed. Two hospital groups in this classification had a much lower incident rate than the balance. The difference between these groups and those in the balance of the classification was that the services provided by these hospitals were limited due to specialization which means that employees could not routinely secure hospital services at their place of employment.

For the reason stated previously, it was assumed that the availability of service has a much stronger effect on utilization or demand than was thought earlier. Measurement of the degree of influence of this factor is practically impossible since a controlled experiment regarding these data is not possible.

The forestated objective factor in the mind of the author works in conjunction with a subjective factor which has never been explored in the field of demand; that is, the association of one's personal physical conditions with that of the hospitalized patient, thus leading to therapeutic or diagnostic treatment of minor or nonexistent conditions. For the general population this association would not exist. The measurement of this assumption is even more remote than that of availability. This subjective factor in all probability is the cause for the tremendously high medical and outpatient incident rate sustained for this classification.

In an attempt to review further mental association as a subjective factor in creating hospital utilization, a review of absenteeism was made using the employees of a leading hospitalization insurance firm. The corporation is divided into several divisions, one of which has the task of reviewing hospital admissions for verification of benefit coverage and bill payment. These employees, although never in physical contact with the patient, do review diagnoses and see the resulting treatment charges. It was found that this division sustained higher absenteeism due to illness than any other division in the firm.

This discovery also created a review of the incident rate of the professional associations which comprise many physician groups who are also subjected to many of the factors relating to medical services. This category yielded on occasion higher incident rates than might be expected although the deviation from the trend is not as great as that of medical services. Physicians, however, do not comprise the percentage of this category's employees as would be necessary to draw any conclusive results.

CONCLUSIONS

The intent of this analysis was to determine whether age and income in consideration of characteristics of particular types of industry in the area of southwest Ohio were influential factors in the demand or utilization of hospital services. The results, limited by the empirical evidence utilized and defined by this report, supply the reader with definite conclusions concerning demand and the individual factors.

Age was found to be a dominant factor in determining the degree of inpatient incidence of hospital utilization. The incidence in relation to the individual types of hospital services varied with age. As age increased the total inpatient incident rate increased. The rate of surgical and maternity incidence declined with increased age, but the increase of medical incidence was more than enough to compensate for this reduction. Conclusive evidence, however, was not obtained in relation to outpatient utilization and age.

Income, the effect of which was reduced by the study population, showed little influence on the demand for hospital service. Although correlation was obtained with most types of hospital service, the dependency of incidence on income was negligible. The conclusion that there is insignificant response of demand to income must be considered valid only within that portion of the general population which has prepaid hospital benefits.

The most outstanding results obtained in this study did not pertain to either of the original factors under consideration, but to the factors which created the high variance from the demand trend sustained by the medical services classification.

Through reviews which were made of individual employee groups, two additional factors were revealed which must be used to explain adequately the variance of demand in the analysis of hospital services.

Of the two factors discovered to have such a positive effect on demand, one was objective while the other was subjective.

The objective factor of demand was availability. The more accessible hospital services, the more they were demanded and utilized. The subjective factor was that of mental awareness of physical conditions that necessitate hospital utilization. The association of personal physical conditions or feelings with those of a particular illness generates the need for diagnostic and/or therapeutic treatment for conditions of minor nature which may have gone unnoticed or untreated.

The two latter factors, although present in any analysis of hospital demand, cannot be adequately measured and the degree of influence must therefore be made by comparison. In this report comparison did exist on an industry basis; however, in a future analytical setting these factors as variables will necessitate more sophisticated techniques than had been anticipated as necessary in this study.

NOTES

1. "Ratio of Personal Consumption Expenditures for Medical Care to Disposable Personal Income," Source Book of Health Insurance Data (New York: Health Insurance Institute, 1967), p. 51.

2. Thomas Paine, "An Overview of Employee Benefit Costs: 'Nowhere to Go But Up,'" Perspective Magazine (July-August 1966), p. 13.

3. "The Nation's Hospitals: A Statistical Profile," Hospitals 42, Part 2 (August 1968):448-49.

4. "The Extent of Coverage Under Health Insurance," Source Book of Health Insurance Data, op. cit., p. 12.

5. Gerald D. Rosenthal, "Factors Affecting the Utilization of Short-Term General Hospitals," Amer. Jour. of Public Health 55 (November 1965): 1734-36.

6. Walter J. McNerney et al., Hospital and Medical Economics, I (Chicago: Hospital Research and Educational Trust, 1962), pp. 122-55.

7. Ibid.

8. For a more detailed discussion see W. S. Robinson, "Ecological Correlations and the Behavior of Individuals," American Sociological Review 15 (June 1950).

SIMPLE, MULTIPLE, AND CANONICAL CORRELATIONS

P. Joseph Phillip
and
Stephen Gibson

In a sense, this is a sequel to an article by Howard R. Garland which appeared in the March 1969 issue of Inquiry under the title: "Hospital Utilization by Characteristic of Industry in Southwestern Ohio" [1]. In that article the author attempts to show the relationship between a set of predictors, Average Age and Average Annual Income, and a set of criteria, Inpatient Incidence, Surgical Incidence, Medical Incidence, Maternity Incidence, and Outpatient Incidence. The statistical tools employed are the simple regression and correlation analyses.

The expressions "regression" and "correlation" are sometimes used synonymously. Strictly speaking, the purpose of the former is prediction, that of the latter analysis or explanation. Together they constitute one of the most direct and powerful statistical tools for the resolution of research problems. They can be applied to a wide variety of situations, and their underlying assumptions are not unduly restrictive. Furthermore, all aspects of these techniques have been fully worked out by theorists and integrated into a unified theory of regression and correlation analysis. Consequently, precise meaningful interpretation of all the measures is possible.

Garland's article is apt to create some misunderstanding about the use and interpretation of the various measures which regression and correlation analyses yield. For instance, he begins by defining $\hat{a}$ as the "Coefficient of Determination," which it is not. The term $\hat{a}$ is the "Regression Constant" or the "Y-Intercept"; it is the value of Y when X is zero. The Coefficient of Determination is, in fact, the square of the correlation coefficient, r. Another questionable method

---

P. Joseph Phillip, Ph.D., is Research Director, division of Research and Development, Blue Cross Association, Chicago.

Stephen Gibson, M.A., is Research Analyst, Michigan Blue Cross.

Reprinted with permission of the Blue Cross Association, from Inquiry 7, No. 2, pp. 55-59. Copyright 1970 by the Blue Cross Association. All rights reserved.

employed by the author is the elimination of certain observations from the original data in an effort to establish relationships between Xs and Ys. This is not objectionable in itself, but when one has only 10 observations to begin with, elimination of two observations is tantamount to eliminating 20 percent of the data, and reducing the working data to a level of extreme unreliability [2]. The result is to force spurious relationships where none exists. Perhaps the most serious weakness is his eclecticism. Throughout the analysis, those measures that seem to lend credence to the author's hypothesis are reported, and those that seem to cast doubt on its validity are avoided.

The purpose of this communication is to present, with some objectivity, the results of regression and correlation analysis performed on the original data reported in Garland's article, and to describe and illustrate the application of a statistical technique most appropriate to test the hypotheses of the author.

SIMPLE AND MULTIPLE REGRESSION AND CORRELATION ANALYSES

Results of simple and multiple regression and correlation analyses performed on the data are presented in Tables 5.2 and 5.3. The measures used and their interpretation are given in the notes to this paper [3, 4].

It should be emphasized that the analyses summarized in Tables 5.2 and 5.3 should be considered as illustrative of a technique rather than statements of the existence (or lack of it) of relationship between variables. The reason is the paucity of observations. With 10 observations, the relationship should be almost overwhelming to be statistically significant. All that can be done is to present certain hypotheses.

Hypotheses

It would appear from Table 5.2 that some positive relationship may exist between the following variables: Surgical Incidence and Average Annual Income; Medical Incidence and Average Age; and Inpatient Incidence and Average Age.

It will be seen from Table 5.3 that when the combined influence of Age and Income on various utilization measures is determined, the size of the correlation coefficients increased, although none of them attained significance level. The partial correlation coefficients indicate possible causal relationship between Surgical Incidence and Average Annual Income ($r_{y_1 \cdot 2} = 0.5607$); Medical Incidence and Average

TABLE 5.2

Simple Regression and Correlation Analyses

Serial Number	Description of Variables	Regression Equation $Y = a + bX$	Coefficient of Correlation r	Coefficient of Determination r^2	Significance at 5 percent Level
1	Inpatient incidence (Y) vs. average age (X)	$Y = 66.0404 + 1.6619X$	0.5288	0.2796	Not significant
2	Surgical incidence (Y) vs. average age (X)	$Y = 39.1937 + 0.3845X$	0.3226	0.1041	Not significant
3	Medical incidence (Y) vs. average age (X)	$Y = 1.3408 + 1.4171X$	0.5459	0.2980	Not significant
4	Maternity incidence (Y) vs. average age (X)	$Y = 25.5059 - 0.1397X$	-0.2731	0.0746	Not significant
5	Outpatient incidence (Y) vs. average age (X)	$Y = 203.7348 - 1.9102X$	-0.3596	0.1293	Not significant
6	Inpatient incidence (Y) vs. average annual income (X)	$Y = 131.0054 + 0.0005X$	0.2086	0.0435	Not significant
7	Surgical incidence (Y) vs. average annual income (X)	$Y = 51.3053 + 0.0005X$	0.5761	0.3319	Not significant
8	Medical incidence (Y) vs. average annual income (X)	$Y = 60.3582 - 0.0001X$	-0.0387	0.0015	Not significant
9	Maternity incidence (Y) vs. average annual income (X)	$Y = 19.3645 + 0.0001X$	0.1352	0.0183	Not significant
10	Outpatient incidence (Y) vs. average annual income (X)	$Y = 116.2315 + 0.0012X$	0.2965	0.0879	Not significant

TABLE 5.3

Multiple Regression and Correlation Analyses

Serial Number	Description of Variables	Regression Equation $(Y = a + b_{y1 \cdot 2}X_1 + b_{y2 \cdot 1}X_2)$	Beta Coefficients $\beta_{yi \cdot j}$	Coefficient of Multiple Correlation $R_{y \cdot ij}$	Coefficient of Multiple Determination $R^2_{y \cdot ij}$	Significance at 5 percent Level	Partial Correlation Coefficients $r_{yi \cdot j}$
1	Inpatient incidence (Y) vs. average age (X_1) and average income (X_2)	$Y = 66.6414 + 1.5976X_1 + 0.0003X_2$	$\beta_{y1 \cdot 2} = 0.5083$ $\beta_{y2 \cdot 1} = 0.1259$	0.5432	0.2951	Not significant	$r_{y1 \cdot 2} = 0.5128$ $r_{y2 \cdot 1} = 0.1464$
2	Outpatient incidence (Y) vs. average age (X_1) and average income (X_2)	$Y = 206.0357 - 2.2250X_1 + 0.0014X_2$	$\beta_{y1 \cdot 2} = -0.4189$ $\beta_{y2 \cdot 1} = 0.3646$	0.5087	0.2587	Not significant	$r_{y1 \cdot 2} = -0.4328$ $r_{y2 \cdot 1} = 0.3855$
3	Surgical incidence (Y) vs. average age (X_1) and average income (X_2)	$Y = 39.9651 + 0.2803X_1 + 0.0005X_2$	$\beta_{y1 \cdot 2} = 0.2351$ $\beta_{y2 \cdot 1} = 0.5379$	0.6211	0.3857	Not significant	$r_{y1 \cdot 2} = 0.2839$ $r_{y2 \cdot 1} = 0.5607$
4	Medical incidence (Y) vs. average age (X_1) and average income (X_2)	$Y = 1.3527 + 1.4619X_1 - 0.0002X_2$	$\beta_{y1 \cdot 2} = 0.5632$ $\beta_{y2 \cdot 1} = -0.1303$	0.5570	0.3103	Not significant	$r_{y1 \cdot 2} = 0.5601$ $r_{y2 \cdot 1} = -0.1542$
5	Maternity incidence (Y) vs. average age (X_1) and average income (X_2)	$Y = 25.6215 - 0.1551X_1 + 0.0001X_2$	$\beta_{y1 \cdot 2} = -0.3030$ $\beta_{y2 \cdot 1} = 0.1845$	0.3282	0.1077	Not significant	$r_{y1 \cdot 2} = -0.3018$ $r_{y2 \cdot 1} = 0.1892$

Age ($r_{y1.2} = 0.5601$); and Inpatient Incidence and Average Age ($r_{y1.2} = 0.5128$). Particularly noteworthy is the fact that the effect of Age on Medical Incidence seems to increase when Income is held constant.

CANONICAL CORRELATION

Rationale

Multiple regression and correlation analyses are designed to establish the relationship between a single criterion, Y, and a series of predictors, $X_1, X_2, \ldots, X_n$. When multiple criteria and multiple predictors are involved, the appropriate technique is the canonical correlation derived by Hotelling [5]. The essential idea behind canonical correlation is as follows: If there are p predictors, $X_1, X_2, \ldots, X_p$ and q criteria, $Y_1, Y_2, \ldots, Y_q$, a linear transformation of the following form is sought:

$$X^* = a_1 X_1 + a_2 X_2 + \cdots + a_p X_p \quad (1)$$

$$Y^* = b_1 Y_1 + b_2 Y_2 + \cdots + b_q Y_q \quad (2)$$

such that the correlation between the transformed variables is the maximum attainable. That is:

$$R_c = \frac{\text{Cov}(X^*, Y^*)}{\sqrt{V(X^*)V(Y^*)}} \quad (3)$$

Here, R_c, the canonical correlation, is the maximum attainable correlation between the predictor and criterion sets. Canonical correlation analysis also yields a set of measures called "canonical variates." These measures indicate the "loading" or impact of each variable on the predictor and criterion sets. In other words, they indicate the extent and nature of the contribution made by the predictor and criterion variables in establishing the relationship epitomized by R_c. A brief description of the mathematics of canonical correlation is provided in the notes to this paper [6].

Despite the power and potentialities of canonical correlation, applications of this technique to research problems have been few because of its computational complexity. With the increasing availability of "canned" computer programs, complexity has ceased to be a deterrent, so that canonical correlation is being used more frequently in contemporary research [7, 8, 9, 10].

Application

For the present research problem the predictor and criterion sets are defined as follows:

1 The Predictor Set

X_1: Average Age
X_2: Average Annual Income

2 The Criterion Set [11]

X_3: Inpatient Incidence
X_4: Outpatient Incidence

The results of canonical analysis performed on the data are presented below:

The Largest Root: $\lambda_1 = 0.6857$

Canonical Correlation Coefficient: $R_c = 0.8281$

The χ^2 value for R_c is significant at 5 percent level.

The canonical variates with the larger coefficients scaled to unity are as follows:

$$X^* = X_1 - 0.000179 X_2$$
$$Y^* = X_3 - 0.565700 X_4$$

Interpretation of Results

The foregoing results may be interpreted as follows: There does exist a significant relationship between Average Age and Average Annual Income of members on the one hand and Inpatient Incidence and Outpatient Incidence on the other. The extent of this relationship may be gauged from the fact that over 68 percent of the variation in Inpatient and Outpatient Incidence is attributable to variations in the members' age and annual income.

The implications of the equations for canonical variates are worth noting: Among the predictor variables the major determinant of the relationship is Average Age (X_1). The effect of Average Annual Income (X_2) is relatively low. Among the criterion variables, Inpatient Incidence (X_3) contributes about twice as much as Outpatient Incidence (X_4) toward the relationship.

NOTES

1. Howard R. Garland, "Hospital Utilization by Characteristic of Industry in Southwestern Ohio," Inquiry 6 (March 1969):60-71.
2. Statisticians call this "arm-twisting" the data. This can best be explained by considering what would happen if a polynomial of the form $Y = bX + cX^2 + \cdots + kX^n$ is fitted to a scatter diagram. If there are as many constants in the equation as there are observations, the trend line will coincide with every point in the scatter diagram, but such a trend equation will be meaningless.
3. The key measures used and their interpretation are as follows:

a : The Regression Constant, or the Y-Intercept. In the prediction equation of the form $Y = a + bX$, "a" is the value of Y when X is zero.

b : The Regression Coefficient. This measure represents the slope of the regression line. If b is not significant, it means that there is no real relationship between X and Y.

r : The Correlation Coefficient. This is a summary measure of the observed relationship between X and Y. If r is not significant, it means that no observed relationship exists. The adjective "observed" is used advisedly. A significant r does not necessarily imply causal relationship between X and Y, for it is possible that the observed relationship is due to the interplay of variables X_2, X_3, etc., not explicitly included in the analysis.

r^2 : The Coefficient of Determination. This measure represents the proportion of variance of Y explained by X.

4. Multiple regression and correlation analysis:

$a_{y.12}$: The Regression Constant. It is the value of Y when X_1 and X_2 are zero.

$\left.\begin{array}{l} b_{y1.2} \\ b_{y2.1} \end{array}\right\}$: The Regression Coefficients. The coefficient $b_{y1.2}$ represents the contribution of X_1 in a setting in which the effect of X_2 is held constant. The coefficient $b_{y2.1}$ should be interpreted similarly.

$\left.\begin{array}{l} \beta_{y1.2} \\ \beta_{y2.1} \end{array}\right\}$: The Beta Coefficients. These are the standardized analogues of the Regression Coefficient. In the equation: $y = \beta_{y1.2}x_1 + \beta_{y2.1}x_2$, the coefficients show the relative contributions of X_1 and X_2 toward the prediction of Y.

$R_{y.12}$: The Coefficient of Multiple Correlation. It is a summary measure of the relationship between Y on the one hand and X_1 and X_2 on the other.

$R^2_{y.12}$: The Coefficient of Multiple Determination. This measure represents the proportion of variance of Y explained by X_1 and X_2.

$\left.\begin{array}{c}r_{y1.2}\\r_{y2.1}\end{array}\right\}$: The Partial Correlation Coefficients. The coefficient $r_{y1.2}$ shows the effect of X_1 on Y holding the effect of X_2 constant. The coefficient $r_{y2.1}$ should be interpreted similarly. The partial correlation coefficients (especially the higher-order variety) are far better indicators of causal relationship than the simple rs.

5. Harold Hotelling, "Relations Between Two Sets of Variates," Biometrika 28 (1936):321-77.

6. The analysis begins by forming R, the zero-order correlation matrix of the p + q variables. This matrix is then partitioned into the following submatrices:

$$R = \begin{bmatrix} R_{11} & | & R_{12} \\ --- & + & --- \\ R_{21} & | & R_{22} \end{bmatrix}$$

R_{11} : The intercorrelations of the p predictors.
R_{22} : The intercorrelations of the q criteria.
R_{12} : The intercorrelations of the predictors and the criteria.
R_{21} : The transpose of R_{12}.

The partitioned portions of R are then substituted into either of the following two canonical equations:

$$(R_{11}^{-1} R_{12} R_{22}^{-1} R_{21} - \lambda_i I) a_i = 0 \tag{1}$$

$$(R_{22}^{-1} R_{21} R_{11}^{-1} R_{12} - \lambda_i I) b_i = 0 \tag{2}$$

In the above equations, the left-hand expression within parenthesis is a nonsymmetrical matrix formed from the partitioned portions of R, λ_i are the canonical roots (eigenvalues), I is an identity matrix, and a_i and b_i are the associated vectors (eigenvectors) representing the coefficients of the canonical equations.

If equation 2 is used the characteristic roots, λ_i, should be found which result in the determinant of the characteristic being equal to zero. That is:

$$| R_{22}^{-1} R_{21} R_{11}^{-1} R_{12} - \lambda I | = 0 \tag{3}$$

Equation 3 states that a quantity, λ, should be deducted from the principal diagonal elements of the matrix such that the determinant of the resulting matrix is zero. There will be m such roots where m is equal to p or q, whichever is smaller. The largest root is the square of the canonical correlation coefficient. That is, $\lambda_{largest} = R^2_c$.

Bartlett has developed a procedure to test the significance of R_c. [See M. S. Bartlett, "The Statistical Significance of Canonical Correlations," Biometrika 32 (1941):29-38.] He defines Lambda:

$$\Lambda = \prod_{i=1}^{q} (1 - \lambda_i), \quad q \leq p$$

The χ^2 approximation to test the null hypothesis that the p predictors are uncorrelated with the q criteria is given by:

$$\chi^2 = -[N - 0.5(p + q + 1)] \log \Lambda$$

where N is the number of observations, p and q are the number of predictors and criteria respectively, and $p \times q$ is the number of degrees of freedom.

The coefficients, a_i, for the predictor set are obtained by solving:

$$a = \frac{R_{11}^{-1} R_{12} b}{(\lambda)^{\frac{1}{2}}}$$

7. Robert P. O'Hara and David V. Tiedman, "Vocational Self Concept in Adolescence," Journal of Counseling Psychology 6 (1959):292-301.

8. J. E. Birren and D. F. Morrison, "Analysis of the WAIS Subsets in Relation to Age and Education," Journal of Gerontology 16 (1961):363-69.

9. M. Perry and B. Curtis Hamm, "Canonical Analysis of Relations Between Socio-economic Risk and Personal Influence in Purchase Decisions," Journal of Marketing Research 6 (1969):351-54.

10. Carl E. Hopkins, "Statistical Analysis by Canonical Correlation: A Computer Application," Health Services Research 4 (Winter 1969):304-12.

11. We could have defined the criterion set as being composed of four variables: Medical Incidence, Surgical Incidence, Maternity Incidence, and Outpatient Incidence. However, we have decided against it because of the paucity of observations. Also, note that the criterion variables are designated X_3 and X_4 instead of Y_1 and Y_2 for convenience.

6

CLUSTERING ANALYSIS

INTRODUCTION

The basic rationale for a classification system is to develop a method of comparison. In the health systems area, federal, state and local health agencies, hospital associations, health service agencies, insurance companies and others are interested in classification as a way of developing criteria for such objectives as rate setting, performance, and planning. Since there is so much variation among hospitals with respect to basic attributes such as size, product mix, and case mix, it would be unrealistic and uninformative to attempt to apply a common evaluative standard to all. A classification scheme that segments the total population into similar groups in respect to basic attributes enables the development of various sets of criteria and measures which can be applied separately to each group of cases. This allows for the most useful information to be drawn from the set of data. Such classification is also useful to the pharmaceutical and equipment supplier who desires valid market segments for development of marketing strategies. Past attempts at classification have been minimal, and where they exist, segmentation has been done on elementary, unidimensional levels. In this paper, Phillip and Iyer suggest that the underlying structure of hospitals is in fact multi-dimensional, and they utilize cluster analysis performed on 5000 hospitals at the national level to develop groupings based on 17 variables. Seventy-one clusters, each with an average size of 64 hospitals, were obtained.

Introduction to Technique

Clustering is an analysis technique whose basic objective is classification. It transforms a heterogeneous set of objects into a set of homogeneous groups, usually for the purpose of ease of handling of data in further analyses. Each group is said to have a distinct profile; that is, within each group the members have similar scores on the set of variables chosen for the analysis, and the group can be described in terms of the average scores of the members on these variables.

There are a variety of ways in which groupings can be determined. For example, based on various distance and criterion functions, individual points can be progressively combined to build up clusters. Or, the process can be performed in reverse; beginning with the entire set, clusters are formed by progressive breakdown, again based on various distance and criterion functions.

The researcher must make a subjective judgment as to which division is most useful. Typically, he is looking for as small a number of clusters as possible that are still clearly distinguishable from each other. Since a small within group variance indicates homogeneity, a decreasing ratio of within group to total variance will indicate an increasing homogeneity. This ratio will decrease as the number of clusters into which the data point are divided increases (that is, as the number of members of each cluster goes to one). Descriptions of the groups, once the number of clusters has been decided, are based on an interpretation of the centroid of each group. The centroid is a theoretical data point representing the mean value, for the objects in the cluster, of each variable in the analysis. Comparisons of coordinates of centroids relative to each other yield a distinctive profile for each group.

REFERENCES

Anderberg, R. M., Cluster Analysis for Applications. New York: Academic Press, 1973.

Ball, H., Classification Analysis, Technical Note. Menlo Park, Calif.: Stanford Research Institute, 1970.

Cooley, W. W., and P. R. Lohnes, Multivariate Data Analysis. New York: Wiley, 1971.

Green, P., and D. Tull, Research for Marketing Decisions. Englewood Cliffs, N.J.: Prentice-Hall, 1970.

Hartigan, J. A., Clustering Algorithms. New York: Wiley, 1975.

Mahajan, V., and M. Agarwal, "A State Level Classification Scheme of Non-federal Hospitals," Working Paper No. 239, State University of New York at Buffalo, Buffalo, N.Y., 1977.

McClain, J. O., and V. R. Rao, "Trade-offs and Conflicts in Evaluation of Health System Alternatives: Methodology of Analysis," Health Services Research, Spring 1974, pp. 35-52.

Overall, J. E., and J. Kleett, Applied Multivariate Analysis. New York: McGraw-Hill, 1972.

Phillip, P. J., and R. N. Iyer, "A Taxonomy of Community Hospitals," Project Report, American Hospital Association, Chicago, Ill., 1975.

CLASSIFICATION OF COMMUNITY HOSPITALS

P. Joseph Phillip
and
Ramani N. Iyer

This article describes the methodology, results, and potential applications of a study conducted by the authors to classify the nation's community hospitals. The classification system is offered as a preferable alternative to the system presently used by the Social Security Administration to implement Section 223 of the Social Security Amendments of 1972 (P.L. 92-603).

Most national health insurance proposals before the Congress of the United States explicitly or implicitly recommend classification

---

Reprinted with permission from Health Services Research 10 No. 4 (Winter 1975). Copyright 1975 by the Hospital Research and Educational Trust, 840 North Lakeshore Drive, Chicago, Ill. 60611.

The authors express their thanks to the referees of an earlier manuscript for their constructive criticism and suggestions.

of the nation's hospitals for performance evaluation. Here, for example, is an excerpt from the Kennedy-Mills [1] proposal:

> For the purpose of comparing similar classes of hospitals . . . the Administration shall develop and utilize a comparison methodology for grouping and comparing similar providers of services.

Recently Senator Talmadge [2], Chairman of the Subcommittee on Health, outlined the salient features of a bill [No. S3205, introduced March 25, 1976—Ed.] to overhaul the current Medicare-Medicaid program. An excerpt from his speech follows:

> The bill will include requirements as to appropriate means of classifying and categorizing health care facilities so that "apples" can be compared with "apples." . . . The key here is to assure comparability of hospitals. The American Hospital Association and the Social Security Administration, as well as other organizations, are working at our request to develop proper methods of classification and comparison.

The purpose of these and other such research efforts is to provide an adequate statistical basis for implementing Section 1861 (v)(1) of the Social Security Act, as amended by Section 223 (a) of P. L. 92-603 (1972), which states that "the reasonable cost of any service shall be the cost actually incurred, excluding therefrom any part of the incurred cost found to be unnecessary in the efficient delivery of needed health services."

At present the Social Security Administration (SSA) classifies the nation's hospitals on the basis of three "discretized" variables: metropolitan vs. nonmetropolitan location (two divisions), per capita income (10 divisions), and hospital size (six or seven divisions). Initial breakdown is by SMSA vs. non-SMSA, followed by state per capita income. Hospitals in each group are then divided into three (and in some cases four) size classes to yield 32 national groups. The limit on routine hospital service costs reimbursable under Medicare is presently set at the 80th percentile of the group distribution plus 10 percent of the median [3]. The rationale behind this approach is that any group of hospitals that are similar with respect to product mix and external environments can be expected to have similar cost per unit of output provided their operations are characterized by similar levels of efficiency and frugality. Hospitals with extremely high costs per unit of output are considered to utilize resources inefficiently and/or extravagantly.

The SSA system presently in use is a crude approach to cost containment for two reasons. First, no classification of hospitals, however refined, can capture all the nuances relating to product mix and environmental characteristics. Second, the approach involves the untested assumption that the levels of efficiency and frugality of the average hospital in the group meet acceptable standards. Nonetheless, as a practical means of identifying hospitals whose performances are out of line with group standards, the approach does have merit if, and only if, the groups established are reasonably homogeneous in terms of carefully chosen criteria. Unfortunately, the SSA classification seems to have failed on both counts—in terms of the criteria chosen and the degree of homogeneity. The failure to produce homogeneous groupings is largely due to the choice of cross-tabulation as the method of classification. In the first place, use of this method places severe restrictions on how refined the classification can be because addition of variables is associated with a sharp proliferation of classification cells and an equally sharp reduction in the number of hospitals per cell. Limiting the classification to three variables meant that many relevant dimensions could not be considered. Second, the "discretization" of continuous variables, an unavoidable requirement of all cross-tabulations, leads to loss of information content. It has been estimated, for example, that the loss of information content associated with the dichotomization of a continuous variable is 36 percent if the variable is normally distributed and the point of division is optimal [4]. Third, the variables chosen for the SSA classification scheme were not the "best" variables. A factor analytic investigation has revealed that per capita income, SMSA vs. non-SMSA dichotomy, and hospital size capture only some aspects of the differences between hospitals. In addition to these problems, inherent in the cross-tabulation approach, the use of such large areas as the state or the SMSA for the income variable conceals vital intraregional differences.

This article describes an alternative classification scheme developed at the American Hospital Association. Although congressional endorsement of classification as a basis for reimbursement provided the initial impetus for this undertaking, the classification system should be useful in a variety of research and evaluative contexts.

PRELIMINARY CONSIDERATIONS

Distinctive Features of the Hospital Industry

Traditional theory of the firm postulates that for any given level of output a firm will attempt to minimize its cost of production in order to maximize profit. Individual firms may differ with respect to technical, economic, and scale efficiency, but differences in efficiency are "aberrations" superimposed on the profit maximizing/cost minimizing process. For a variety of reasons, this picture of the typical firm hardly fits hospitals [5, 6]. In addition, there is a potential source of variation in "social" efficiency that is peculiar to hospitals. It is well known that major decisions concerning the admission, treatment, and disposition of patients are made by physicians, who are not members of the hospital management. In addition, the patient is often a passive recipient of care, and his out-of-pocket expenses are typically minimal. In this situation the patient may well receive services in excess of or less than what is warranted by his condition. Indeed, the assumption that incidents of overutilization and underutilization of services (especially the former) are prevalent in the hospital industry is implicit in the establishment of utilization review committees, professional standards review organizations, and quality assurance programs.

The crucial question is how to identify hospitals that utilize resources inefficiently and/or extravagantly. This is by no means easy, since the hospital industry is a highly heterogeneous aggregation of institutions, differing both in product characteristics and external characteristics. At one end of the product spectrum are institutions providing a narrow range of basic services, while at the other end are institutions specializing in complex, sophisticated services such as open heart surgery, organ transplants, renal dialysis, and cobalt therapy.

The socioeconomic characteristics of the areas in which hospitals are located also differ widely. A New York City hospital, for example, faces an entirely different factor price situation than a rural hospital. Also, the demographic composition of the area served by a hospital influences the product mix of the hospital. For instance, if the service area of a hospital has a high proportion of older people, the hospital will tend to be more oriented toward the care of chronic and degenerative diseases.

Possible Approaches to Hospital Classification

Because of the differences in the product characteristics and external characteristics of hospitals, standard tests of efficiency such as cost per unit of output and average length of stay cannot simply be applied across the board to identify "deviant" hospitals. A method of classification must be used that brings together hospitals that are, as far as possible, similar with respect to product and external characteristics.

One possible approach would be to use a monothetic classification method, simply classifying hospitals on one dimension. In such a classification scheme, "the classes established differ by at least one property which is uniform among members of each class" [7]. The alternative approach is to use polythetic classification, in which the classes established "are groups of individuals or objects that share a large proportion of their properties but do not necessarily agree on any one property" [7]. That is, the differences among groups extend along several dimensions so that a group is definable in terms of its locus in a multidimensional variate space. Unlike monothetic groups, the differences among polythetic groups cannot be adequately expressed by the concept of "distance"; they can only be expressed by the concept of "configuration" except in the rare case in which group centroids are collinear [8]. In an operational context, monothetic classifications may be optimal for a single purpose but would be unlikely to be of general use. In contrast, polythetic classifications may be useful for a great variety of purposes although they are unlikely to be optimal for any single purpose.

Polythetic classification was used here for two reasons: First, hospitals can be evaluated in terms of several criteria such as cost per day, per case, or per specific services, or average length of stay. Second, as discussed in the previous section and in greater detail in Phillip and Iyer [9], the underlying structure of hospital differences is multidimensional. In the light of these considerations, use of monothetic classification would have been both inadequate and inappropriate.

Selection of Variables

Since a classification is only as good as the variables on which it is based, the selection of variables is critical. Actually the problem has three parts: What kinds of variables should be considered, how many variables should be chosen, and what weight (if any) should be assigned to the variables chosen?

Biological taxonomists are inclined to include as many variables as possible [10, 11], but in the present study we decided to use a limited subset of variables for two reasons: First, inclusion of a large number of variables would create a formidable feasibility problem, particularly since the classification system needs to be updated on a periodic basis. Second, the impact of a variable is inversely related to the total number of variables used. Consequently, inclusion of too many variables, some of which may be of marginal importance, could swamp the effect of the more important variables.

Weighting of Variables

The selection of variables may be regarded as an extreme form of weighting in the sense that the excluded variables are implicitly given a weight of zero. There are two types of explicit weighting—subjective weighting and the weighting introduced by the proximity (similarity) or distance (dissimilarity) measure employed to assess similarity between pairs of entities (hospitals). Experts are generally against subjective weighting [7, 12-17].

Some variables may exert more weight than others depending upon the measure used to assess similarity. Consider, for example, the familiar product moment correlation coefficient, r. Traditionally this measure is computed between pairs of variables as, for instance, between columns 1 and 2 of matrix M below. Sometimes, however, the correlation coefficient is used as a measure of similarity between

	Matrix M					Matrix M'			
	Variables					Entities			
	X_1	X_2	...	X_p		E_1	E_2	...	E_n
E_1	x	x	...	x	X_1	x	x	...	x
E_2	x	x	...	x	X_2	x	x	...	x
:	:	:	: :	:	:	:	:	: :	:
E_n	x	x	...	x	X_p	x	x	...	x

(left: Entities; right: Variables)

pairs of entities as, for example, between columns 1 and 2 of matrix M'. A correlation coefficient computed in this way will weight the variables in an irrational manner, so this kind of correlation has been rejected by most taxonomists as an unsuitable measure of similarity [18-21]. Or consider the Euclidean distance between entities i and j, written as follows:

$$d_{ij}^2 = \sum_{k=1}^{p} (X_{ki} - X_{kj})^2$$

where k is an index of variables 1 through p. This measure assigns higher weights to variables with large scale values and ignores the redundancy implicit in intercorrelations. The scale disparities can be corrected by first standardizing the variables (i.e., by dividing each variable by its standard deviation) and then computing the Euclidean distance on standard scores, but the problem introduced by intercorrelations will persist.

Establishing Group Boundaries

Since hospitals do not fall neatly into clear-cut groups, one must use some system for establishing group or cluster boundaries. If the boundaries are drawn too tightly, the result will in all probability be a large number of tiny clusters and several nonclusterable entities. If the boundaries are drawn too loosely, some internal (intragroup) homogeneity and external (intergroup) distinctiveness will be sacrificed.

In establishing group boundaries one must strike a balance between the conflicting demands of internal homogeneity and the requirement that, as far as possible, all entities be brought within a manageable number of groups. In the present study the balance was tilted somewhat toward the latter objective.

METHODS

Variables Selected

The variables initially selected are listed in Table 6.1. The first 14 variables are proxies for product mix. The two personnel variables (NURSES and NONMED) were included in this category on the basis of findings of a concurrent study [22] indicating that level of staffing is closely related to two aspects of hospital product, degree of sophistication and patient turnover rate, both of which raise per diem cost. Exclusion of these variables would have had the effect of penalizing institutions with complex, sophisticated services and fast patient turnover rates. The remaining 11 variables in the list are proxies for external socioeconomic, demographic, and related characteristics over which hospitals have no control.

As the first step toward classification, hospitals were stratified into five size classes as shown in Table 6.2. Within each stratum a factor analysis (quartimax rotation) was performed. The manner in which a subset of key variables was chosen for each stratum is illustrated in Table 6.3, an excerpt from the factor structure matrix of stratum I. The first four variables chosen were those that correlated maximally with the factors, thus ensuring that the major dimensions along which hospitals in stratum I differ were represented by their best surrogates. In adding to these variables, two aspects of

TABLE 6.1

Variables Initially Selected

Acronym	Description
	Product Characteristics
SERVICES	Total number of facilities/services
TECH SERV	Number of "advanced" technology facilities/services (incl. intensive care unit, cardiac care unit, open-heart surgery, x-ray therapy, cobalt therapy, radium therapy, radioisotope facility, and organ bank)
LONGTERM	Long-term care facilities (coded 1 if present, 0 otherwise)
LT CARE	Long-term care facilities as a fraction of total facilities/services
TEACH	Teaching hospital (coded 1 if teaching hospital, 0 otherwise)
GOVT	Government, nonfederal (coded 1 if government, nonfederal; 0 otherwise)
NONPROFIT	Nongovernment, nonprofit (coded 1 if nongovernment, nonprofit; 0 otherwise)
BEDS	Average number of licensed beds during the year
NURSES	Number of RNs and LPNs per 100 beds
NONMED	Number of personnel not involved in direct patient care per 100 beds
PAY	Average yearly salary per full-time employee
ASSETS	Net assets per bed
SURGERY	Surgical operations per inpatient admission
OPD VISITS	Outpatient visits per inpatient admission
	External Characteristics
SMSA	Hospital located in an SMSA (coded 1 if SMSA, 0 otherwise)
POP	Population per square mile for the county [23]
$INCOME_f$	Median family income for the county [23]
$INCOME_{pc}$	Average per capita income for the county [23]
POOR	Percent families in the county below poverty level [23]
INSURED	Percent of residents of the state under 65 with hospital expense coverage [24]
PHYSICIANS	Number of physicians per 1000 county residents [25]
WHITE	Percent white population for the county [23]
MALE	Percent male population for the county [23]
OVER 64	Percent population in the county 65 and over [23]
UNDER 15	Percent population in the county under 15 [23]

TABLE 6.2

Stratification of Hospitals by Number of Beds

Stratum	Number of Licensed Beds	Number of Hospitals
I	6-49	1378
II	50-99	1271
III	100-299	1666
IV	300-499	508
V	500 and over	211

the factor structure were considered: (1) The relative importance of the factors. For example, since factor 1 was more than twice as important as factor 2, and more than four times as important as factor 5, additional variables representing factor 1 were chosen. (2) The loading of a variable on several factors. An instance in point is SERVICES, which had significant correlations (loadings) with factors 1, 2, 3, and 5.

The variables excluded from Table 6.3 either had minimal loading on the significant factors or were highly correlated with the variables already chosen (e.g., $INCOME_f$, whose correlation with $INCOME_{pc}$ was over 0.9). Subsets of variables chosen in this way for each stratum are displayed in Table 6.4.

Table 6.5 shows means and coefficients of variation of the 17 selected variables. Four performance measures—not used for cluster analysis—appear at the bottom of the table. They are included to provide some idea of the variability of the measures under a stratification scheme and to serve as bases for evaluating the homogeneity of clusters formed within each stratum.

The Distance Measure

The distance measure used to assess the similarity between hospital groups was the Mahalanobis distance [26-30], written

$$D_{12}^2 = (\bar{x}_1 - \bar{x}_2)C^{-1}(\bar{x}_1 - \bar{x}_2)' \qquad (1)$$

TABLE 6.3

Excerpt from Factor Structure Matrix: Stratum I (Quartimax Rotation)

Variable	Socio-economic (1)	Long-term Care (2)	Factor Loading Organizational Structure (3)	Demographic (4)	Product Configuration (5)	Communality	Uniqueness
INCOMEpc	0.934	0.025	0.014	−0.082	0.027	0.955	0.045
LT CARE	0.003	0.925	−0.003	−0.032	−0.052	0.903	0.097
NONMED	0.064	0.024	0.815	0.024	0.100	0.783	0.217
UNDER 15	−0.081	−0.023	0.009	0.840	0.004	0.773	0.227
TECH SERV	0.095	0.007	0.175	−0.009	0.686	0.528	0.472
PHYSICIANS	0.714	−0.001	0.041	−0.089	0.052	0.705	0.295
BEDS	0.065	0.014	0.725	−0.005	0.114	0.691	0.309
SERVICES	0.159	0.150	0.353	0.050	0.378	0.735	0.265
POP	0.331	−0.022	0.040	−0.011	−0.034	0.282	0.718
PAY	0.344	−0.065	−0.012	0.055	0.041	0.391	0.609
SURGERY	0.292	−0.048	0.201	0.059	0.049	0.334	0.666
ASSETS	0.052	0.046	0.211	0.028	0.048	0.195	0.805
NURSES	0.200	−0.061	0.188	0.052	0.080	0.352	0.648
% variance explained	39.2	18.5	17.7	13.7	9.4		
Cumulative % variance explained	39.2	57.7	75.4	89.1	98.5		

TABLE 6.4

Subsets of Variables Selected for Cluster Analysis

Variable	Stratum				
	I	II	III	IV	V
SERVICES	X	X	X	X	X
TECH SERV	X	X	X	X	X
LT CARE	X	X	X	X	X
BEDS	X	X	X	X	X
OPD VISITS				X	X
SURGERY	X	X	X	X	X
PAY	X	X	X	X	X
ASSETS	X	X	X	X	X
NURSES	X	X	X	X	X
POP	X		X	X	X
OVER 64				X	X
WHITE		X	X		
UNDER 15	X	X			
INCOME$_f$			X	X	X
INCOME$_{pc}$	X	X			
PHYSICIANS	X	X	X		X
NONMED	X	X	X	X	X

where $(\bar{x}_1 - \bar{x}_2)$ is a row vector of mean differences between groups 1 and 2 with respect to all variables (k = 1, 2, ..., p), $(\bar{x}_1 - \bar{x}_2)'$ its transpose, and C^{-1} the inverse of the within-group covariance matrix.

Mahalanobis distance is equivalent to (1) Euclidean distance computed on standard scores if the variables used to compute the distance are uncorrelated, (2) Euclidean distance computed on orthogonal factor scores, and (3) Sibson's normal information radius [17] in the special case of normal distributions with equal covariance. Mahalanobis distance is related to (1) Fisher's linear discriminant function [31] which provides maximum separation between groups, (2) the multiple correlation coefficient, R, computed with a binary-coded dependent variable, (3) Hotelling's T^2 [32] and (4) Wilks' Λ [33]. Finally, the Mahalanobis distance statistic can be used to test

TABLE 6.5

Means and Coefficients of Variation of 21 Characteristics, by Stratum

	All		Stratum								
			I		II		III		IV		V	
Characteristics	Mean	Coef. of Var.*	Mean	Coef. of Var.*	Mean	Coef. of Var.*	Mean	Coef. of Var.*	Mean	Coef. of Var.*	Mean	Coef. of Var.*
Variables												
SERVICES	10.431	0.639	4.269	0.553	7.470	0.402	13.065	0.314	20.112	0.198	24.644	0.164
TECH SERV	2.179	1.017	0.379	1.821	1.056	1.107	3.048	0.569	5.300	0.262	6.420	0.190
LT CARE	0.025	2.040	0.011	4.545	0.025	2.480	0.027	1.630	0.045	0.800	0.069	0.362
BEDS	155.690	1.113	33.994	0.301	74.297	0.198	177.864	0.314	381.120	0.144	732.207	0.417
OPD VISITS	3.900	1.625	3.577	2.348	3.145	1.812	4.013	1.277	4.980	0.890	7.143	0.761
SURGERY	0.373	0.566	0.231	0.818	0.337	0.674	0.454	0.333	0.521	0.236	0.532	0.318
PAY ($)	5 301.230	0.259	4 642.982	0.279	5 070.410	0.246	5 668.742	0.228	6 067.874	0.188	6 260.240	0.209
ASSETS ($)	17 780.869	0.690	13 120.730	0.754	15 838.197	0.733	20 135.994	0.637	24 639.292	0.482	24 944.092	0.460
NURSES	53.486	0.407	41.179	0.418	48.886	0.416	61.900	0.340	65.350	0.250	66.831	0.344
POP	1 615.362	4.170	204.122	5.856	769.007	5.668	2 232.475	3.496	3 010.661	2.630	7 496.964	2.141
OVER 64	11.046	0.321	12.419	0.327	11.408	0.317	10.175	0.281	10.662	0.889	10.094	0.291
WHITE	89.582	0.175	90.631	0.152	90.451	0.135	88.788	0.132	86.522	0.133	82.239	0.142
UNDER 15	28.654	0.190	28.497	0.127	28.514	0.149	28.484	0.144	28.540	0.194	28.219	0.237
INCOMEf ($)	8 741.418	0.232	7 550.437	0.238	8 322.638	0.228	9 413.141	0.194	10 255.400	0.160	10 120.087	0.126
INCOMEpc ($)	2 861.121	0.245	2 493.951	0.229	2 701.194	0.240	3 054.307	0.220	3 374.209	0.177	3 472.880	0.164
PHYSICIANS	1.251	1.306	0.793	0.667	1.028	0.855	1.424	0.692	1.955	0.606	2.536	0.800
NONMED	255.440	1.414	41.154	0.511	96.875	0.376	273.538	0.489	689.695	0.336	1 440.565	0.512
Performance measures												
Expenses/day ($)	68.860	0.391	59.075	0.376	62.681	0.366	73.174	0.315	84.351	0.303	98.513	0.527
Expenses/day, adj. ($)	63.200	0.359	53.747	0.341	57.976	0.339	67.732	0.319	76.395	0.262	88.889	0.373
Expenses/visit, adj. ($)	16.030	1.004	13.844	0.835	15.596	0.808	16.252	0.657	14.362	0.791	17.258	0.552
Average length of stay	7.960	0.412	7.015	0.357	7.785	0.364	8.327	0.483	8.594	0.190	10.820	0.383

*Standard deviation divided by group mean.

the discriminatory power of a set of variables [34] and the sufficiency of a subset of variables [35].

The Clustering Algorithm

The clustering algorithm (CLASF) developed for the study proceeds as follows: In cycle 1 the "distances" between all pairs of hospitals are computed using a variant of Mahalanobis distance written

$$\hat{D}^2_{ij} = (x_i - x_j)\hat{C}_t^{-1}(x_i - x_j)'$$

where $(x_i - x_j)$ is a row vector of differences between hospitals i and j with respect to all variables, $(x_i - x_j)'$ its transpose, and C_t^{-1} the inverse of the covariance matrix of the entire stratum. Since the classification system should strike a compromise between the conflicting demands of intracluster homogeneity and the requirement that the clusters established be reasonably large, some trial runs are made to determine a suitable threshold value. Having chosen this value (10.00), the program searches for the smallest distance, say, D^2_{jk} in the entire matrix of distances. Then it searches for entities closest to j and k and links them with the first pair provided their $\hat{D}^2$ values do not exceed the threshold value. This process is continued until all linkage possibilities are exhausted. All entities linked so far constitute the elements of the first cluster. These are removed from the matrix of distances, and the linking procedure is repeated until all clustering possibilities are exhausted. At this stage there are many small "nuclear" clusters and several nonclusterable entities.

In cycle 2, regular Mahalanobis distances (Eq. 1) between clusters established in the preceding cycle are computed and the linking procedure described above is repeated in order to collapse similar clusters into a smaller number of large clusters.

RESULTS

The results of cluster analysis are summarized in Table 6.6. There were 71 hospital clusters with an average size of 64 hospitals. A few clusters were smaller than one would have hoped for. There were, for example, four clusters with fewer than 15 hospitals and 11 clusters with fewer than 20 hospitals. Attempts to eliminate such small clusters through mergers or reassignment of hospitals were abandoned because within-group homogeneity dropped sharply.

The clustering process also identified 484 "nonclusterable isolates," that is, hospitals whose characteristics were so atypical

TABLE 6.6

Number of Hospitals in Each Cluster and Number
of Nonclusterable Isolates, by Stratum

Cluster	Stratum					
	I	II	III	IV	V	All
A	91	84	76	56	15	
B	160	80	5	130	18	
C	86	92	10	62	15	
D	86	85	29	173	63	
E	77	133	173	25	29	
F	239	17	199		21	
G	124	106	113			
H	89	87	133			
I	52	97	10			
J	99	32	126			
K	39	36	75			
L	22	38	54			
M	45	48	81			
N	18	24	25			
O	21	36	46			
P	20	29	21			
Q		37	98			
R		15	46			
S		34	61			
T		36	43			
U		21	51			
V		19	14			
Total no. of hospitals clustered	1268	1186	1489	446	161	4550
Nonclusterable isolates	110	85	177	62	50	484
Total no. of hospitals	1378	1271	1666	508	211	5034*

*627 hospitals were excluded due to lack of complete data.

TABLE 6.7

Nonclusterable Isolates in Stratum I

Cluster	No. of Nonclusterable Isolates Closest to Cluster	Average Distance from Cluster Centroid
A	11	559.27
B	4	29.00
C	4	101.50
D	0	—
E	2	59.50
F	9	70.67
G	3	39.67
H	1	38.00
I	16	100.63
J	1	44.00
K	5	141.80
L	10	42.90
M	26	256.85
N	9	165.44
O	3	59.00
P	6	60.50

that they could not be assigned to any cluster. Some idea of the atypical attributes of these hospitals can be gained from Table 6.7, which shows the average Mahalanobis distances between them and the centroids of the clusters to which they were closest.

"Closest clusters" were identified in the event group evaluation of all hospitals becomes mandatory. Most of these isolates had extremely high scores on the variables, although there were a few with extremely low scores. As an illustration, Table 6.8 displays the characteristics of five isolates, one in each stratum. Their scores may be compared to the corresponding stratum averages shown in Table 6.5. A, C, and E are isolates with high scores on most of the variables positively correlated with per diem expenses, whereas B and D are isolates with low scores. The expense measures of A, C, and E are significantly higher than the corresponding stratum averages, and those of B and D significantly lower.

TABLE 6.8

Profiles of Five Selected Nonclusterable Isolates

Characteristic	A (Stratum I)	B (Stratum II)	Isolate C (Stratum III)	D (Stratum IV)	E (Stratum V)	Correlation with Adj. Expenses Per Day
Variables						
SERVICES	5.00	8.00	23.00	3.00	31.00	0.51
TECH SERV	1.00	0.00	6.00	1.00	8.00	0.47
LT CARE	0.00	0.00	0.04	0.00	0.07	-0.13
BEDS	35.00	86.00	242.00	338.00	1 152.00	0.39
OPD VISITS	—	—	—	2.52	8.63	0.27
SURGERY	0.00	0.19	0.59	0.51	0.64	0.47
PAY ($)	5 066.67	2 511.63	8 093.84	3 180.77	—	0.65
ASSETS ($)	51 095.06	13 674.34	35 284.87	15 056.99	31 889.88	0.41
NURSES	42.86	16.28	71.07	67.75	59.38	0.48
POP	620.90	—	15 903.90	228.90	66 923.20	0.27
OVER 64	—	—	—	10.40	14.00	-0.29
WHITE	—	99.56	71.43	—	—	-0.09
UNDER 15	24.17	30.40	—	—	—	-0.04
INCOMEf ($)	—	—	10 503.00	7 259.00	8 983.00	0.55
INCOMEpc ($)	3 467.00	2 385.00	—	—	—	0.59
PHYSICIANS	2.48	0.62	5.06	—	7.82	0.49
NONMED	102.00	72.00	531.00	550.50	2 797.00	0.52
Performance measures						
Expenses/day ($)	143.36	23.33	199.77	56.05	162.86	
Expenses/day, adj. ($)	106.74	23.20	189.95	54.96	145.49	
Expenses/outpatient visit, adj. ($)	17.55	5.23	13.43	3.92	27.42	
Average length of stay	7.23	8.00	7.54	8.18	16.31	

VALIDATION

Since the central purpose of this classification is to bring together hospitals that are, as far as possible, similar with respect to product and external characteristics, its validity may be defined as the extent to which it has succeeded in minimizing within-group variations with respect to product and external characteristics. Results of validity tests are presented in succeeding sections.

The Generalized Mahalanobis Distance

The generalized Mahalanobis distance, V, is written as follows:

$$V = \sum_{i=1}^{k} n_i \underset{1 \times p}{(\bar{x}_i - \bar{\bar{x}})} \underset{p \times p}{C^{-1}} \underset{p \times 1}{(\bar{x}_i - \bar{\bar{x}})'}$$

where k = number of groups

p = number of variables

n_i = number of hospitals in the ith group

$\bar{x}_i$ = mean vector of the ith group

$\bar{\bar{x}}$ = grand mean vector

C^{-1} = inverse of covariance matrix

TABLE 6.9

Generalized Mahalanobis Distances

Stratum	V	Degrees of Freedom
I	47 123	195
II	53 157	273
III	295 521	273
IV	2 032	52
V	1 066	65

TABLE 6.10

Coefficients of Variation: First Cluster in Each Stratum vs. Randomly Selected Group of Same Size within Same Stratum

Characteristic	Stratum I Clstr. A N = 91	Stratum I Group N = 91	Stratum II Clstr. A N = 84	Stratum II Group N = 84	Stratum III Clstr. A N = 76	Stratum III Group N = 76	Stratum IV Clstr. A N = 56	Stratum IV Group N = 56	Stratum V Clstr. A N = 15	Stratum V Group N = 15
Organizational Structure Variables										
BEDS	0.114	0.300	0.142	0.209	0.297	0.323	0.112	0.149	0.124	0.299
ASSETS	0.371	0.594	0.470	0.587	0.594	0.571	0.428	0.422	0.453	0.438
NURSES	0.301	0.398	0.143	0.403	0.274	0.356	0.174	0.203	0.265	0.286
NONMED	0.214	0.437	0.292	0.350	0.394	0.447	0.250	0.249	0.250	0.429
Product Configuration Variables										
SERVICES	0.274	0.500	0.273	0.376	0.234	0.295	0.165	0.183	0.149	0.191
TECH SERV	0	1.945	0.775	1.288	0.504	0.578	0.198	0.241	0.121	0.163
LT CARE	0	6.723	0	2.356	0	2.084	0.510	0.827	0	0.572
SURGERY	0.419	0.519	0.336	0.432	0.218	0.352	0.148	0.252	0.189	0.279
OPD VISITS	—	—	—	—	—	—	0.502	0.638	0.647	0.557
Socioeconomic and Demographic Variables										
POP	1.748	1.928	—	—	0.189	3.981	0.806	1.349	1.272	1.717
INCOMEpc	0.150	0.219	0.162	0.198	—	—	—	—	—	—
INCOMEf	—	—	—	—	0.078	0.215	0.111	0.193	0.086	0.124
WHITE	—	—	0.043	0.129	0.098	0.148	—	—	—	—
UNDER 15	0.118	0.135	0.112	0.126	—	—	—	—	—	—
OVER 64	—	—	—	—	—	—	0.189	0.245	0.205	0.194
PHYSICIANS	0.547	0.591	0.354	0.568	0.136	0.723	—	—	0.270	1.248
PAY	0.181	0.200	0.184	0.209	0.117	0.179	0.139	0.179	—	—
Performance Measures										
Expenses/day	0.346	0.532	0.228	0.274	0.153	0.268	0.218	0.236	0.143	0.406
Expenses/day, adj.	0.275	0.286	0.209	0.262	0.166	0.265	0.216	0.222	0.159	0.395
Expenses/outpatient visit, adj.	0.583	1.395	0.517	0.899	0.453	0.709	0.771	0.392	0.335	2.518
Mean length of stay	0.242	0.410	0.219	0.287	0.195	0.262	0.148	0.152	0.247	0.242

This statistic may be thought of as the multivariate analogue of the familiar t-test, and its significance is evaluated by the χ^2 test [36]. The results are displayed in Table 6.9. All V values are significant beyond the 6×10^{-7} level; therefore the null hypothesis of equality of cluster means is rejected categorically. Putting it differently, the within-cluster variation relative to between-cluster variation is extremely low.

Visual Inspection

Presented in Table 6.10 are the within-cluster coefficients of variation of the first cluster (cluster A) formed in each stratum. For comparison purposes, similar statistics were computed for a group of identical size selected at random from each stratum after removing the nonclusterable isolates. In virtually every case, cluster coefficients of variation are substantially smaller than the corresponding measures for the randomly selected group.

Supplementary Test

The aim of this classification method is not to minimize within-group variations with respect to performance; that could easily have been accomplished by arraying hospitals in terms of, say, observed expenses per day. Then clusters could have been established simply by dividing the array into several segments. But such a classification system would have little operational significance; it would serve only to legitimize and perpetuate the status quo. Nonetheless, the question may be posed: Is it logical to expect that the within-cluster variations in performance will be smaller than the corresponding measures of a group of similar size drawn at random? The answer is a qualified "yes" because the cluster analysis was designed to minimize that part of performance variations stemming from product and external differences. The lower segment of Table 6.10, which displays comparative performance measures within each stratum, indicates that the coefficients of variation for the "A" clusters are indeed smaller than the corresponding measures of the randomly selected groups.

UPDATING THE CLASSIFICATION SYSTEM

Like most industries, the hospital industry is dynamic. New hospitals enter the industry; some existing ones go out of business or undergo change. Therefore a classification system based on charac-

TABLE 6.11

Classification Matrix for Stratum I

								Predicted								
		A	B	C	D	E	F	G	H	I	J	K	L	M	N	O	P
Actual	A	86	0	1	0	1	0	2	0	0	0	0	0	1	0	0	0
	B	0	153	1	0	1	0	2	0	0	3	0	0	0	0	0	0
	C	0	0	84	0	0	0	1	1	0	1	0	0	0	0	0	0
	D	0	0	0	81	0	0	3	1	0	1	0	0	0	0	0	0
	E	0	0	0	1	76	0	0	0	0	0	0	0	0	0	0	0
	F	0	0	0	0	0	239	0	0	0	0	0	0	0	0	0	0
	G	0	0	0	1	0	0	124	0	0	0	0	0	0	0	0	0
	H	0	0	0	0	0	0	0	87	0	0	0	1	0	0	0	0
	I	0	1	0	0	0	1	0	0	51	0	0	0	0	0	0	0
	J	0	0	0	0	0	0	0	0	0	98	0	0	0	0	0	0
	K	0	0	0	0	0	0	0	0	0	0	38	0	0	0	1	0
	L	0	0	0	0	0	0	0	0	0	0	0	22	0	0	1	0
	M	0	0	0	0	0	0	0	0	0	0	0	0	45	0	0	0
	N	0	0	0	0	0	0	0	0	0	0	1	0	0	17	1	0
	O	0	0	0	0	0	0	0	0	0	0	0	0	0	0	20	0
	P	0	0	0	0	0	4	0	0	0	0	0	0	0	0	0	16

TABLE 6.12

Performance of Discriminant Functions

Stratum	No. of Clusters	No. of Hospitals	Correct Assignments		Incorrect Assignments	
			No.	%	No.	%
All	71	4550	4399	96.7	151	3.3
I	16	1268	1237	97.6	31	2.4
II	22	1186	1168	98.5	18	1.5
III	22	1489	1400	94.0	89	6.0
IV	5	446	437	98.0	9	2.0
V	6	161	157	97.5	4	2.5

teristics observed at any point in time will eventually become outdated. Completely reclassifying hospitals on a periodic basis would be both costly and time-consuming. A relatively inexpensive and expeditious alternative should, therefore, be found if the classification system developed is to have enduring usefulness. Discriminant analysis suggests itself as such an alternative.

We have constructed a set of discriminant equations for the clusters established within each stratum. These equations are based on Rao's generalization of the linear discriminant function to the multigroup case [28], the equation for the jth group being

$$\gamma_j = \sum_{i=1}^{p} c_i x_i - \frac{1}{2} \sum_{i=1}^{p} c_i \bar{x}_{ij} + \log_e \pi_j$$

where γ_j is the discriminant score of the jth group, x_i is an observed score on the ith variable for the jth group, and c_i is the associated coefficient; $\bar{x}_{ij}$ is the jth group's mean on the ith variable, and π_j is the relative size of the jth group. Of course the usual assumptions—multivariate normality, common covariance, and equal cost of misclassifications—are made.

Performance of the discriminant function pertaining to stratum I is displayed in Table 6.11. The diagonal entries are the correct assignments, and the off-diagonal entries are the incorrect assignments. Since the misclassified hospitals are those that lie in the overlapping segments of adjacent groups, it is a matter of indifference to which of these groups they are assigned. (One must distinguish between misclassifications due to overlaps and misclassifications resulting from an unsound classification system; the consequences of the former are far less serious than those of the latter.) The performance of the discriminant functions constructed within all strata are summarized in Table 6.12. Out of 4,550 clusterable hospitals, 4,399 hospitals (96.7 percent) were correctly classified using the discriminant equations. Few applications of discriminant functions to empirical data have attained a comparable level of predictive accuracy [37]. We plan to use these discriminant functions to update the classification system on a periodic basis.

DISCUSSION

This study was based on the entire universe of community hospitals. Obviously, in an undertaking as large as this, one could not hope to capture all the peculiar circumstances surrounding the operation of individual hospitals. Feasibility considerations imposed constraints on the number and kinds of variables that could be used for cluster analysis. The need to update the classification system on a periodic basis introduced an additional constraint because variables obtainable through a one-shot survey could not be considered. For these reasons, certain variables were not included at the outset and certain variables used for cluster analysis were not available in a form that would have been ideal for the study.

These limitations underscore the need for a cautious, judicious application of the present classification system as a cost control mechanism. It is recommended that the system be used as a basis for making tentative identifications of hospitals whose operations call for closer scrutiny. Thus the real merit of this system in a cost control context would be its ability to narrow down the number of institutions that need closer scrutiny to a manageable number.

Identification of "nonclusterable isolates" is both useful and necessary. Placing atypical hospitals in groups with which they have nothing in common would force them to conform to standards that are at least partially inappropriate for them. Furthermore, since group standards are based on the performance of all members, the standards themselves are apt to be distorted. Therefore the best approach would be to treat them on an individual basis. If this is not feasible, identification of these isolates should be helpful to regulatory agencies such as the Social Security Administration and Blue Cross plans in their handling of exception appeals.

In addition to rate review, the classification system should be useful for self-evaluation, for use by fiscal intermediaries, and for experimental purposes.

Self-Evaluation. Programs such as the Hospital Administrative Services, the Professional Activity Study, and the Health Services Data System generate individual and peer group statistics to enable member hospitals to evaluate themselves against peer group norms. Since these programs define peer groups as hospitals belonging to specific size classes and/or regions, many distinguishing attributes are ignored. Consequently, many participants and users of these programs have expressed the need for a more homogeneous classification system.

Reimbursement by Intermediaries. A number of Blue Cross plans across the country have classified hospitals in their service areas for the purpose of setting rates, but since their classification systems generally have been rather crude, the plans are unable to enforce their standards with any degree of rigor because "deviant" hospitals are often able to show that they are quite different from the rest of the members of the group. Perhaps the classification system developed in this study can be adopted by Blue Cross plans, or the methodology presented can be applied to develop more refined classification systems of their own.

Experimental Design. Since the classification system identifies clusters of similar hospitals, one can construct experimental and control groups through random assignment of members of a given cluster. The role of classification in studies on index numbers, production functions, macro relations, input-output analysis, and so on, may be best illustrated by an example. A hospital price index for Greater New York recently developed by Michael Gort and associates was reviewed by three health economists and a consulting firm. A major criticism leveled against the index was the apparent failure of the authors to establish homogeneous hospital groups. The reviewers recommended cluster analysis to minimize within-group variations [38].

Research applications of the classification system are discussed in detail in A Taxonomy of Community Hospitals [9]. This report also includes listings of community hospitals belonging to each cluster and nonclusterable isolates and describes the clustering program.

REFERENCES

1. Kennedy, E. M., and W. D. Mills, The Comprehensive National Health Insurance Act of 1974 (HR13870 and S3286), April 2, 1974.

2. Talmadge, H. E., "Medicare-Medicaid Administrative and Reimbursement Reform," Congressional Record—Senate, June 20, 1975, pp. S11122-25.

3. Social Security Administration, "Hospital Costs," Federal Register 40 (April 17, 1975):17190.

4. Cochran, W. H., and C. Hopkins, "Some Classification Problems with Multivariate Qualitative Data," Biometrics 17 (March 1961):10.

5. Berki, S. E., Hospital Economics. Lexington, Mass.: Heath, 1972.

6. Pauly, M., and M. Redisch, "The Not-for-Profit Hospital as a Physician Cooperative," Am. Econ. Rev. 63 (March 1973):87.

7. Sokal, R. R., "Classification: Purposes, Principles, Progress, Prospects," Science 185 (September 27, 1974):1115.

8. Tatsouka, M. M., and D. V. Tiedman, "Discriminant Analysis," Rev. Educ. Res. 24 (December 1954):402.

9. Phillip, P. J., and R. N. Iyer, A Taxonomy of Community Hospitals. Project report. American Hospital Association, Chicago, 1975.

10. Anderberg, R. M., Cluster Analysis for Applications. New York: Academic Press, 1973. P. 12.

11. Sokal, R. R., and P. H. A. Sneath, Principles of Numerical Taxonomy. San Francisco: Freeman, 1963. Pp. 85-91.

12. Cain, A. J., and G. A. Harrison, "Phyletic Weighting," Proc. Zool. Soc. (London) 135 (September 1960):1.

13. Gilmour, J. S., "A Taxonomic Problem," Nature 139 (June 1937):1040.

14. Gilmour, J. S., "The Development of Taxonomic Theory Since 1851," Nature 168 (September 1951):400.

15. Jardine, N., and R. Sibson, Mathematical Taxonomy. New York: Wiley, 1971. Chap. 4.

16. Michner, C. D., and R. R. Sokal, "A Quantitative Approach to the Problem of Classification," Evolution 11 (June 1957):130.

17. Verheyen, R., "Outline of Procedure in Basic Avian Systematics," Gerfaut (September 1960), p. 223.

18. Anderberg, R. M., Cluster Analysis for Applications. New York: Academic Press, 1973. P. 114.

19. Eades, D. C., "The Inappropriateness of the Correlation Coefficient as a Measure of Taxonomic Resemblances," Syst. Zool. 14 (June 1965):98.

20. Jardine, N., and R. Sibson, Mathematical Taxonomy. New York: Wiley, 1971. P. 31.

21. Minkoff, E. C., "The Effects on Classification of Slight Alterations in Numerical Techniques," Syst. Zool. 14 (September 1965):196.

22. Phillip, P. J., and A. Hai, "Hospital Costs: An Investigation of Causality." In Hospital Research and Educational Trust, The Nature of Hospital Costs: Three Studies. Chicago: HRET (in press).

23. U. S. Bureau of the Census, County and City Data Book, 1972. Washington, D.C.: U.S. Government Printing Office, 1973.

24. Health Insurance Institute, Source Book of Health Insurance Data. 1971-1972. New York: Health Insurance Institute, 1970.

25. American Medical Association, Distribution of Physicians in the United States, 1970. American Medical Association, 1971.

26. Mahalanobis, P. C., "On the Generalized Distance in Statistics," Proc. Natl. Inst. Sci. (India) 12 (1936):49.

27. Rao, C. R., "On the Use and Interpretation of Distance Functions in Statistics," Bull. Inst. Int. Stat. 34 (1954):90.

28. Rao, C. R., Advanced Statistical Methods in Biometric Research. Darien, Conn.: Hafner, 1952. Chap. 8.

29. Rulon, P. J., and W. D. Brooks, "On Statistical Tests of Group Differences." In D. K. Whitla (ed.), Handbook of Measurement and Assessment in Behavioral Sciences. Reading, Mass.: Addison-Wesley, 1968. Pp. 60-99.

30. Cacoullos, T., "Distance, Discrimination and Error." In T. Cacoullos (ed.), Discriminant Analysis and Applications. New York: Academic Press, 1973. Pp. 61-75.

31. Fisher, R. A., "The Use of Multiple Measurements in Taxonomic Problems," Ann. Eugenics 7 (June 1936):179.

32. Hotelling, H., "The Generalization of the Student Ratio," Ann. Math. Stat. 2 (August 1931):360.

33. Wilks, S. S., "Certain Generalizations in the Analysis of Variance," Biometrika 24 (November 1932):471.

34. Rao, C. R., Advanced Statistical Methods in Biometric Research. Darien, Conn.: Hafner, 1952. P. 247.

35. Rao, C. R., Linear Statistical Inference and Its Applications. New York: Wiley, 1965. P. 484.

36. Rao, C. R., Advanced Statistical Methods in Biometric Research. Darien, Conn.: Hafner, 1952. P. 257.

37. Cochran, W. G., "On the Performance of the Linear Discriminant Functions," Technometrics 6 (May 1964):179.

38. Rossman, J., J. Chang, M. Ram, J. Shaw, J. Birchhollz, R. Latham, and C. Lefebvre, "Comments on 'Report on the Hospital Price Index of Greater New York' by Consultant Economists, New York," Hospital Association of New York State, May 1975.

7

AUTOMATIC INTERACTION DETECTOR ANALYSIS (AIDS)

INTRODUCTION

The purpose of the article that follows is presentation of a model to assist health planners in the identification of needy subpopulations and to suggest some of the reasons why these subpopulations have differing utilization patterns. The authors interviewed 2,171 households in a five county area located in the states of New York and Pennsylvania. The data generated were used in a two-stage process to test dental utilization rates and behavior patterns.

In the first stage, the authors used automatic interaction detection analysis (AID) to obtain clusters of households with homogeneous utilization patterns. Results showed that predictors of utilization in order of importance were income, dentist/population ratio, and social class.

In the second stage, multiple regression analysis was used to test eighteen independent variables including need, predisposing, and enabling factors simultaneously. Separate regressions were also run for each of the AID identified subgroups. Need was, of course, found to be the strongest factor in all groups, with varying significance found over the other factors.

Introduction to Technique

AID (Automatic Interaction Detector) is a multivariate analysis technique developed by J. A. Sonquist and J. N. Morgan, sociologists from the University of Michigan. The technique embodied in a computer program provides a solution to the problem of considering simultaneously the effects of a large number of variables. The analysis employs a nonsymmetrical branching process, based on variance analysis techniques, that divides the sample into a series of nonoverlapping subgroups. The approach reduces the error and avoids subdivisions that are either unreliable because of insufficient observations or irrelevant because of inability to explain the dependent variable.

AID proceeds sequentially, in a series of binary splits, to develop a set of subgroups that best explain the dependent variable. At each step AID finds the split of an independent variable that will explain as much of the unexplained sums-of-squares as possible. The process produces a predictor tree, which looks like a decision model tree, that shows which independent variables are most important, how they interact, the size of the subgroups, and how much of the error is reduced at each stage. The terminal branches are then considered the significant groups and are used as the logical opportunity set for further study.

REFERENCES

Anderson, R., S. Bjorn, and S. Gunnar, "Automatic Interaction Detector Program for Analyzing Health Survey Data," Health Services Research 6 (Summer 1971): 165-83.

Einhorn, H., and J. Zieber, "An Examination of the AID Technique" (available from University of Chicago School of Business).

Gooch, L., and G. Wagner, "Modelling of Configural Judgment Processes as a Series of Subspace Hyperplanes," Decision Sciences 7 (October 1976):759-70.

Kimbel, L., and J. Lorant, "Methods for Systematic and Efficient Classification of Medical Practices," Health Services Research 8 (Spring 1973):46-60.

Reinke, W. A., "Analysis of Multiple Sources of Variation: Comparison of Three Techniques (AID, multisort and multiple regression)," Health Services Research 8 (Winter 1973):309-21.

Sonquist, J. A., and J. N. Morgan, "The Detection of Interaction Effects," Monograph No. 35, Ann Arbor, University of Michigan, Survey Research Center, Institute for Social Research, 1964.

PREDICTION OF DENTAL SERVICES UTILIZATION:
A MULTIVARIATE APPROACH

Thomas T. H. Wan
and
Ann Stromberg Yates

Public health officials and health planners concerned with promoting dental health are faced with the fact that dental services utilization rates are generally deficient relative not only to other medical services but also to dental needs. Despite some one billion unfilled cavities and large quantities of untreated periodontal disease [1], Americans do not seem to give high priority to their dental problems. They are spending a decreasing proportion of their health dollar on dental care and in recent years have only maintained their average annual number of visits at 1.4 to 1.6 [2].

This would not be alarming if the persons who rarely utilize dental services enjoyed good dental health but, in fact, the opposite is true. Utilization rates are lowest among groups with greatest need: nonwhites, rural residents, and persons with little education, low status jobs, and small incomes [3].

Local and areawide planning agencies concerned with increasing services to the "dentally-indigent" in their own communities need, of course, more precise data on utilization patterns than national averages. The purpose of this paper is to present a model and techniques that can 1) help planners to identify needy subpopulations with considerable precision, and 2) suggest at least some of the reasons why these groups have differential utilization patterns.

Dental services utilization may be thought of in terms of the following general model: beginning with the need for care, a person's

---

Thomas T. H. Wan, Ph.D., is Associate Professor of Sociology, University of Maryland Baltimore County (Baltimore, Md. 21228).

Ann Stromberg Yates, M.A., is Assistant Professor of Sociology, Pitzer College (Claremont, Calif. 91711).

This is a revised version of a paper presented to the Dental Health Section of the American Public Health Association at the annual meeting in New Orleans, Louisiana, October 22, 1974. Reprinted, with permission of the Blue Cross Association, from Inquiry 12, No. 2, pp. 143-56. Copyright 1975 by the Blue Cross Association. All rights reserved.

decision to use services may be conceptualized as being influenced by predisposing factors and enabling factors (Figure 7.1). This process takes place in the context of the social, cultural, and economic values and traditions of the society [4].

In this paper it is impossible to examine the entire model. Rather, an attempt will be made to review the variables that previous research has found predictive of differential utilization patterns, to verify the relative importance of these variables, and finally, to ascertain their interaction and predictive power for utilization. We shall proceed first to a brief review of some of the previous research on dental care utilization and then turn to our analysis of data on dental services use in five counties in New York and Pennsylvania.

The literature on dental services utilization is not as abundant as that on the use of physician services. Nevertheless, a number of studies have been devoted entirely or in part to dental care utilization, and several broad statements may be made about these studies. First, there has been little refinement of or consistency in the definition of the dependent variable, dental services utilization. Simple measures of volume or recency of dental visits predominate. Second, although the National Opinion Research Center (NORC) and the National Health Interview Survey have provided national data on dental practices, many of the other studies are limited to specific groups [5]. Their generalizability is therefore somewhat limited. Third, the retrospective design of most of the studies raises the problem of respondent error in recall. One study that compared reported dental visits with clinic records for a one-year period found that less than half of the interviewees reported their visits accurately [6]. A closely related difficulty is the heavy reliance of dental services utilization research on data from cross-sectional surveys. While this approach has provided much valuable information, it could be usefully supplemented by greater use of dentists' records and by longitudinal data. Fifth, many of the studies on dental services utilization employ very simple analytical techniques. The majority use simple cross tabulations of selected independent variables and utilization without attempting to assess the relative importance of the independent variables or their interaction.

Finally, the research on dental services utilization generally fails to consider structural features of the dental services themselves that may influence utilization. More work is needed concerning the impact on dental services utilization of such factors as methods of payment, type of practice (solo, group, public clinics), characteristics of dentists, and presence of auxiliaries [7].

Despite the shortcomings of dental care utilization research to date (and this study shares many of them), much has been learned with regard to differential utilization, as will be seen.

FIGURE 7.1

A Schematic Model of Dental Services Utilization with Examples of Operational Specifications

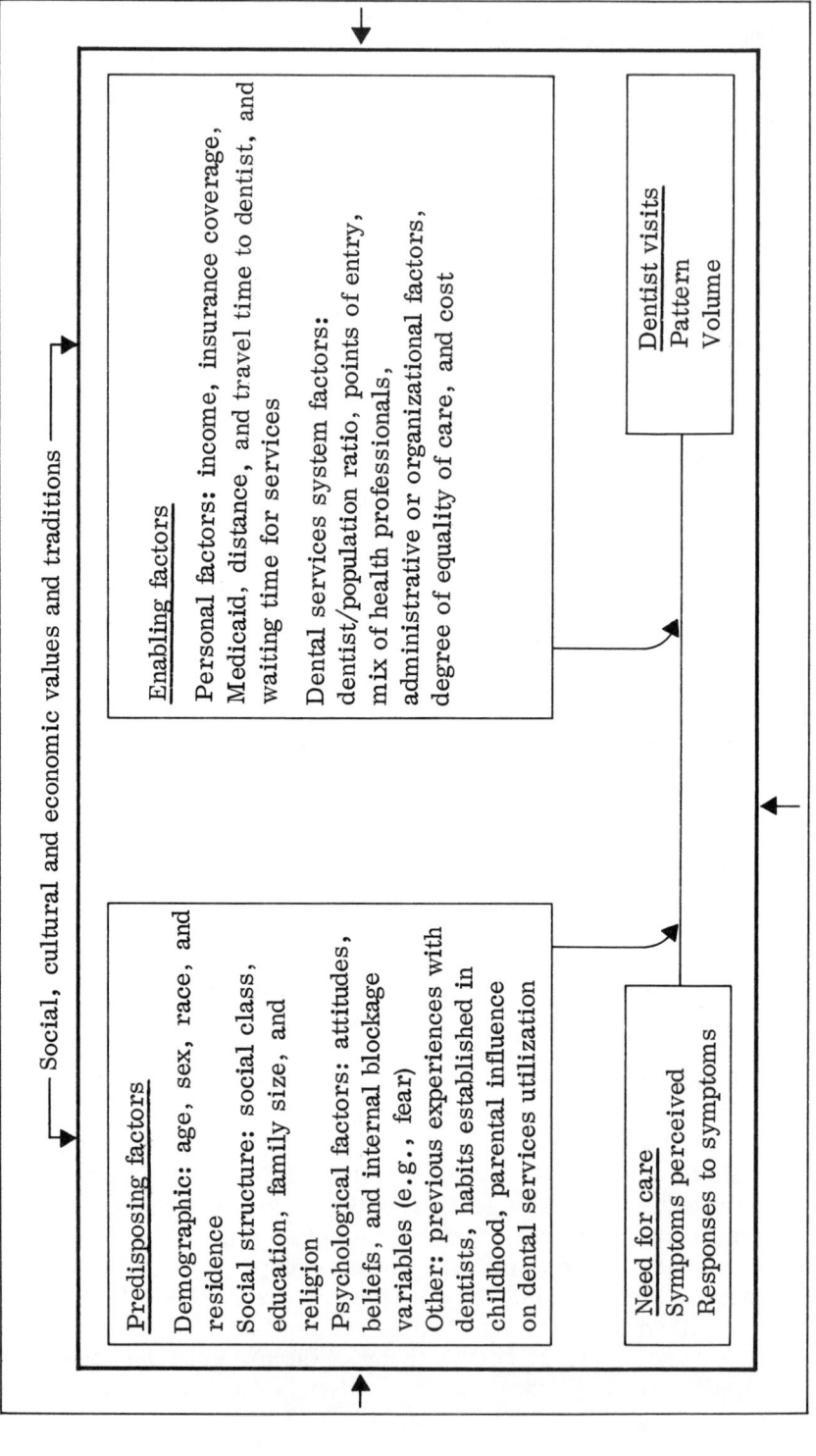

DENTAL SERVICES UTILIZATION

Utilization could be operationally defined in a variety of ways, but most studies employ convenient if somewhat crude indicators of the volume and/or types of dental visits. The dimension of quality, for example, has received almost no attention; and virtually no efforts have been made to study dental care utilization as a series of events or episodes.

Volume of dental care has been measured by annual expenditures on dental services, number of dental visits in the previous year, and recency of last visit [8]. Recency and number of visits are employed more frequently than expenditures, however, because it is thought that patients can recall dental visits more accurately than expenditures. Furthermore, expenditures may not accurately reflect use because free services and sliding income scales are thus ignored and because charges for comparable services vary from one practitioner to another [9].

Many studies distinguish between dental visits made for preventive purposes, such as check-ups, fluoride treatments, and cleaning, and those made for restorative work [10]. This is an important distinction because different predictors of utilization behavior may be relevant in each case. When need is great, as in the case of a severe toothache, almost everyone tries to see a dentist. Predisposing and enabling factors, such as attitudes or income, however, are more crucial in determining preventive visits. Many investigators concentrate exclusively on preventive visits, apparently finding them to be the only ones of much sociological interest [11].

The research to date has employed attributes of both the individual and the family as predictors of dental services utilization. These characteristics have been categorized into three major dimensions: need for care, predisposing factors, and enabling factors.

Need for Care

Need—usually measured by the symptoms perceived by the individual and his response, or by clinical assessment of dental conditions—presumably represents the most immediate and the most important factor affecting the likelihood of a person's going to the dentist [12]. Nonetheless, many studies of dental services utilization, particularly those on preventive care, do not examine the need for care. The investigations that have attempted to assess this factor and its relationship to utilization of services have shown mixed results. Newman and Anderson's analysis of NORC data suggested that need, measured by interviewees' response to both a dental symptoms index and to a question about tartar or stains on teeth, was positively associated with utilization [13]. An American Dental Association survey, however, found dental needs, which were clinically defined, to be negatively correlated with recency of last visit [14]. Freeman and Lambert found that, among low income teenagers, low rates of utilization were associated with relatively large numbers of decayed surfaces; Tyroler and colleagues' research yielded similar results [15].

The inconsistencies in these findings may be due in part to the differences in self-assessment and dentist's assessment of need. There is evidence that these two measures show very little correlation with each other [16]. The concept of need, in short, requires more clarification and exploration than it has received to date in dental services utilization research.

Predisposing Factors

The propensity or predisposition to use specific dental services varies from person to person and is influenced by various social, demographic, and psychological factors which may be classified as follows:

Demographic Factors

A number of demographic variables appear to influence dental services utilization. Females have higher rates than males, and teenagers and young adults use more services than young children or older persons. The precise age group of highest utilization varies from study to study (14-24, 5-24, 6-34), but the general pattern of an inverted U-shaped curve always holds [17]. Residence also seems to influence utilization. Rates are higher in urban areas than in rural ones [18], and within metropolitan areas they are highest in non-poverty districts. Hochstim's research shows that the handicap of poverty-area residence is significant even when income and race are controlled [19]. Finally, data from the 1965 NORC survey reveal that families with six or more members have somewhat lower utilization rates than do smaller families [20].

Social Status

Research on variables that reflect the position of the household in the social structure reveals low utilization rates among disadvantaged groups. These findings show a generally inverse relationship between occupational rank and education on the one hand, and utilization on the other [21], although the relationship may not be completely linear. Studies by Andersen and by Butler on occupational differentials suggest that there may be a threshold above which increasingly higher standing makes relatively little difference [22]. Investigators who have examined the influence of occupation, education, and income simultaneously have found that each factor makes an independent contribution [23]. Some writers have also attempted to specify the mechanisms by which socioeconomic class is linked to utilization [24].

Race has been found to have a significant influence on utilization, with blacks and Puerto Ricans showing lower rates than whites [25]. Exceptions to this pattern may be due to the unique circumstances of the population studies [26]. Jews have shown consistently higher rates of utilization than Protestants and Catholics in studies that examine religion [27].

Beliefs and Attitudes

A variety of attitudes and beliefs have been examined with regard to dental services utilization. Several attempts have been made to relate general personal orientations to utilization. Kriesberg and Treiman, for example, explored orientations toward planning, time perspectives, and self-control, but did not find them to be associated with utilization in any systematic way [28]. Suchman and Rothman, however, found utilization rates to be positively correlated with a general preventive health orientation [29]. Freeman and Lambert, on the other hand, were unable to identify a generalized preventive orientation in their research, although the variables they selected differed from those of Suchman and Rothman [30].

Research on the influence of specific dental health beliefs and knowledge has also produced mixed results. Studies that have sought to examine beliefs such as those suggested in the social-psychological models of Rosenstock [31] and Kegeles [32] (e.g., belief in one's own susceptibility to dental disease, belief in the seriousness and relative importance of the disease, and belief in or skepticism about the efficacy of dental treatment) have produced inconsistent findings regarding the significance of these factors for utilization [33]. Likewise, knowledge of dental health and proper care appears to have a significant influence on utilization in some studies [34], but not in all [35]. Perceived barriers to dental services have also received occasional attention in the literature; and perceived cost and perceived pain appear to be associated with differential utilization [36].

It is clear that the attitudinal measures employed in the literature lack comparability and that the findings are inconsistent. Beyond that, the value of studying attitudes for their ability to predict dental services use may be questionable. Critics have argued that attitudes do not determine but are determined by behavior [37], and that a sizeable discrepancy exists between what people say they should do about health care and what they actually do [38].

Other Factors

Parents' dental health behavior has been examined in a number of studies and found to be significantly correlated with children's utilization behavior [39]. Likewise, early childhood training in dental care apparently encourages preventive visits later in life [40].

Enabling Factors

Enabling factors refer to conditions that facilitate or impede the use of services by an individual who is predisposed to seek care. These factors include family or individual resources (e.g., income, health insurance coverage, proximity to dentist), and characteristics of the dental care system (e.g., availability of dental services, type of practice—solo, group, public clinic, methods of payment).

Personal Factors

An inverse although not entirely linear relationship between family income and dental services utilization is one of the most pervasive and consistent findings in the literature [41]. There is also some evidence that insurance coverage boosts utilization rates among beneficiaries [42]. Other data, however, suggest that the importance of income for differential utilization should not be exaggerated. A number of studies show that when income is held constant, or even when economic barriers to services are eliminated, differences in behavior persist among racial, occupational, and educational groups and among persons whose parents differ in dental practices [43].

Distance to the dentist's office is another personal enabling factor that has been studied. Some research has found that distance has a significant influence on utilization rates [44], but other studies do not show this to be the case [45].

Dental Services System Factors

A number of studies have sought to study the influence of the availability of dentists on utilization. Although a far from perfect measure of the supply of dentists, the dentist/population ratio has often been employed for this purpose because of its convenience [46]. The results generally show that higher utilization rates accompany more favorable ratios [47], although there is some contrary evidence [48]. The higher ratio of dentists to population found in cities may help to explain the correlation noted earlier between high utilization rates and urban residence.

Other characteristics of dental services would seem to merit more attention than they have received to date. Kriesberg and

Treiman's work, for example, shows that high utilization rates are associated with selected characteristics of dental practice, such as the use of high speed drills, mailed reminders, and the dentist's frequent performance of certain specific tasks, such as taking x-rays and cleaning teeth [49]. Lambert and Freeman have found the use of a public dental clinic by young children to be associated with lower adolescent utilization rates than are found among teenagers who have always used private practitioners. These differential rates could not be accounted for by differences in income [50]. Finally, Soricelli has shown that cancellation rates fall remarkably when dental teams including highly trained auxiliaries are used, and that cancellation rates vary considerably from dentist to dentist [51].

DATA AND METHODS

In August 1972, a community health survey using a multistage sampling procedure was conducted by the New York-Pennsylvania Health Planning Council, Inc. The purpose of this study was to identify the health status, health needs, and health care utilization patterns of the residents of a five-county area (Broome, Chenango, and Tioga in New York, and Bradford and Susquehanna in Pennsylvania) in order to formulate rational health services programs and to improve the care received by community members. The population of each county was divided into towns or townships and then subdivided into urban, rural farm, and rural nonfarm areas. These three types of areas, identified by aerial photographs, yielded mutually exclusive area segments covering the five counties in their entirety.

A total sample of 2,966 households was systematically selected from 1) a sample of area clusters in the urban areas; and 2) rural households stratified into farms and nonfarms. Of the original sample, 2,171 interviews were completed and 795 were not completed because of refusals, vacancies, etc. The present study uses the data from 2,168 households on which information on dental care was complete. The household is used as the unit of analysis in keeping with the focus of the original survey.

The analytic technique used in this study is a two stage multivariate analysis that identifies the differential effects of various predictor variables on dental services use. In the first stage of analysis, the automatic interaction detector (AID) analysis is employed to partition the total sample under study into clusters of households having dental services utilization patterns that are more or less homogeneous. This analysis employs a nonsymmetrical branching process, based on variance analysis techniques, to subdivide the sample into a series of nonoverlapping subgroups, which reduce the errors in predicting the dependent variable [52]. In partitioning households through sequential identification and dichotomous splits into the subgroups, the AID analysis provides a predictor tree that clearly shows the relative influence of the significant independent variables.

This method has several advantages over other techniques. Perhaps the most important is that it can identify interaction between various independent variables. It is also useful because of its ability to handle nominal as well as ordinal and interval data. Finally, because of its identification of homogeneous subgroups, which may have special needs for services, AID is helpful in policy-oriented research.

In this study multiple classification analysis (MCA) is employed to supplement the AID analysis of differentials in dental services utilization. MCA, a multivariate technique that can accommodate nominal data, examines the interrelationships between several predictor variables and a dependent variable. It provides information about the effects of each predictor taken by itself, and of each predictor after adjustment for its intercorrelations with other predictors. The results are presented in the form of subclass deviations from the grand mean of the sample. Unadjusted deviations show the difference between subclass means and the grand mean; adjusted deviations reflect the differences between the two means when other factors on the analysis are simultaneously controlled [53].

The second stage uses multiple regression analysis to investigate the relative influence of an expanded number of independent variables (18) on dental services use, taking all factors into account simultaneously. Separate regressions are done for each subgroup identified by the AID analysis, as well as for the total sample.

The dependent variable, dental services use, is operationally defined as the annual average number of dental visits per person. It is calculated by dividing the total number of annual dental visits in each household by the number of household residents.

RESULTS

Table 7.1 presents subclass means of per capita dental visits with respect to seven social and demographic predictors—residence (urban, rural nonfarm, and rural farm), duration of residence in the community, religion, income, race, social class, and dentist/population ratio in the county where dental services are obtained. The rate of dental services use increases with income (excepting income unknown) and with the dentist/population ratio. Urban residents report more dental visits than residents of rural farm and rural nonfarm areas. Jews and Catholics have greater use than Protestants, and whites show slightly higher rates than blacks. Inconsistent patterns emerge

TABLE 7.1

Annual Average Number of Dental Visits per Person per Household ($\bar{Y}$) for Seven Independent Variables in Automatic Interaction Detector (AID) Analysis

Category	Independent Variables						
	Residence	Residency Duration	Religion	Income	Race	Dentist/Population Ratio[a]	Social Class[b]
1	Urban (1.42)	No response (1.56)	No response (1.48)	Unknown (1.12)	No response (.91)	Unknown (.77)	No response (1.01)
2	Rural nonfarm (1.21)	<1 year (1.22)	Protestant (1.22)	$0-2,899 (.59)	White (1.28)	High (1.59)	I (1.81)
3	Rural farm (1.09)	1-2 years (1.18)	Catholic (1.46)	$2,900-$4,899 (1.02)	Black (1.07)	Medium (1.33)	II (1.81)
4		3-5 years (1.43)	Jewish (1.97)	$4,900-$6,999 (1.14)		Low (1.23)	III (1.31)
5		6-10 years (1.37)	Other (1.14)	$7,000-$9,999 (1.31)			IV (1.50)
6		11+ years (1.21)		$10,000-$14,999 (1.66)			V (1.02)
7				$15,000+ (1.74)			VI (1.16)
8							VII (.96)

[a] Dentist/population ratio refers to the number of dentists per 10,000 persons in a county. The ratios for the three categories are: 5.4; 3.8–3.9; and 1.2–2.1, respectively.
[b] Social class is measured by the Hollingshead Index of Social Positions.

FIGURE 7.2

Predictor Tree for Analysis of Dental Visits

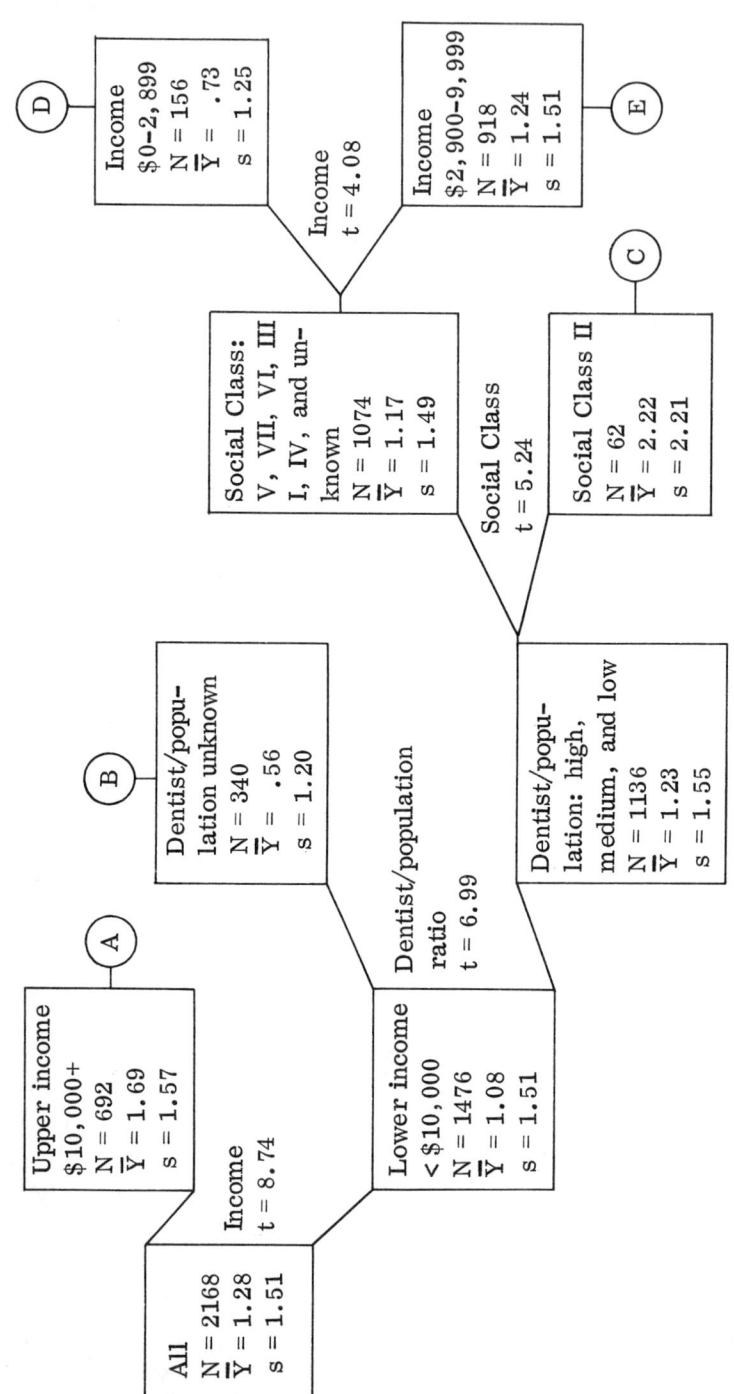

Note: N = number of households; $\bar{Y}$ = average number of dental visits per person; s = standard deviation; and t = t-value for split.

TABLE 7.2

Relative Importance of Seven Social and Demographic Variables in Predicting Dental Visits of 2,168 Households: AID Analysis

Variable	Proportion of Variance Explained*	
	Gross B^2	Partial B^2
Residence	.0073	
Residency duration	.0033	
Religion	.0054	
Income	.0341	.0409
Race	.0008	
Dentist/population ratio	.0278	.0206
Social class	.0267	.0124
Total (R^2)		.0739

*Gross B^2, or the maximum proportion of variance that can be explained by each variable by one split of the first group into two subgroups, denotes the relative importance of one predictor while the other variables are not controlled. Partial B^2 is the actual proportion of variance explained by each predictor in AID analysis. A blank indicates the variable was not used in the splits of the AID analysis.

by residency duration and by social class (measured by the Hollingshead Index of Social Positions).

Figure 7.2 and Table 7.2 report the results of the AID analysis (a split reducibility criterion of .006 and a minimum group size criterion of 40 were used in partitioning the subgroups). The predictor tree shows income to be the most powerful determinant of dental care utilization. The dentist/population ratio is the second most important factor, and social class follows. The final split shows income to be important in accounting for differential dental care utilization rates even within the lower income group identified at the first split.

Table 7.2 presents the gross and net variance in dental care utilization rates that can be explained by the seven selected social and demographic variables in the AID analysis. The effect of income is greater than that of any other predictor, accounting for 4 percent

TABLE 7.3

Multiple Classification Analysis of Dental Services Utilization for 2,168 Households

Selected Predictors	Number	Deviations		Percent Deviations	
		Unadjusted	Adjusted	Unadjusted	Adjusted
Residence					
Urban	998	.144	.047	11.3	3.7
Rural nonfarm	616	-.067	-.015	-5.2	-1.2
Rural farm	554	-.184	-.068	-14.4	-5.3
Residence duration					
Less than 1 year	142	-.054	.014	-4.2	1.1
1-2 years	205	-.091	-.112	-7.1	-8.8
3-5 years	319	.151	.105	11.8	8.2
6-10 years	446	.097	.013	7.6	1.0
11+ years	1,049	-.064	-.018	-5.0	-1.4
No response	7	.282	.108	22.0	8.4
Religion					
Protestant	1,400	-.058	-.035	-4.5	-2.7
Catholic	541	.180	.095	14.1	7.4
Jewish	14	.696	.571	54.4	44.6
Other	202	-.139	-.064	-10.9	-5.0
No response	11	.197	.271	15.4	21.2
Income					
$0-2,899	243	-.681	-.535	-53.2	-41.8

	N				
$2,900–4,899	212	−.256	−.121	−20.0	−9.5
$4,900–6,999	274	−.136	−.088	−10.6	−6.9
$7,000–9,999	435	.033	.031	2.6	2.4
$10,000–14,999	408	.385	.295	30.1	23.0
$15,000+	285	.467	.330	36.5	25.8
Unknown	311	−.153	.015	−12.0	1.2
Race					
White	2,128	.006	.006	.5	.5
Black	12	−.200	−.213	−15.6	−16.6
No response	28	−.365	−.373	−28.5	−29.1
Dentist/population ratio					
High	693	.319	.223	24.9	17.4
Medium	504	.059	.065	4.6	5.1
Low	517	−.043	−.021	−3.4	−1.6
Unknown	454	−.504	−.388	−39.4	−30.3
Social class					
I	128	.532	.242	41.6	18.9
II	170	.667	.418	52.1	32.7
III	481	.035	.092	2.7	7.2
IV	266	.226	.151	17.7	11.8
V	338	−.258	−.261	−20.2	−20.4
VI	288	−.111	−.077	−8.7	−6.0
VII	152	−.312	−.200	−24.4	−15.6
No response	345	−.267	−.132	−20.9	−10.3
Total	2,168				
Grand mean	1.28				
R^2					.084

of the total variance in dental visits. The dentist/population ratio accounts for 2 percent of the variance, and social class accounts for 1 percent. The effects of residence, residency duration, religion, and race on dental visits are negligible.

Although the total variance explained is small, the AID technique identifies the most important determinants of dental care utilization and identifies subgroups with relatively homogeneous utilization behavior. The MCA analysis, reported in Table 7.3, adds further detail by providing information on utilization rates within each subclass of each predictor under study.

Urban residents, with an unadjusted deviation of .144 from the average have 11 percent more dental visits than the average for the entire sample. When the effects of the other predictors included in the analysis are controlled, the deviation is reduced to .047 and the percent deviation to percentage points above average. The adjusted percent deviation for rural farm residents is 5 percent below the average and for nonfarm residents it is 1 percent lower. The relationship between residency duration and dental visits appears to be a reverse U-shaped one. Persons living in the area for 3-5 years are 8 percent above the average in their utilization of dental services, while residents of less than 2 years or more than 11 years have lower than average rates. Jews have substantially more dental visits (45 percent above average) than do the other religious groups, and the rates of whites greatly exceed those of blacks. The positive effect of income on dental services utilization is consistent and marked. The relationship between social class and dental visits, however, is somewhat erratic. Nonetheless, classes I and II apparently have higher utilization than do the lower social classes. Finally, there is a positive association between dental visits and dentist/population ratios.

In the second stage of the analysis we attempt to further our understanding of utilization patterns still more by adding a number of new predictor variables that represent the need, predisposing, and enabling dimensions of our model (Figure 7.1). These variables are used in multiple regression analysis on each of the homogeneous population clusters identified by the AID analysis as well as on the entire sample. The operational definitions of these predictors follow:

Need Dimension

- Percent responding to symptoms—proportion of persons in households having dental visits for curative purposes. (This variable is used as an indicator of demand for dental care for a household as a whole. The assumption is that the more persons in each household who have a curative visit to a dentist, the greater the need for care.)

- Percent reporting dentist not needed—proportion of persons in household reporting no need for dentist because of dentures.

Predisposing Factors

- Education level—highest level of schooling completed by household head.
- Occupational score—Duncan occupational prestige score of household head.
- Percent aged 5-24—proportion of persons in each household aged 5-24.
- Percent female—proportion of persons in each household who are females.
- Residence—urban residence coded as 1 and all others as 0.
- Race—whites coded as 1 and nonwhites as 0.
- Religion—Catholics and Jews coded as 1 and others as 0.
- Percent reporting internal barriers—proportion of persons in household reporting fear and skepticism with regard to dentists and dental visits.
- Percent perceiving unavailability of dental services—proportion of persons in household reporting that dental services were not available in the community or that dentists did not take new or Medicaid patients.

Enabling Factors

- Dentist/population ratio—the number of dentists available per 10,000 population in a county where the respondents received dental services.
- Income—total annual household income.
- Distance—log score of the distance in miles between dentist's office and home.
- Travel time—log score of time in minutes in travel from home to dentist's office.
- Waiting time—log score of time in minutes from the time of arrival at the dentist's office until the time dentist is seen.
- Cost—per capita cost per dental visit in each household.
- Percent reporting other external barriers—proportion of persons in household who were prevented from visiting the dentist in the past due to no time to go to a dentist, lack of transportation and money to pay.

Table 7.4 presents summary statistics including the regression coefficient (B), the standardized regression coefficient (beta), and the

TABLE 7.4
Multiple Regression Analysis of Dental Services Utilization for Total and Subgroups

Independent Variables	Total			A Upper Income $10,000+			B Lower Income Dentist/Population Ratio Unknown			C Lower Income Dentist/Population Ratio Known Social Class II			D Dentist/Population Ratio Known Mixed Social Class $0-2,899			E Dentist/Population Ratio Known Mixed Social Class $2,900-$9,999		
	B	Beta	t	B	Beta	t	B	Beta	t	B	Beta	t	B	Beta	t	B	Beta	t
Need																		
Percent responses to symptoms	.019	.484	17.5[a]	.022	.476	9.6[a]	.019	.563	8.1[a]	.037	.543	2.2[a]	.019	.580	7.9[a]	.016	.404	9.7[a]
Percent dentist not needed	-.002	-.036	-1.1[b]	-.001	-.022	-.5	-.001	-.026	-.4	.007	.079	.4	.000	.004	.1	-.001	-.029	-.7
Predisposing factors																		
Educational level	-.004	-.008	-.4	-.002	-.003	-.1	-.033	-.082	-1.7[c]	.068	.164	1.0	.035	.087	1.5[b]	-.015	-.029	-.9
Occupation score	.003	.054	2.7[a]	.002	.044	1.2	.004	.060	1.3[b]	-.020	-.070	-.5	.005	.079	1.4[b]	.003	.039	1.3[b]
Percent aged 5-24	.002	.037	1.6[b]	.001	.015	.3	.002	.038	.6	-.001	-.019	-.1	.012	.238	3.6[b]	.003	.045	1.1
Percent female	.001	.020	1.1	-.003	-.027	-.8	.003	.068	1.4[b]	-.010	-.135	-.6	-.001	-.022	-.4	-.003	.040	1.3[b]
Residenced	.002	.001	.0	-.112	-.036	-.9	.101	.039	.8	.919	.233	1.5[b]	-.155	-.062	-1.0	.051	.017	.5
Raced	.181	.016	.9	.012	.001	.0	.007	.001	.0	—	—	—	.740	.123	2.2[a]	.363	.031	1.0
Religiond	.008	.002	.1	-.085	-.024	-.7	-.070	-.023	-.5	.466	.094	.7	-.317	-.116	-2.0[a]	.162	.046	1.5[b]
Percent internal barriers	-.002	-.008	-.4	.002	.007	.2	-.001	-.005	-.0	.043	.064	.4	-.006	-.017	-.3	-.003	-.018	-.6
Percent perceived unavailability of services	.005	.083	3.9[a]	.008	.077	1.8[c]	.001	.023	.4	.010	.151	.6	.009	.237	3.8[a]	.004	.060	1.5[b]
Enabling factors																		
Dentist/population ratio	.052	.038	1.9[c]	.090	-.064	1.8[c]	—	—	—	.504	.195	1.4[b]	.288	.185	3.1[a]	.071	.039	1.3[b]
Income	.015	.045	2.2[a]	-.029	-.009	-.3	-.031	.010	.031	.6	.083	.150	1.1	-.005	-.003	-.1	.006	.015	.5
Log 10 [distance]	.049	.016	.5	.168	.054	1.0	-.121	-.065	-.4	.273	.067	.3	-.332	-.132	-1.7[c]	.072	.023	.5
Log 10 [travel time]	.114	.037	1.2	.024	.006	.1	.250	.154	1.0	.652	.117	.5	.217	.072	1.0	.140	.035	.8
Log 10 [waiting time]	.020	.009	.5	.036	.015	.4	.094	.053	1.0	.216	.189	1.4[b]	-.148	-.107	-1.9[c]	.026	.012	.4
Average cost/visit	-.011	-.025	-1.3[b]	-.040	-.078	-2.3[a]	-.018	-.044	-.9	-.033	-.096	-.7	.052	.148	2.5[a]	.001	.003	.1
Percent other external barriers	.000	.002	.0	.002	.012	.3	.001	.016	.3	-.011	-.060	-.4	.000	.006	.1	-.002	-.023	.7
Coefficient of multiple determination (R^2)	30.2			24.5			40.6			36.8			63.5			21.2		

[a]Significant at 99 percent level on basis of two-tailed t-test.
[b]Significant at 80 percent level on basis of two-tailed t-test.
[c]Significant at 90 percent level on basis of two-tailed t-test.
[d]Dummy variable is used: urban residents coded 1 and rural residents coded 0; white coded 1 and nonwhite coded 0; and Catholics and Jews coded 1 and Prostestants and other coded 0.

t-value and its level of significance for each variable in the regression equation. The coefficient of multiple determination (R^2), which indicates the total variance explained by all independent variables, is also provided for each homogeneous subgroup as well as for the total sample.

It is apparent that the proportion of persons in each household responding to symptoms by seeking dental care is the most significant variable in predicting dental services utilization. It has a strong positive effect in both the total sample and in the subgroups. The second predictor, the proportion reporting no need for dental care because of dentures, has a very weak influence on dental visits in the total sample but does not appear to be statistically significant in any of the subgroups.

A review of the predisposing factors shows that education exerts an effect on utilization in only two groups, B and D. The beta coefficients reveal, however, that the direction of the influence is in the opposite direction in the two cases. This finding may be attributable to a high intercorrelation between education and occupation in Group B but not in Group D. The effect of occupation on dental use is statistically significant in Groups B, D, and E and the total sample. Its net effect appears to be stronger than that of education in Group E and in the total sample. The age variable (percent of household aged 5-24) exerts an important positive effect on dental use only in the total sample and Group D. Urban residents show a high utilization rate in Group C; indeed, with the exception of the first independent variable, the residence variable is the most important one in predicting dental care in this subgroup. The effect of race is significant only in Group D where being white exerts a positive net effect (.123). Religion exerts a strong impact in Group D (-.116), and a weak effect in Group E (.046). In this analysis, the internal barriers examined—fear and skepticism toward dental services—do not appear to influence dental services utilization. This finding may perhaps be attributable to the crude measurement available for this variable. Finally, perceived unavailability of dental services shows a strong effect on utilization in Groups A, D, and E and in the total sample. The beta coefficients reveal that its influence on dental use is a positive one.

In examining the influence of the enabling factors, we find that travel time to the dentist is not statistically significant in explaining the variation of dental visits in any subgroups or in the total sample. In contrast, the dentist/population ratio, an indicator of availability of dentists in the county where people seek care, appears to have a positive effect on dental visits in all clusters (excepting B where the ratio is unknown) and in the total sample. Consistent with the findings of the AID analysis, household income plays an important role in explaining the variations of dental use in the total sample. Its influence within each cluster, however, is negligible because income had already been employed in splitting the sample into subgroups. Proximity to the dentist is a significant factor in Group D. Within this lowest income group living close to a dentist apparently facilitates the use of his services. Waiting time at the dentist's office is somewhat of an important factor only in Groups C and D. The negative effect (-.107) found in Group D is not surprising for it implies that persons who experience long waits are discouraged from seeking services. An explanation for the positive effect in Group C is not readily available. The cost per dental visit exerts a significant negative effect (-.078) on dental use in Group A (the upper income cluster), but a positive effect in Group D (the lowest income group). The somewhat unexpected finding in Group D may reflect the fact that the poor have access to public dental services or that Medicaid covers their bills. The other external barriers (e.g., transportation) have no apparent influence on dental services use.

Finally, it is worth noting that the coefficients of multiple determinations (R^2) range from 24.5 to 63.5. In every case there is still considerable variance left unaccounted for, and it should be the work of future analysis to try to develop better measures and select other pertinent indicators which might increase the total amount of variance explained by the model.

CONCLUSIONS

The findings of this study may be summarized as follows:

1 The automatic interaction detector (AID) analysis showed that income, the dentist/population ratio, and social class have significant influence on dental services utilization. In addition, it clarified the interaction between these variables and identified subgroups with more or less homogeneous dental utilization behavior.
2 The multiple classification analysis (MCA) identified high dental utilization rates among households which were: urban, living in the community an intermediate length of time (3-5 years), Jewish, white, with an annual household income of $10,000 or more, falling in social class I or II, and using dentists located in areas of high dentist/population ratios.
3 A multiple regression analysis performed on each AID-identified subgroup, and on the entire sample, showed that the effects of 18 different predictors (categorized in three dimensions—need for care, predisposing factors, and enabling factors) varied from group to group. Table 7.5 summarizes the variables found to be significant in each cluster.

TABLE 7.5

Significant Predictors of Dental Services Utilization in the Total Sample and in Subgroups, Identified by Multiple Regression Analysis

Independent Variables	Total	A	B	C	D	E
Need						
Percent responses to symptoms	a	a	a	a	a	a
Percent dentist not needed	b					
Predisposing factors						
Educational level			c		b	
Occupation score	a		b		b	b
Percent aged 5–24	b				a	
Percent female			b			b
Residence				b		
Race					a	
Religion					a	b
Percent perceived unavailability of services	a	c			a	b
Enabling factors						
Dentist/population ratio	c	c		b	a	b
Income	a					
Log 10 [distance]					c	
Log 10 [waiting time]				b	c	
Average cost/visit	b	a			a	

aSignificant at 99 percent level on basis of two-tailed t-test.
bSignificant at 80 percent level on basis of two-tailed t-test.
cSignificant at 90 percent level on basis of two-tailed t-test.

A study of this type may be useful to a health planner by helping him to identify groups in need of care and to understand the barriers that limit their ability to obtain that care. The findings concerning income, perceived unavailability of services, and dentist/population ratios suggest useful courses of action. These might include insurance plans or sliding scale schemes to ease the financial burden that adequate dental care places on low income families, publicity campaigns to make community residents more aware of the available services and facilities, public education to reinforce the value of preventive dental care, and attempts to attract more dentists to areas where they are few in number. We know from earlier attempts that it is not easy to alter patients' patterns of utilization or practitioners' mode of delivering care, but a considered and concerted effort along the lines suggested here would undoubtedly improve the care of at least some groups.

The two stage analysis performed in this study indicates that AID is a very useful analytic technique, especially in conjunction with other multivariate methods, for studying dental services utilization in subpopulations and for identifying impediments to care. It could be further developed to estimate unmet dental health needs in different subpopulations.

NOTES

1. National Center for Health Statistics, Decayed, Missing, and Filled Teeth, Series 11, No. 23 (Washington, D.C.: U.S. Government Printing Office, 1967); National Center for Health Statistics, Periodontal Disease in Adults, U.S. 1960-1962, Series 11, No. 12 (Washington, D.C.: U.S. Government Printing Office, 1965); D. A. Soricelli, "Implementation of the Delivery of Dental Services by Auxiliaries: The Philadelphia Experience," American Journal of Public Health 62 (August 1972):1077-87.

2. National Center for Health Statistics, Dental Visits, Volume, and Interval Since Last Visit, Series 10, No. 76 (Washington, D.C.: U.S. Government Printing Office, 1972); J. F. Newman and O. W. Anderson, Patterns of Dental Service Utilization in the United States: A Nationwide Social Survey, Research Series 30 (Chicago: University of Chicago Center for Health Administration Studies, 1972).

3. National Center for Health Statistics, Need for Dental Care Among Adults, U.S. 1960-1962, Series 11, No. 36 (Washington, D.C.: U.S. Government Printing Office, 1970); Newman and Anderson, Patterns of Dental Service Utilization.

4. D. L. Rabin et al., "Methods," in: "International Comparisons of Medical Care," Milbank Memorial Fund Quarterly 50 (1972):19;

R. Andersen, A Behavioral Model of Families' Use of Health Services, Research Series 25 (Chicago: University of Chicago Center for Health Administration Studies, 1968); A. Antonovsky and R. Kats, "The Model Dental Patient: An Empirical Study of Preventive Health Behavior," Social Science and Medicine 4 (1970):367-80; T. W. Bice and K. L. White, "Cross-National Comparative Research on the Utilization of Medical Services," Medical Care 9 (1971):253-71; W. R. Posnick, "Dentistry in a Neighborhood Health Center: An Evaluation," Journal of Public Health Dentistry 34 (1974):42-49; P. J. Frazier, J. Jenny, and R. A. Bagramian, "Parents' Descriptions of Barriers Faced and Strategies Used to Obtain Dental Care," Journal of Public Health Dentistry 34 (1974):22-38.

5. See: J. Moosbruker and A. Jong, "Racial Similarities and Differences on Family Dental Care Patterns," Public Health Reports 84 (August 1969):721-27; E. A. Powell and K. J. Roghmann, "Use of Dental Services in an Urban Area Before Medicaid and an OEO Health Center," Health Services Research 88 (March 1973):260; D. Sarda, R. W. Stallard, and H. J. Goldberg, "Dental Utilization of a Neighborhood Health Center," Journal of Public Health Dentistry 32 (1972): 175-79.

6. J. V. P. Chatwin, F. N. Delaquis, and C. B. Walker, "Accuracy of Recall of Dental Care Received During the Preceding Year," Journal of the Canadian Dental Association 34 (1968):409-12.

7. Bice and White, "Cross-National Comparative Research"; J. B. McKinlay, "Some Approaches and Problems in the Study of the Use of Services: An Overview," Journal of Health and Social Behavior 13 (1972):115-52; T. H. Wan and S. Soifer, "Determinants of Physician Utilization: A Causal Analysis," Journal of Health and Social Behavior 15 (1974):100-08.

8. Andersen, A Behavioral Model; Newman and Anderson, Patterns of Dental Service Utilization; H. E. Freeman and C. Lambert, "Preventive Dental Behavior of Urban Mothers," Journal of Health and Social Behavior 6 (1965):141-47; D. G. Hay, O. F. Larson, and D. Jutton, "Utilization of Dental Services by Rural People in Selected New York Counties," Journal of the American Dental Association 47 (1953):423-30; R. H. Tash, R. M. O'Shea, and L. K. Cohen, "Testing a Symptomatic Theory of Dental Health Behavior," American Journal of Public Health 59 (1969):514-21.

9. American Dental Association, Bureau of Economic Research and Statistics, "National Dental Fee Survey, 1970," Journal of American Dental Health 83 (1971):57-63; Newman and Anderson, Patterns of Dental Service Utilization.

10. Ibid.; Antonovsky and Kats, "The Model Dental Patient"; C. Lambert and H. E. Freeman, The Clinic Habit (New Haven, Conn.: College and University Press, 1967); Moosbruker and Jong, "Racial Similarities."

11. Antonovsky and Kats, "The Model Dental Patient"; Freeman and Lambert, "Preventive Dental Behavior"; D. P. Haefner, S. S. Kegeles, J. Kirscht, and I. M. Rosenstock, "Preventive Action in Dental Disease, Tuberculosis and Cancer," Public Health Reports 82 (1967):451-59; R. M. O'Shea and S. B. Gray, "Dental Patients' Attitudes and Behavior Concerning Prevention: National Survey," Public Health Reports 83 (1968):405-10; Tash et al., "Testing."

12. Andersen, A Behavioral Model; L. Kriesberg and B. R. Treiman, "Socioeconomic Status and the Utilization of Dentists' Services," Journal of the American College of Dentists 27 (1960): 147-65.

13. Newman and Anderson, Patterns of Dental Service Utilization.

14. American Dental Association, Bureau of Economic Research and Statistics, "Survey of Needs for Dental Care, 1965: Dental Needs According to Length of Time Since Last Visit to Dentist," Journal of the American Dental Association 74 (1967):145-50.

15. Freeman and Lambert, "Preventive Dental Behavior"; H. A. Tyroler, A. L. Johnson, and J. T. Fulton, "Patterns of Preventive Health Behavior in Populations," Journal of Health and Human Behavior 6 (1965):128-40.

16. J. S. Bulman, G. L. Slack, N. D. Richards, and A. J. Willcocks, "A Survey of the Dental Health and Attitudes Towards Dentistry in Two Communities. Part III: Comparison of Dental and Sociological Data," British Dental Journal 125 (1968):102-06.

17. Haefner et al., "Preventive Action"; Hay et al., "Utilization of Dental Services"; Tash et al., "Testing"; National Center for Health Statistics, Dental Visits; Newman and Anderson, Patterns of Dental Service Utilization.

18. National Center for Health Statistics, Dental Visits; Newman and Anderson, Patterns of Dental Service Utilization.

19. J. R. Hochstim, D. A. Athanasopoulos, and J. H. Larkins, "Poverty Area Under the Microscope," American Journal of Public Health 58 (1968):1815-27.

20. Newman and Anderson, Patterns of Dental Service Utilization.

21. L. Kriesberg and B. R. Treiman, "Preventive Utilization of Dentists' Services Among Teenagers," Journal of the American College of Dentists 29 (1962):28-45; Kriesberg and Treiman, "Socioeconomic Status"; National Center for Health Statistics, Dental Visits; O'Shea and Gray, "Dental Patients' Attitudes"; Newman and Anderson, Patterns of Dental Service Utilization; S. S. Kegeles, "Some Motives for Seeking Preventive Dental Care," Journal of the American Dental Association 67 (1963):90-98; S. S. Kegeles, "Why People Seek Dental Care: A Test of a Conceptual Framework," Journal of Health and Human Behavior 4 (1963):166-73.

22. Andersen, A Behavioral Model; J. R. Butler, "Studies in the Use of Dental Services," Social and Economic Administration 1 (1967):5-18.

23. A. S. Metz and L. G. Richards, "Children's Preventive Dental Visits: Influencing Factors," Journal of the American College of Dentists 34 (1967):204-12; E. A. Suchman and A. A. Rothman, "The Utilization of Dental Services," Milbank Memorial Fund Quarterly 47 (1969):56-63.

24. Kriesberg and Treiman, "Preventive Utilization"; Kriesberg and Treiman, "Socioeconomic Status"; L. Kriesberg, "The Relationship Between Socioeconomic Class and Behavior," Social Problems 10 (1963):334-53; J. F. Rayner, "Socioeconomic Status and Factors Influencing the Dental Health Practices of Medical Care," American Journal of Public Health 60 (1970):1250-58.

25. Hochstim et al., "Poverty Area"; M. K. Nikias, "Trends and Patterns of Dental Care in an Urban Area Before Medicaid," HSMHA Health Reports 86 (1971):52-65; Suchman and Rothman, "The Utilization"; Tash et al., "Testing."

26. Moosbruker and Jong, "Racial Similarities."

27. Nikias, "Trends"; O'Shea and Gray, "Dental Patients' Attitudes."

28. Kriesberg and Treiman, "Socioeconomic Status."

29. Suchman and Rothman, "The Utilization."

30. Freeman and Lambert, "Preventive Dental Behavior."

31. I. M. Rosenstock, "Why People Use Health Services," Milbank Memorial Fund Quarterly 44 (1966):94-124.

32. S. S. Kegeles, "Why People Seek Dental Care: A Review of Present Knowledge," American Journal of Public Health 51 (1961): 1306-11.

33. Kegeles, "Some Motives"; Kegeles, "A Test"; O'Shea and Gray, "Dental Patients' Attitudes"; Tash et al., "Testing."

34. Ibid.

35. Kriesberg and Treiman, "Preventive Utilization"; Kriesberg and Treiman, "Socioeconomic Status"; Tash et al., "Testing."

36. Ibid.

37. McKinlay, "Some Approaches"; Rayner, "Socioeconomic Status."

38. R. Pomeroy, Studies in the Use of Health Services by Families (New York: The City University of New York Center for the Study of Urban Problems, 1969).

39. Kriesberg and Treiman, "Preventive Utilization"; Metz and Richards, "Children's Preventive Visits"; Rayner, "Socioeconomic Status"; Tyroler et al., "Patterns of Preventive Health Behavior."

40. Kriesberg and Treiman, "Socioeconomic Status."

41. R. Andersen and O. W. Anderson, A Decade of Health Services (Chicago: University of Chicago Press, 1967); Newman and Anderson, Patterns of Dental Service Utilization; Kriesberg and Treiman, "Socioeconomic Status"; Haefner et al., "Preventive Action"; Hay et al., "Utilization"; O'Shea and Gray, "Dental Patients' Attitudes"; Tash et al., "Testing."

42. Health Information Foundation, "Patterns in Use of Health Services," Journal of the American College of Dentists 33 (1966): 243-44; N. D. Richards, "Dentistry in Great Britain," Milbank Memorial Fund Quarterly 49 (1971):133-69.

43. M. K. Nikias, "Social Class and the Use of Dental Care Under Prepayment," Medical Care 6 (1968):381-93; Richards, "Dentistry in Great Britain"; Metz and Richards, "Children's Preventive Visits"; Haefner et al., "Preventive Action"; Nikias, "Social Class"; Kriesberg and Treiman, "Socioeconomic Status."

44. Kegeles, "Some Motives."

45. Hay et al., "Utilization"; C. H. McCormick, "Availability and Utilization of Dental Services by Rural Manitoba Children," Journal of the Canadian Dental Association 32 (1966):280-85.

46. R. B. Cole and L. K. Cohen, "Dental Manpower: Estimating Resources and Requirements," Milbank Memorial Fund Quarterly 49 (1971):29-62.

47. Butler, "Studies"; Hay et al., "Utilization"; Newman and Anderson, Patterns of Dental Service Utilization.

48. Nikias, "Trends."

49. Kriesberg and Treiman, "Preventive Utilization"; Kriesberg and Treiman, "Socioeconomic Status."

50. Lambert and Freeman, The Clinic Habit.

51. Soricelli, "Implementation."

52. J. A. Sonquist, Multivariate Model Building (Ann Arbor: University of Michigan Institute for Social Research, 1970); J. A. Sonquist and J. N. Morgan, The Detection of Interaction Effects (Ann Arbor: University of Michigan Institute for Social Research, 1964).

53. F. M. Andrews, J. N. Morgan, and J. A. Sonquist, Multiple Classification Analysis (Ann Arbor: University of Michigan Survey Research Center, 1967).

8

CONJOINT MEASUREMENTS

INTRODUCTION

The authors report that a survey indicates that more than 50 percent of the admissions to a hospital were based on the patient's decision or the recommendations of a friend rather than from a physician's referral. Given this finding, hospital administrators could benefit from understanding the factors which influence the consumer in his hospital selection decision. Conjoint measurement was viewed appropriate for the analysis of this hospital selection problem, given the multi-attribute nature of the problem which involves trade-offs among various cost/benefit options.

Six basic factors were selected as important predictors in this selection decision. Each factor was considered on three separate levels. The factors or attributes are as follows: type of hospital, physical appearance of hospital, proximity, assignment of physician, prestige of physician, and the price of room per day. The number of possible combinations of factors and levels is 3^6 or 729. To simplify the process, a fractional factorial design was developed involving only 27 profiles. These 27 profiles were evaluated under two distinct scenarios:

1) Simple surgery with expected rapid recovery
2) Serious surgery and an expected longer hospitalization

Content analysis was used to analyze reasons given by respondents for selecting a hospital. Conjoint measurement using the MONANOVA algorithm was conducted on the total sample data, to determine the relative importance of the various hospital characteristics. The results of the two conjoint measurement analyses were compared and a multivariate analysis of variance program was applied to assess the effect of the consumer's age, sex, and history.

Introduction to Technique

Borrowed from recent developments in mathematical psychology and psychometrics, conjoint measurement is a technique to measure consumers' judgments based on the perceived characteristics of goods and services. This technique examines the joint effect of two or more independent variables on the ordering of a dependent variable. A respondent is presented with a set of multi-attribute alternatives and is asked to make an overall judgment about the relative value of various combinations of attributes. The dependent variable, on which the attribute combinations are evaluated, might be the respondents' preference, liking, intention to buy, and so on. The respondents' rank order the attribute alternatives, and conjoint measurement converts these rank orderings into interval scale estimates of utilities for the attributes.

Attribute utility scales computation, which determines how influential each attribute is in the consumers' evaluations, is performed by various computer programs. A number of algorithms are available for scaling the ranking data by means of conjoint measurement. One such algorithm, Kruskal's MONANOVA, appears to be the most popular, and was used in all of the applications. This algorithm assumes that the overall utility for a product or service is the sum of the utilities for the characteristics and that deficiencies in one characteristic can be compensated for with additional utility from other characteristics. This is known as the additive main-effect model. The computed range of utilities for each attribute indicates the relative importance of each attribute, that is, the larger the range the more important the attribute.

The mathematical model is expressed as

$$U(X) = U_1(X_1) + U_2(X_2) + \cdots + U_n(X_n)$$

where $U(X)$ is the utility to a consumer of a product or a service "X."

The product or service X is represented as a vector of n characteristics,

$$X = (X_1, X_2, \ldots, X_n)$$

The additive model states that the total utility, $U(X)$, is simply the sum of the individual utilities. For large samples, the number of respondents may be reduced into subgroups through the use of clustering analysis before conjoint measurement techniques are applied.

REFERENCES

Acito, F., "Consumer Preferences for Health Care Services: An Exploratory Investigation," Ph.D. Dissertation, State University of New York at Buffalo, March 1976.

Green, P. E., and V. R. Rao, "Conjoint Measurement for Quantifying Judgmental Data," Journal of Marketing Research 8 (August 1971):355-63.

Green, P. E., and Y. Wind, "New Way to Measure Consumers' Judgments," Harvard Business Review 53 (July-August 1975): 107-17.

Green, P. E., Y. Wind, and A. K. Jain, "Benefit Bundle Analysis," Journal of Advertising Research 12 (April 1972):31-36.

ANALYTICAL APPROACH TO MARKETING DECISIONS
IN HEALTH-CARE ORGANIZATIONS

Yoram Wind
and
Lawrence K. Spitz

We discuss the potential applicability of a new choice model and scaling procedure to the marketing decisions of health-care organizations. After a brief exposition of this analytical procedure the paper focuses on an illustrative application to

---

Reprinted, with permission of the Operations Research Society of America, from Operations Research 24, No. 5 (September-October 1976):973-90.

This research was supported by the Department of Community Medicine of the University of Pennsylvania through a grant from the Johnson Foundation Clinical Scholar program. An earlier version of the paper was delivered at the TIMS College of Marketing seminar on "Marketing, Management Science and Non-Profit Organizations," August 12, 1974, Portland, Oregon.

the hospital selection decision under two scenarios—
surgery with a rapid recovery period and serious surgery that requires a long hospitalization period. The
paper concludes with some suggestions for future use
of conjoint measurement and related techniques in
marketing studies of health care organizations.

Marketing in nonprofit organizations has emerged as a popular topic in the recent marketing literature [12, 13]. The two basic implicit premises of these efforts are that (a) the survival and growth of nonprofit organizations require the adoption of a marketing orientation and (b) the implementation of the marketing orientation calls for the use of appropriate marketing concepts, approaches, and techniques (including marketing research and marketing applications of the management and behavioral sciences).

Given these premises and the large repertoire of marketing techniques, one of the questions facing managers of nonprofit organizations is which specific marketing approaches and techniques they should use. Although no single technique can be appropriate for all marketing decisions, it is hoped that the experience gained in the application of marketing research and management science to the solution of marketing problems (and guidance of marketing decisions) in profit-oriented firms could be of some help to the marketing managers of nonprofit organizations.

Thus our objective is to propose, as a research tool for guiding marketing decisions of health care organizations, the use of a relatively new analytical approach to the quantification of utilities (for multi-attribute alternatives).

In particular, we focus on the potential applicability of conjoint measurement procedures to the marketing decisions of health care organizations. After a brief discussion of this analytical procedure we describe an illustrative application to the hospital selection decision. The paper concludes with some suggestions for future use of conjoint measurement and related techniques in marketing studies for health care organizations.

ON MEASUREMENT OF MULTI-ATTRIBUTE ALTERNATIVES

The approach we suggest for quantifying the utilities of multi-attribute alternatives differs considerably from traditional attitude measurement procedures. It is based on recent developments in mathematical psychology concerning conjoint measurement techniques, which have been applied to such diverse areas as psychiatric diagnosis

[5], common stock appraisals [15], job performance [3], a number of marketing problems including product and package design [9], retail discount card evaluations [6], benefit segmentation [10], and one health-care related study on physician selection of a clinical laboratory [17].

As the name suggests, conjoint measurement is concerned with measuring the joint effect of two or more independent variables (such as product attributes) on the ordering of a single response (dependent) variable or a categorical response variable. In a prototypic experiment a respondent is presented with a set of multi-attribute alternatives and is asked to make an overall judgment about the relative value of various combinations of attributes. By evaluating (for example, ranking or rating) combinations of attributes on some desired dependent variable (preference, liking, intention to buy, and so forth), the respondent is not asked to indicate directly the relative importance of each attribute (as in the case of the traditional attitude measurement approaches) but rather to provide his overall evaluation of a "product"—a combination of various attributes. This more realistic task provides insights into the respondent's trade-off among the various attributes, and supplies the input data for the conjoint measurement algorithm.

Conjoint measurement provides a model and scaling procedure for constructing, from these data, utility functions whose arguments are represented by stimulus dimensions. Using a variety of algorithms (such as those in [1] or [14]) the overall evaluations of a set of multi-attribute alternatives are "decomposed" into derived utilities (interval scale values) of the various factors—the components of the multi-component alternatives—and levels. This "decomposition" of the respondents' overall evaluations into separate compatible utility scales enables the researcher to reconstruct the original global judgments or predict the respondent's evaluation of new combinations of attributes.

These utilities provide unbiased information about the relative importance of the various attributes, the value of various levels of each of the attributes, and an estimate of the psychological trade-offs respondents make when they evaluate several attributes together. (For further discussion of conjoint measurement see [7-9].)

One of the simplest and most commonly used conjoint measurement models is the additive main effect model. This model, in an illustrative case of a stimulus set composed of three attributes (factors) each at three levels, is:

$$U(X) = F(X) = \beta_0 + \beta_1(X_{21}) + \beta_2(X_{31}) + \beta_3(X_{22}) + \beta_4(X_{32}) + \beta_5(X_{23}) + \beta_6(X_{33}) + e$$

where β_0 is the contribution to overall utility in which each of the three factors is at its first (lowest) level; $\beta_1, \beta_2, \ldots, \beta_6$ are the incremental contribution of level i (i = 2, 3) of factor j (j = 1, 2, 3); F(X) is a monotonic increasing function of X; and e is the error term.

Conjoint measurement algorithms, such as Kruskal's MONANOVA [14], establish scale values—utilities—(β_{ij}) for the independent variables whose ranking of the additive utilities of each combination best preserves the respondent's original ranking of the stimulus combination.

ILLUSTRATIVE APPLICATION OF CONJOINT MEASUREMENT TO HOSPITAL SELECTION PROBLEM

The specific pilot application we consider here is the use of conjoint measurement in marketing problems of health care organizations. The problem setting is the hospital selection decision of individuals. A recent study on the referral chain of an urban hospital [2] suggests that more than 50 percent of the admissions to a hospital were based on the patient's decision or the recommendations of a friend (as distinct from physician referral). This finding suggests that hospital administrators should try to understand the factors that determine the consumer's hospital selection decision. Current research approaches to the problem (primarily open-ended direct questioning or simple importance rating of various attributes) were viewed by a number of hospital administrators as unacceptable. Open-ended approaches, although useful for identifying the relevant factors, could not provide insight into the relative importance of the various attributes. Traditional attitude measurement approaches tended to stress price, while indicating that other factors are also very important.

Given the multi-attribute nature of the problem, which involves trade-offs among various cost/benefit options, the conjoint measurement model was viewed as most appropriate for the analysis of the hospital selection problem.

Study Objectives

The objectives of the study can be stated in terms of the following research questions:
1. What factors do consumers consider in selecting a hospital?
2. What is the relative importance of the various hospital characteristics in the hospital selection decision?
3. To what extent is the relative importance of the various hospital characteristics a function of the type and length of hospitalization required?
4. Do the age, sex, and hospitalization history of consumers affect their evaluation of the various hospital characteristics?

TABLE 8.1

Sample Composition

Hospitalization History	Respondent				
	Under 35		Over 35		
	Male	Female	Male	Female	Total
Previously hospitalized	7	7	7	7	28
Never hospitalized	7	7	7	7	28
Total	14	14	14	14	56

Personal in-home interviews were conducted with a convenient quota sample of 56 respondents from the Philadelphia suburban area. The sample was drawn from a relatively homogeneous socioeconomic area following a balanced factorial design based on age, sex, and hospitalization history. The sample composition is summarized in Table 8.1.

Stimulus Set and Respondents' Tasks

An exploratory study among physicians and hospital administrators suggested six factors as possible determinants of the hospital selection decision—the type of hospital affiliation, the physical appearance of the hospital, the proximity of the hospital to the patient's home, the reputation of the attending physician, the familiarity with the attending physician, and the cost per day. The six factors and their corresponding levels are summarized in Table 8.2.

A fractional factorial design [5] was developed for the 3^6 design involving 27 profiles (of the 729 possible combinations) of hypothetical hospitals. The 27 combinations are presented in Table 8.3.

Each stimulus of a hypothetical hospital was presented as a card describing different levels of all six factors. Table 8.4 presents one of the stimuli. This verbal description seemed appropriate in this case, although at least one of the factors—physical appearance of the hospital—could have been presented pictorially. Cost considerations, however, precluded the development of color photographs of the three levels involved. The description of the hypothetical hospitals as various combinations of levels of all six factors is only one of the possible ways of presenting the stimuli. The alternative two-factors-at-a-time approach [11] does not control for the frame of reference

TABLE 8.2

Stimulus Set

A.	Type of hospital	1.	Teaching hospital affiliated with a medical school of a major university.
		2.	Teaching hospital not associated with a medical school.
		3.	Non-teaching community hospital.
B.	Physical appearance of hospital	1.	Very modern.
		2.	Average facilities.
		3.	Poor condition, old.
C.	Proximity	1.	Downtown area—easy parking and access.
		2.	Downtown area—difficult access and parking.
		3.	In your neighborhood.
D.	Assignment of physician	1.	A physician recommended by your doctor.
		2.	A physician recommended by a friend.
		3.	A physician assigned to you by the hospital.
E.	Prestige of physician	1.	World-renowned.
		2.	Highly respected in his field.
		3.	A specialist.
F.	Price of room per day	1.	$60.
		2.	$90.
		3.	$120.

used by the respondents in the evaluation of each pair of factors. Given this limitation of the two-factors-at-a-time approach and our favorable experience with the "total-combination" approach (see [6-10, 19]), we decided to use the latter one.

In addition, two scenarios were identified on the basis of the type and length of hospitalization. One was a simple surgery with expected rapid recovery, while the other was serious surgery and an expected longer hospitalization. Each respondent was asked to

TABLE 8.3

Fractional Factorial Design for 3^6 Stimulus Set

Stimulus Combination	Factor					
	A	B	C	D	E	F
1	1	3	3	3	1	2
2	1	1	3	3	3	1
3	2	1	1	3	3	3
4	1	2	1	1	3	3
5	2	1	2	1	1	3
6	3	2	1	2	1	1
7	2	3	2	1	2	1
8	2	2	3	2	1	2
9	3	2	2	3	2	1
10	1	3	2	2	3	2
11	2	1	3	2	2	3
12	2	2	1	3	2	2
13	2	2	2	1	3	2
14	1	2	2	2	1	3
15	1	1	2	2	2	1
16	3	1	1	2	2	2
17	1	3	1	1	2	2
18	3	1	3	1	1	2
19	2	3	1	3	1	1
20	3	2	3	1	3	1
21	3	3	2	3	1	3
22	2	3	3	2	3	1
23	1	2	3	3	2	3
24	3	1	2	3	3	2
25	3	3	1	2	3	3
26	3	3	3	1	2	3
27	1	1	1	1	1	1

TABLE 8.4

Illustrative Stimulus Card

A. Type of hospital
   Teaching hospital affiliated with a major university
B. Physical appearance of hospital
   Poor condition, old
C. Proximity
   In your neighborhood
D. Attending physician
   A physician assigned to you by the hospital
E. Prestige of physician
   World renowned
F. Price per day
   $90

---

carefully examine the stimulus set of 27 descriptions of the hypothetical hospitals and, assuming that he (she) were to go through a surgery with a rapid recovery period (Scenario 1) and had to choose a hospital, evaluate the various hospitals and assign them to four categories: "definitely would select it," "probably would select it," "probably would not select it," and "definitely would not select it." Once this task was completed, the respondent was asked to repeat it with respect to the second scenario—going to a hospital for a more severe surgery that requires a long hospitalization period.

These two tasks provided the major thrust of the study and the required input for the conjoint measurement analysis. In addition, each respondent was asked to indicate (at the beginning of the interview) his major considerations in selecting a hospital. This open-ended task was designed to ensure that the relevant factors were included in the subsequent conjoint measurement tasks. In addition, the subjects responded to a short battery of demographic questions and repeated the conjoint measurement task under Scenario 1 for eight additional combinations. These new stimulus combinations were selected at random and screened to exclude all clearly dominant combinations. It provided the basis for testing the predictive power of the conjoint measurement procedure.

Plan of Analysis

The major analytical technique used in this study was Kruskal's MONANOVA algorithm. To test whether the additive main effect model underlying this algorithm does hold in this study, the utilities were developed at the individual level and the stress (badness of fit) measures examined. All respondents had relatively low stress (which is analogous to high correlation between the raw data and the calculated utilities), suggesting the appropriateness of the additive main effect conjoint measurement for the study of the hospital selection decision by this group of respondents.

The specific plan of analysis followed the four key research questions and included the following steps:

1. To establish the factors consumers use in the hospital selection decision, a content analysis was conducted on reasons given by the respondents for selecting a hospital.

2. To determine the relative importance of the various hospital characteristics, conjoint measurement analysis using the MONANOVA algorithm was conducted (separately for each scenario) on the total sample data.

3. To determine the effect of the type of hospitalization required on the evaluation of the six hospital characteristics, the results of the two conjoint measurement analyses (under Scenarios 1 and 2) were compared.

4. To assess the effect of consumers' age, sex, and hospitalization history on their evaluation of the six hospital characteristics, the individual utility scores for respondents in each of the 8 cells (of the $2 \times 2 \times 2$ design—Table 8.1) were submitted to the BMD 12V- Multivariate Analysis of Variance—MANOVA—program.

In addition, we established the predictive power and validity of the additive conjoint measurement model by comparing the respondent's actual evaluation of the eight validation stimuli (which were not used in the calculation of the utilities) with their predicted position based on the utility scores derived from the conjoint measurement analysis.

Results

The discussion of the results follows the four research questions that motivated this study.

1. Factors considered in consumers' hospital selection decision.
   The analysis of the free response data suggests that the six factors included in the stimulus set are the major characteristics

FIGURE 8.1

Utility Scores for the Six Hospital Characteristics under the Two Scenarios:* Total Sample

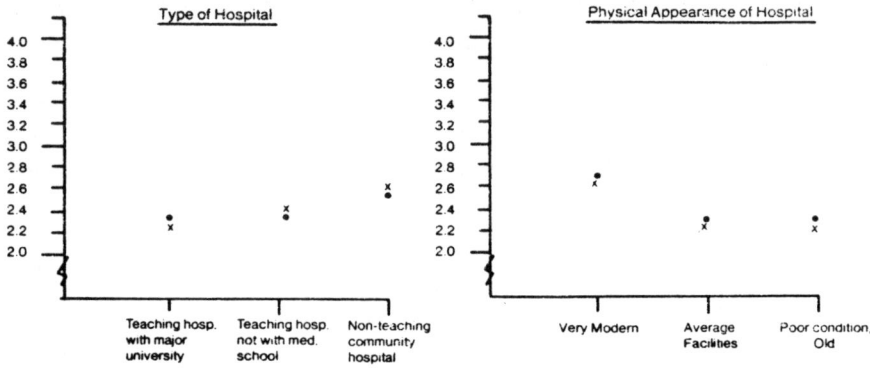

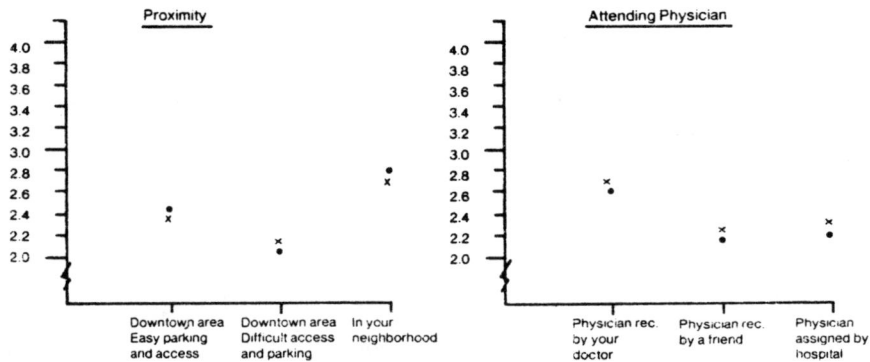

(continued)

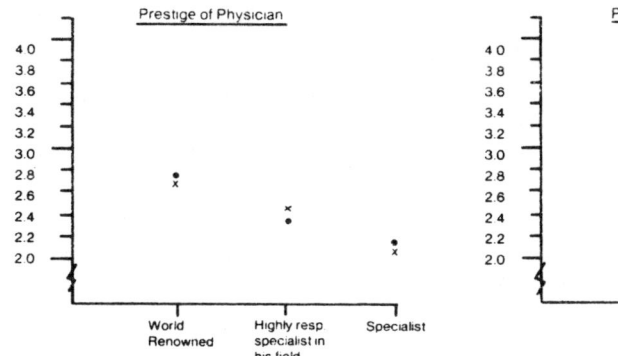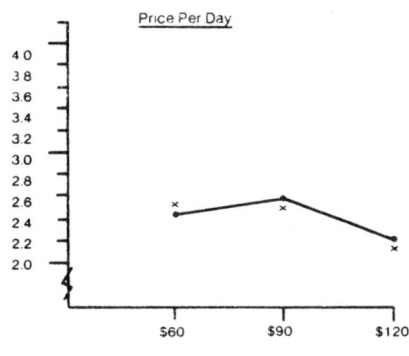

*× = Scenario 1—a surgery with rapid recovery period;
● = Scenario 2—severe surgery which requires long hospitalization period.

considered in selecting a hospital. The only additional factor (not included in our stimulus set) is nursing care—quality and speed—which was mentioned by all groups but somewhat more frequently by those who have been hospitalized before.
2. <u>Relative importance of six hospital characteristics in consumers' hospital selection decision</u>. Figure 8.1 presents the results of the conjoint measurement analysis for the total sample (under both scenarios). An examination of these results suggests the following order of importance for the six factors (determined by the range of utilities for each factor, that is, the larger the range the more important the factor). Under both scenarios proximity of the hospital is the most important factor (26 percent for Scenario 1 and 24 percent for Scenario 2), followed by prestige of physician (21 and 22 percent), physical appearance of the hospital (17 and 16 percent), price per day (14 percent for both scenarios), type of hospital affiliation (13 and 11 percent). Least important under Scenario 1 and second to last under Scenario 2 is who recommended or assigned the attending physician (9 percent for Scenario 1 and 13 percent for Scenario 2).
3. <u>Impact of type of required hospitalization on respondents' evaluation of hospital characteristics</u>. An examination of Figure 8.1 suggests little difference between the utility scores under the two hospitalization scenarios. Under Scenario 2 the respondents have a slightly higher utility for physicians who are recommended by their doctor. Yet this difference is not statistically significant.

TABLE 8.5

Summary of Multivariate Analysis of Variance

Source of Variation	Approximate F Statistic
A. Hospitalization vs. nonhospitalization history	1.69
B. Male vs. female	0.71
C. Over 35 vs. under 35	1.24
Interaction AB	1.52
AC	0.97
BC	1.49
ABC	0.67

4. *Effect of sex, age, and hospitalization on respondents' utility scores.* To examine the differences in evaluation of the six hospital characteristics among the age, sex, and hospitalization experience groups, the individual utilities were analyzed via multivariate analysis of variance procedure [18]. The results of this analysis, presented in Table 8.5, suggest that the age, sex, and hospitalization history had no statistically significant effect on consumers' utilities for the six hospital characteristics. Hospitalization history, although not statistically significant, is the most important factor in explaining the respondents' utility scores (highest omega square value) and is therefore subjected to further analysis.

Figure 8.2 provides a direct comparison of the utility scores of the previously hospitalized respondents and those who have never been hospitalized. (Given the similarity in responses across the two scenarios, the results are presented only for Scenario 1.) An examination of this exhibit suggests the following conclusions:

   i. Respondents with no prior hospitalization tend to have greater utility for all the factors associated with hospital selection. For the nonhospitalized group the range of the utilities for the six factors is from a high of 0.69 (27 percent important) to a low of 0.24 (9 percent important), compared to a 0.41 to 0.12 range (23 to 7 percent important) for the respondents with prior hospitalization experience. This may reflect a somewhat greater anxiety on the part of the nonhospitalized respondents.

FIGURE 8.2

Utility Scores for the Six Hospital Characteristics under Scenario 1:
Hospitalized vs. Nonhospitalized Group*

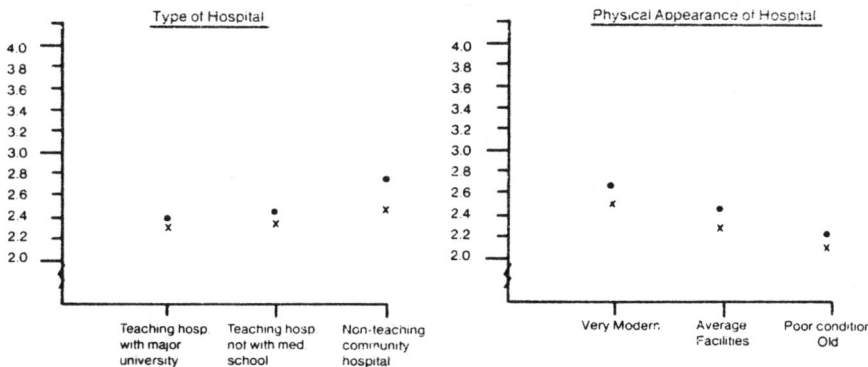

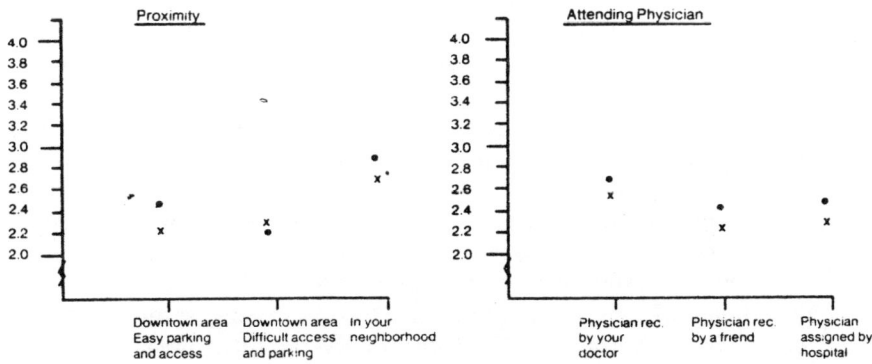

(continued)

Figure 8.2 (continued)

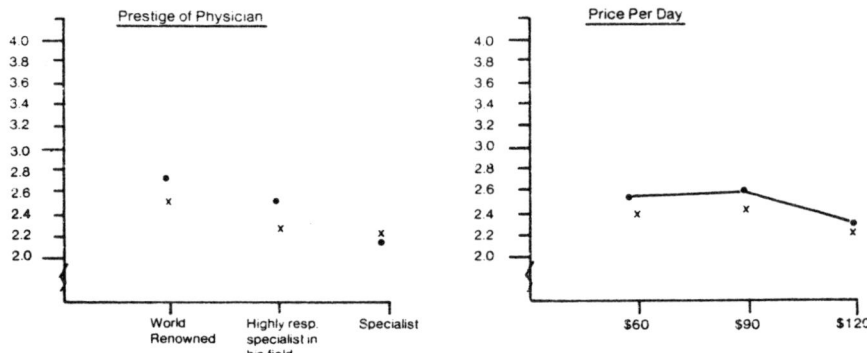

*x = hospitalized; ● = nonhospitalized

ii. The most important hospital characteristic for both groups is the geographical proximity of the hospital—23 percent (range of 0.41 out of total range of 1.78) for the hospitalized group and 27 percent for the nonhospitalized group. This finding is consistent with a number of previous studies that emphasized the desirability of minimizing the travel distance of time traveled to a health-care facility. Yet, despite its importance, the geographical proximity of the hospital is only one of a number of relevant factors. For the hospitalized group the importance of the other factors is: physical appearance of hospital (22 percent), prestige of physicians (21 percent), familiarity with attending physician (16 percent), price per day (11 percent), and the type of hospital affiliation (7 percent). The rank order of importance of the five remaining hospital characteristics for the nonhospitalized group is: prestige of physician (21 percent), physical appearance of hospital (19 percent), type of hospital affiliation (11 percent), price per day (13 percent), and the familiarity with the attending physician (9 percent).

iii. The hospital with the highest likelihood of being selected is the same for both groups. The total utility for this "best" hospital is 15.20 for the previously hospitalized group and 16.37 for the nonhospitalized group. The specific characteristics of such a hospital are shown in Table 8.6. Concerning the cost per day, it seems that both respondent groups are not price sensitive. For both groups price is among the least important factors

TABLE 8.6

Characteristics (and Their Associated Utilities) of "Best" Hospital for Two Respondents Groups

Factor	Utility Score For	
	Hospitalized	Nonhospitalized
Hospital characteristic		
A neighborhood hospital	2.64	2.90
Very modern appearance	2.56	2.71
Non-teaching Community hospital	2.44	2.77
Physician		
A world renowned physician	2.59	2.74
Recommended by your doctor	2.56	2.60
Cost		
$60 or $90 a day	2.41	2.60

(reflecting perhaps the respondents' hospital/medical insurance). The respondents are almost indifferent between $60 and $90 a day, and when the price increases to $120 a day the loss in utility is only 0.20 for the hospitalized group and 0.35 for the nonhospitalized group. (This loss in utility can easily be recovered by shifting most other factors from a less preferred to the most preferred position.)

Validation

In the use of conjoint measurement or any other analytical procedure for assessing consumers' responses to a set of attributes, the key question is "How valid is the procedure?" Ideally, one would like to compare the predictions of the conjoint measurement study with the respondent's subsequent behavior, that is, the actual choice of a specific hospital. Given the obvious difficulties (with respect to cost and time) involved in collecting such data, the validation procedure chosen in this study was based on a comparison between consumers' responses to a validation set of hypothetical hospital profiles (this set included the eight additional randomly selected combinations that were not included in the computation of the utility scores) and

TABLE 8.7

Comparison of Actual Evaluation of New Hypothetical Hospitals with
Predicted Evaluation Based on Additive Conjoint Measurement Results

Rank Order Analysis			Pair Comparisons of Actual vs. Predicted Dominance (at the aggregate level)		
	Stimulus		Actual Evaluation of Pairs of 8 New Stimuli	Predicted Evaluation of Pairs of 8 New Stimuli	
Rank Position	Actual	Pre-dicted		$i > j$	$i < j$
1st	2 ↔ 2				
2	8 ↔ 8				
3	5 ↗ 1				
4	1 ↗ 6		$i > j$	86%	14%	28 = 100%
5	6 ↗ 5				
6	4 ↔ 4		$i < j$	14%	86%	28 = 100%
7	7 ↗ 3				
8	3 ↗ 7				

the calculated scores for these combinations (based on the results of the conjoint measurement analysis).

The comparison was conducted at both the aggregate and individual levels and included at the aggregate level a comparison of the rank order of the eight stimuli based on the actual and predicted results. The rank order was quite similar, as can be seen in the left-hand panel of Table 8.7. A more detailed analysis of the relations among all possible pairs of the eight new items was also undertaken and is reported in the right-hand panel of Table 8.7. An examination of the actual vs. predicted pairwise relationships indicates a high degree of agreement between the two (86 percent of the cases were correctly predicted), suggesting relatively high validity for the conjoint measurement model. An examination at the individual level suggested that for over 90 percent of the respondents, 85 percent or better of the predicted relations between all pairs of the validation set were correct.

Discussion

The hospital selection study was presented not for its immediate implications for hospital management but rather as an illustration for an application of conjoint measurement to the study of a health care marketing problem. Given the small size and the nonprobability nature of the sample, no substantive implications can be suggested from this exploratory study. Yet a number of conclusions and suggestions for future research can be drawn:

1. The hospital selection problem (and other similar health care problems) can be approached as a marketing problem using standard marketing research techniques.

2. The additive conjoint measurement model seems to be a good descriptor of consumers' choices among various hospital characteristics. More complex interactive models do not seem to be required, although any subsequent study utilizing conjoint measurement should test, for each respondent, whether the additive model holds.

3. This research approach to health-care problems can be extended to cover other respondents, such as physicians or even hospital administrators.

4. In designing conjoint measurement or other studies of the hospital selection decision, other attributes should not be ignored. New factors (for example, nursing care) and new levels for the existing six factors (for example, higher prices than the $120 per day) should be examined by management and, if relevant, included in the stimulus set.

TABLE 8.8

Illustrative Set of Multi-attribute Decision Problems of Various Health Care-Organizations

Decision	Health Care Organizations					
	Hospital	Health Maintenance Organization (HMO)	Private Physician and Group Practice	Health Related Organizations	Medical Schools and Basic Research Organizations	Government and Regulatory Organizations
Establishing decision criteria	How to allocate resources among competing objectives—profits vs. expansion vs. staffing pattern vs. prestige vs. social consideration	Criteria for ordering, screening, and diagnostic procedures; cost vs. utility for various age groups	Establishing criteria for type and nature of practice—profits vs. social considerations vs. research, etc.	Objectives for new product—profits vs. market share vs. growth vs. cash flow, etc.	Criteria for funding—short vs. long-run benefits; applied vs. basic research	Degree and type of government financing and regulating
Selecting target markets	What patient groups to select—poor	What target markets and physicians	What target market to appeal to?	What target groups of physicians	Who should be funded?	Who should be regulated and who should

198

	Hospital	HMO	Private Practice	Pharmaceutical	Research	Government
	vs. paying patients, etc.	should the HMO try to attract?		and patients to appeal to?—different benefits segments		receive the benefits?
Determining product/service mix	What departments and services should the hospital offer?	What should be the services offered by HMO?	What mix of specialties to offer?	What product benefits should a product offer?	What type of training and research programs should be established?	What central mechanism should be established to assure quality and appropriateness of health care?
Establishing pricing strategy	How much should the hospital charge for various services?	What should be the prepayment charge?	What should the fee be?	What should the price of the products be?	What incentive system can be designed to attract the "right" type of researchers?	What price controls and guidelines to establish?
Determining distribution/location mix	Where should a hospital be located and what transportation system	Should an HMO establish peripheral clinics?	Where to locate?	How to distribute the products—detail men vs. direct selling; drug-	Where to locate?	How to redistribute health care services geographically and by subspecialty

(continued)

Table 8.8 (continued)

		Health-Care Organizations				
Decision	Hospital	Health Maintenance Organization (HMO)	Private Physician and Group Practice	Health Related Organizations	Medical Schools and Basic Research Organizations	Government and Regulatory Organizations
	should be offered?			stores vs. supermarkets; etc.		
Determining the communication mix	How and what to "advertise" without using advertising	How to "sell" the HMO concept	How to "advertise" without advertising	How and what to advertise—physician vs. patient advertising	How to improve the flow of information among researchers	How to communicate effectively preventive health campaigns (smoking, cancer)
Other (non-marketing areas)	How to design attractive subspecialty training programs		How does a physician make a clinical decision?			Establish testing procedures for physicians on realistic, multi-attribute patient characteristics

5. The descriptive stimulus (Table 8.4) and respondent's task (rating on an "intention to select" scale) were easily comprehended by the respondents and easy to administer. Yet, in future hospital selection and other health-care studies, attention should be given to alternative mode of stimulus definition (for example, pictorial presentation) and respondent's task (for example, "preference" or some other evaluative dimension instead of "intentions to select") and strict ranking or a combination of rating and ranking instead of the rating scale used here.

SOME FURTHER APPLICATIONS OF CONJOINT MEASUREMENT IN MARKETING STUDIES OF HEALTH-CARE ORGANIZATIONS

Most marketing decisions of health-care organizations are multi-attribute in nature, requiring trade-offs between cost, efficiency, political expediency, and consumer and provider satisfaction without sacrificing the fundamental quality of health care. As such, conjoint measurement and its related techniques provide an extremely useful analytical approach to marketing decision in health care organizations.

More specifically, conjoint measurement can be applied to three major decision areas:

1. Determining the objectives, criteria, and decision rules [9] for various health care decisions.
2. Selecting target markets [10] for the given health care organization.
3. Determining the most appropriate marketing strategy [9]—what product/service mix to offer, what price to charge, how to select an appropriate location, what distribution system to employ, and how to communicate with the relevant audience.

Specific illustrative examples of multi-attribute decisions in each of these areas for each of the relevant health care organizations—hospitals, HMOs, physicians (private and group practice), health related organizations (for example, pharmaceutical companies) and government and other regulatory agencies—are presented in Table 8.8.

These and similar decisions lend themselves to conjoint measurement study, which can provide management with quantifiable information on the relevant audience utilities for various options. These studies can be supplemented by a computer simulation model that provides management with share of choices information (similar to brand switching matrices) for various alternative strategies. Such simulations have been developed for a number of companies (see [9] and [19]) and can be used by health-care organizations.

In addition to these marketing problems, a number of nonmarketing health care problems, such as the understanding of physician's clinical judgments, can benefit from research using conjoint measurement procedures (see [16]).

CONCLUSIONS

Most marketing problems of health care and other nonprofit organizations are basically multi-attribute in nature. As such, conjoint measurement analysis may be an extremely useful analytical procedure for the quantification of respondents' utilities for various multi-attribute alternatives.

Although this paper illustrated the applicability of conjoint measurement techniques to a pilot study of consumers' hospital selection decision and speculated on a number of other possible applications, the study of the marketing problems of nonprofit organizations in general, and of health-care organizations in particular, should not be limited to the use of this procedure. Other choice models at both the individual and group level should be developed and tested. Similarly, other data analytical procedures and especially multivariate statistical techniques and multidimensional scaling procedures can and should be considered, when appropriate, among the tools available to the marketing researcher of nonprofit organizations.

REFERENCES

1. J. D. Carroll, "Categorical Conjoint Measurement," Meeting of Mathematical Psychology, Ann Arbor, Michigan, August 1968.

2. C. Creditor and V. K. Creditor, "The Ecology of an Urban Voluntary Hospital, the Referral Chain," Med. Care 10 (1972):88-92.

3. D. L. Ford, G. P. Huber, and D. H. Gustafson, "Predicting Job Choices with Models that Contain Subjective Probability Judgments: An Empirical Comparison of Five Models," Organizational Behav. Hum. Performance 7 (1972):397-416.

4. L. R. Goldberg, "Man Versus Model of Man: A Rationale Plus Some Evidence for a Method of Improving on Clinical Inferences," Psychol. Bull. 73 (1970):422-32.

5. Paul E. Green, "On the Design of Choice Experiments Involving Multifactor Alternatives," J. Consumer Res. 1 (1974):61-68.

6. Paul E. Green, Frank J. Carmone, and Yoram Wind, "Subjective Evaluation Models and Conjoint Measurement," Behav. Sci. 17 (1972):288-99.

7. Paul E. Green and Vithala R. Rao, "Conjoint Measurement for Quantifying Judgmental Data," J. Marketing Res. 8 (1971):355-63.

8. Paul E. Green and Yoram Wind, Multi-Attribute Decisions in Marketing: A Measurement Approach. New York: Dryden Press, 1973.

9. Paul E. Green and Yoram Wind, "New Way to Measure Consumers' Judgment," Harvard Business Rev. 53 (1975):107-17.

10. Paul E. Green, Yoram Wind, and Arun K. Jain, "Benefit Bundle Analysis," J. Advertising Res. 12 (1972):31-36.

11. Richard M. Johnson, "Trade-Off Analysis of Consumer Values," J. Marketing Res. 11 (1974):121-27.

12. Philip Kotler, Marketing for Non-Profit Organizations. Englewood Cliffs, N.J.: Prentice-Hall, 1975.

13. Philip Kotler and Sidney J. Levy, "Broadening the Concept of Marketing," J. Marketing 33 (1969):10-15.

14. Joseph B. Kruskal, "Analysis of Factorial Experiments by Estimating Monotone Transformations of the Data," J. Roy. Statistical Soc. B. 27 (1965):251-63.

15. Paul Slovic, D. Fleissner, and W. S. Bauman, "Analyzing the Use of Information in Investment Decision Making: A Methodological Proposal," J. Business 45 (1972):283-301.

16. Lawrence Spitz, Ronald Daniele, and Yoram Wind, "Multivariate Decision Making in the Settling of Pulmonary Outpatient Clinic," paper presented at the American College of Physicians, San Francisco, April 1975.

17. Yoram Wind, "Recent Approaches to the Study of Organizational Buying Behavior," in T. V. Greer (ed.), Combined Proceedings of the 1973 American Marketing Association Conferences, Chicago, 1974, pp. 203-06.

18. Yoram Wind and Joseph Denny, "Multivariate Analysis of Variance in Research on the Effectiveness of TV Commercials," J. Marketing Res. 11 (1974):136-42.

19. Yoram Wind, Stuart Jolly, and Arthur O'Connor, "Concept Testing as Input to Strategic Marketing Simulations," in E. Mazzie (ed.), Proceedings of the 58th International AMA Conference, Chicago, 1975, pp. 120-24.

PART II
MANAGEMENT SCIENCE/ OPERATIONS RESEARCH

9

DECISION THEORY

INTRODUCTION

In the first article the authors applied decision theory techniques to determine the number of hospital beds required in a particular region. A decision to allow the construction of too many beds places a financial burden on the community. On the other hand, a decision to allow the construction of too few beds may result in some patients' not receiving timely medical care. The authors constructed a normative model under uncertainty. Several techniques were used to arrive at a strategy, and from there possible outcomes were determined.

In the second article a decision theory approach is used to develop an index of illness severity, which in turn is used to analyze the costs and benefits of burn care systems. The severity index model developed by the authors is basically a multi-attribute utility model. Five criteria (size of full-thickness burn, the patient's age, the patient's medical history, size of partial-thickness burn, and burn site) were selected for evaluating the severity of a burned patient's condition. The model was tested for predictive and content validity. The results suggest that although continued validation is required, the model appears to have the potential to provide an illness severity index which may aid in health policy decisions.

Introduction to Technique

Decision theory is a modeling technique to analyze decisions and to improve the decision process especially under conditions of risk and uncertainty. Decision theory enables the decision maker to analyze a set of complex situations with many alternatives and many possible outcomes. Decision models are formulated through matrices or decision trees. Decision trees are normally used when the decision maker must make a sequence of decisions rather than a single one. Matrix formulation is usually used when there are several alternatives with numerous different outcomes. Decision models are classified as normative and descriptive. In the normative model, the decision maker faces a known set of alternatives and selects a course of action by a rational selection process. Normative decision models are used for recurring decisions with a historical background. Descriptive models are concerned with how decisions are actually made. Their framework incorporates learning features and acts or choices which span over many behavioral dimensions. Descriptive models are widely used on one-time, nonrecurring decisions.

REFERENCES

Bierman, H., Jr., C. P. Bonini, and W. H. Hausman, Quantitative Analysis for Business Decisions. Homewood, Ill.: R. D. Irwin, 1973.

Esogbue, A. O., and A. J. Singh, "A Stochastic Model for an Optimal Priority Bed Distribution Problem in a Hospital Ward," Operations Research 24 (September-October 1976):884-98.

Schweitzer, S. O., "Cost-effectiveness of Early Detection of Disease," Health Services Research 9 (Spring 1974):22-32.

Turban, E., and P. N. Loomba, Readings in Management Science. Dallas, Texas: Business Publications, 1976.

USE OF DECISION THEORY IN REGIONAL PLANNING

Richard M. Grimes
Catherine L. Allen
Ted R. Sparling
Gerald Weiss

The Houston-Galveston Area Council (HGAC), the local comprehensive health planning agency for a 13-county area in southeast Texas, was faced with the task early in 1973 of setting a limit on the number of short-term general hospital beds in the region. Approximately 5500 new beds had been proposed for construction in the area, and there was a general feeling among the HGAC board that many of these beds were not needed.

HGAC requested the assistance of the authors in setting bed limits within the following framework: First, bed need projections were to be made for the period from 1974 through 1980. Second, a set of population forecasts were specified to be used in determining demand. Third, the areas for which limitations would be set were to be the service areas defined by the Texas Hill-Burton agency; these were a mixture of county, multicounty, and subcounty areas believed to reflect the usage patterns of area residents. Fourth, bed limitation was to be based on projections of hospital days/population/year (converted to number of beds by dividing by 365 and by an 85 percent occupancy factor). Finally, the projections of bed use were to be based on one of four extrapolations of past utilization rates. The extrapolations were based on the assumptions that (1) the trend of the use rate over the last seven years would continue, or (2) the last-four-year trend would continue, or (3) the last-two-year trend would continue, or (4) the use rate of the most recent year would remain constant.

With these decisions as background, the authors began seeking a method that would allow the HGAC board to evaluate the impact of basing the bed limitation on one of the four extrapolations of use rates. The critical problem was that a decision to allow the construction of

---

Reprinted with permission from Health Services Research 9, No. 1 (Spring 1974). Copyright 1974 by the Hospital Research and Educational Trust, 840 North Lakeshore Drive, Chicago, Ill. 60611.

TABLE 9.1

Sample Decision Matrix

		Outcome			
		I Low Use Rate	II Medium–Low Use Rate	III Medium–High Use Rate	IV High Use Rate
Decision	I Construct 100 beds	OK	100 beds short	200 beds short	300 beds short
	II Construct 200 beds	100 beds over	OK	100 beds short	200 beds short
	III Construct 300 beds	200 beds over	100 beds over	OK	100 beds short
	IV Construct 400 beds	300 beds over	200 beds over	100 beds over	OK

too many beds would place a financial burden on the community, while a decision to allow the construction of too few beds would mean that the sick would not receive care. But simply saying that this was the case was not adequate information for the HGAC board; they would need firmer data on which to base their decision. With the use of a decision matrix as shown in Table 9.1 it was possible to show the board what the potential excess or shortage of beds would be if they decided on one of the extrapolations and then one of the other extrapolations turned out to be correct. It was then relatively simple to project 1980 demand under each extrapolation for the 15 service areas and to array them in matrixes similar to the one shown in Table 9.1.

After review of the service-area matrixes, it was decided that the matrixes would be more useful if they showed the dollar costs of excess beds. In order to do this it was necessary first to project the average daily cost of an occupied bed for 1974-80, by extrapolating the line that best described the 1966-72 average daily cost for Texas hospitals (taken from AHA data). This line was determined by use of a least-squares method. The projected average daily cost for 1974-80, read off the line at the intersection of 1977, was approximately $113 per day. Average daily cost for an unoccupied bed was estimated by multiplying the average projected daily cost of an occupied bed by 0.7. (While various investigators have estimated the cost of an unoccupied bed at from 45 percent to 80 percent of the cost of an occupied bed [1-3], most estimates center at approximately 70 percent.) Average yearly cost of an excess bed was then calculated by multiplying daily cost by 365 days and by 7 years. The total operating cost for one excess bed for the 1974-80 period was thus estimated to be approximately $202,000.

Multiplying this rather sizable figure by the number of excess beds (projected on the basis of utilization rates) gave the HGAC board members an idea of the potential costs of various decisions. Table 9.2 is an example of the 1974-80 decision matrix for the Houston service region, showing the board members the range of error that might occur. For example, if they made decision II they would know that the bed shortage would not exceed 983 and the cost to the community would not be over $75,300,000. By analyzing each of the decisions they could find a strategy of minimizing dollar cost or bed shortage to their liking. In addition, they would discover the maximum penalty associated with such a strategy. For example, if they decided to minimize bed shortage (decision IV), they would know that over the next seven years such a strategy might cost Houston consumers up to $273,900,000.

But the matrix shown in Table 9.2 still leaves a great deal of latitude in the decision-making process. For example, the range of cost outcomes of decision IV is over a quarter of a billion dollars—not a

TABLE 9.2

Decision Matrix for Houston Service Area under Four Decision Alternatives (cost of outcomes in millions)

Decision	Outcome			
	I Low Use Rate	II Medium-Low Use Rate	III Medium-High Use Rate	IV High Use Rate
I Major reduction in beds	OK	373 beds short	1095 beds short	1356 beds short
II Slight reduction in beds	373 beds over $75.3M	OK	722 beds short	983 beds short
III Slight increase in beds	1095 beds over $221.2M	722 beds over $145.8M	OK	261 beds short
IV Major increase in beds	1356 beds over $273.9M	983 beds over $198.6M	261 beds over $52.7M	OK

very precise estimate. Certain theorists have proposed using the expected-values technique as a means of reducing broad ranges such as these [4-6]. The basic idea behind this technique is the calculation of the average result of a decision if it is repeated a large number of times under situations of varying outcome. For example, if a given decision were to result in a gain of $1000 in one-third of the cases, a $500 gain in one-third of the cases, and a $750 loss in one-third of the cases, then the expected value of that decision is $250 (the sum of $1000/3 and $500/3 minus $750/3).

Application of this technique requires some knowledge of the probability distribution of the outcomes. Most authors in this field suggest using past experience as the guide to ascertaining these probabilities, but since this was not possible in the present study, Bayes' rule was used for calculating expected values in the face of unknown probabilities [4]. This rule simply states that when the probabilities of various outcomes are unknown one should proceed as if all outcomes were equally likely. Applying Bayes' rule to the Houston situation allowed the creation of the matrix shown in Table 9.3. This matrix showed the planning council members what the average cost of a given decision would be if they were willing to accept the equal probability of outcomes. Although several of the council members were not satisfied with the equal-probability theory, they could see the utility of the matrix and were particularly taken by the ability to do marginal analysis. For example, Table 9.3 shows that reducing the expected bed shortage from 427 to 65 (going from decision II to decision III) would raise expected dollar cost during the period by about 73 million.

After some discussion concerning the bed situation in the area, members of the council agreed that decision I appeared to be the best alternative. At the time of the study about one-third of the hospital beds in Houston were not occupied, so it seemed that there would be ample room to absorb unexpected increases in use rates. In addition it was recognized that a decision not to allow construction of beds could be corrected later, whereas a decision to allow construction would be very difficult to correct.

However, as already mentioned, there was some discomfort with the use of equal probabilities. This centered around the fact that both extrapolations that called for reductions in beds were based on short-term projections. It seemed intuitively to some of the HGAC board members that a projection based on a seven-year trend was more likely to be accurate than a projection based on one year, and there was some concern that this technical point could be legitimately seized upon by applicants whose certificates of need had been denied. The probabilities were therefore weighted according to the length of time on which the projections were based. This, of course, gave greater weight to decisions allowing more construction. Projections

TABLE 9.3

Expected Values for Various Decision Alternatives Using Bayes' Procedure (cost of outcomes in millions)

		Outcome			Expected Value of Various Decisions (Sum of Various Outcomes × Their Probabilities)
	I Low Use Rate (P = 1/4)	II Medium–Low Use Rate (P = 1/4)	III Medium–High Use Rate (P = 1/4)	IV High Use Rate (P = 1/4)	
I Major reduction in beds	OK	93 beds short	274 beds short	339 beds short	706 beds short
II Slight reduction in beds	$18.8M	OK	181 beds short	246 beds short	$18.8M and 427 beds short
III Slight increase in beds	$55.3M	$36.5M	OK	65 beds short	$91.8M and 65 beds short
IV Major increase in beds	$68.5M	$49.7M	$13.2M	OK	$131.4M

214

TABLE 9.4

Expected Values for Various Decision Alternatives Using Unequal Probabilities (cost of outcomes in millions)

		Outcome				Expected Value of Various Decisions (Sum of Various Outcomes × Their Probabilities)
		I Low Use Rate (P = 2/14)	II Medium-Low Use Rate (P = 1/14)	III Medium-High Use Rate (P = 7/14)	IV High Use Rate (P = 4/14)	
Decision	I Major reduction in beds	OK	27 beds short	548 beds short	387 beds short	962 beds short
	II Slight reduction in beds	$10.8M	OK	361 beds short	281 beds short	$10.8M and 642 beds short
	III Slight increase in beds	$31.6M	$10.4M	OK	75 beds short	$42.0M and 75 beds short
	IV Major increase in beds	$39.1M	$14.2M	$26.4M	OK	$79.7M

215

based on seven years were given a weight of 7, projections based on four years were given a weight of 4, and so on.

With the assignment of these probabilities, it was possible to create the matrix shown in Table 9.4. Again the HGAC board found it useful to do marginal analysis, and once more it could be seen that even a modest reduction in expected bed shortages would have a high economic cost. For example, reducing the bed shortage from 75 (decision III) to zero (decision IV) would raise the expected dollar cost by about 38 million.

After deliberation the full council elected to support decision I, but with the provision that the occupancy rate be lowered from 85 percent to 75 percent, which had the effect of increasing the number of allowable beds by approximately 13 percent. Unless use rates rise rapidly, no hospital will receive a certificate of need to construct short-term beds in Houston before 1980, assuming that no existing beds are removed from service.

In the entire 13-county area, fewer than 700 beds were approved for construction. Since some hospitals decided to forgo federal funds and since some came under a grandfather clause in P. L. 92-903 [7], the number of beds constructed will exceed the number approved by HGAC. It is thus impossible to estimate accurately the dollar savings, but even if half the originally proposed 5500 beds are not built, the capital expenditure saving will be over 100 million dollars, with an estimated saving in operating costs of approximately 500 million over seven years.

The council will monitor bed use rates closely to see if they differ from the projections, and an information system is being considered that will allow for sophistication of the model by more clearly delineating service areas and by determining which hospital services will be directed toward certain population groups and diseases.

REFERENCES

1. P. Feldstein, "An Empirical Investigation of the Marginal Cost of Hospital Services," Graduate Program in Hospital Administration, Center for Health Administration Studies, University of Chicago, 1961.

2. R. E. Berry, Jr., "Returns to Scale in the Production of Hospital Services," Health Serv. Res. 2 (Summer 1967):123.

3. J. R. Lave and L. B. Lave, "Hospital Cost Functions," Amer. Econ. Rev. 60 (June 1970):379.

4. H. E. Thompson, "Management Decisions in Perspective." In
   W. E. Schlender et al. (eds.), Management in Perspective.
   Boston: Houghton-Mifflin, 1965.

5. H. Raiffa, Decision Analysis. Reading, Mass.: Addison-Wesley,
   1970.

6. R. Levin and C. A. Kirkpatrick, Quantitative Approaches to
   Management. New York: McGraw-Hill, 1971.

7. Social Security Act Amendments of 1973, P. L. 92-603, Sec. 221,
   96 Stat. 1386; 42U. S. C. 1320a-1 (October 30, 1972).

A DECISION THEORY APPROACH TO
MEASURING SEVERITY IN ILLNESS

David H. Gustafson
and
Donald C. Holloway

The purpose of this study was to evaluate the applicability
of a multiattribute utility model for measuring the severity
of a patient's illness. A single medical problem (an analysis of the costs and benefits of different burn care systems)
was used to test the model. Physicians estimated the

Research supported by Public Health Service Grant No. HS-0031-05. Reprinted with permission from Health Services Research 10, No. 1 (Spring 1975). Copyright 1974 by the Hospital Research and Educational Trust, 840 North Lakeshore Drive, Chicago, Ill. 60611.
The authors wish to express their appreciation to the physicians and staff of the burn research centers of the University of Michigan, University of Wisconsin, and St. Mary's Hospital, Milwaukee, for their cooperation in this effort. We also wish to acknowledge the valuable contributions to this work of Dr. I. Feller and Mr. K. Crane of the University of Michigan and Mr. R. Lerner of the University of Wisconsin.

relative importance of and severity functions for criteria influencing severity. The model's estimates of severity were compared with survival rates of more than 6000 actual patients and with physicians' rankings of hypothetical patients. Although continued validation is needed, the multiattribute utility model appears to have potential as an index for illness severity and, possibly, health status.

Burn research units have been established in many locations around the country. New approaches in burn treatment are expensive, though, and their cost/benefit ratios do not clearly demonstrate their worth. A national information system on burn treatment has been established in order to facilitate comparison of different treatment methods and systems, but since the case mix of patients treated in the new centers differs markedly from that encountered in traditional settings, it is still quite difficult to compare the efficacy of new treatment techniques.

The study reported here was conducted in an attempt to provide cost and benefit information about the patient care systems in one of these centers. So that treatment effectiveness could be compared, it was necessary to rate patients according to severity of condition, using some stratification mechanism that would be acceptable to a broad range of medical care providers. A number of statistical attempts at developing an index of illness severity had failed in the past, and it was clear that even if these attempts had worked the indexes would not have been accepted by the providers because they did not understand the techniques used. A decision theory approach was therefore selected because it required that providers of care be actively involved in developing the severity index and estimating its parameters. This meant that the index would likely be acceptable if it were shown to perform well. This article describes the development and evaluation of the index.

THE SEVERITY INDEX MODEL

Assuming that the severity of a patient's illness is some aggregate of individual criteria, illness severity (S) may be represented as follows:

$$S = \sum_{i=1}^{n} w_i B(x_i) + \sum_{j=n+1}^{n+m} w_j R_j$$

where
  i = quantitative variable (1, 2, ..., n)
  j = qualitative variable (n + 1, n + 2, ..., n + m)
  w = relative weight
  x = extent to which a quantitative variable is present
  $B(x_i)$ = severity function associated with the ith variable
  R = presence or absence of the jth variable

All variables are assumed to be independent of one another. The term severity is used to represent the extent to which a patient is perceived by physicians to meet illness criteria. It differs from the term utility in that it does not possess any risk or trade-off considerations. Although the decision-theory model used here [1] has not been used in assessing severity of illness, this approach has proved useful in evaluating other complex problems. Gustafson used a multiattribute utility model to choose research projects [2]. A similar model has been used in a computerized job-selection system for rating job desirability [3]. The decision theory approach has also been validated in experimental contexts [4]. MacCrimmon's review article on subjective decision-making models [5] suggests other possible applications and reports on his attempt to develop such a model for selection of students. Huber has also reviewed field studies using multiattribute utility models [6].

DEVELOPMENT OF THE INDEX

In developing the index, (1) criteria were selected that were considered to be important in evaluating severity of illness, (2) measures of each criterion were developed, (3) the severity function associated with each criterion was determined, (4) the relative importance of each criterion was estimated, and (5) the evaluations of all physicians were aggregated. Each of these steps is described in detail in the following sections.

Selection of Criteria

Criteria for evaluating the severity of a burned patient's condition were selected on the basis of a review of the literature and structured problem identification sessions [7]. Four physicians, one nurse, and one industrial engineer were involved in these sessions. The following criteria were selected as the most important: size of full-thickness burn, the patient's age, the patient's medical history, size of partial-thickness burn, and burn site.

FIGURE 9.1

Relative Contribution of Size of Burn to Severity of Full-Thickness Burn, As Independently Conceptualized by Four Physicians

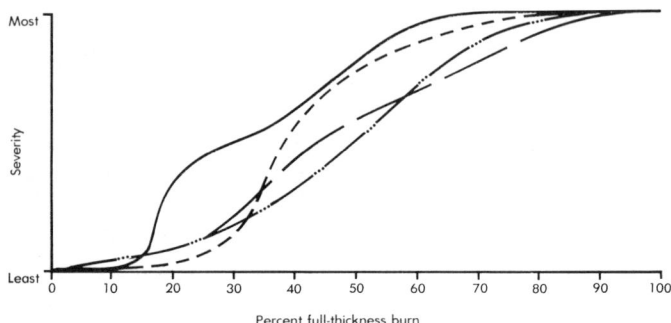

FIGURE 9.2

Relative Contribution of Size of Burn to Severity of Partial-Thickness Burn, As Independently Conceptualized by Four Physicians

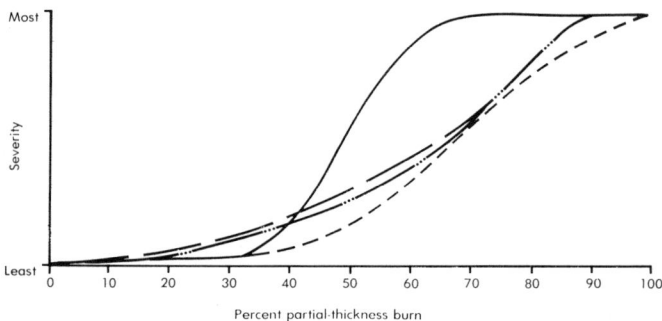

FIGURE 9.3

Relative Contribution of Age to Severity of Burn, As Independently Conceptualized by Four Physicians

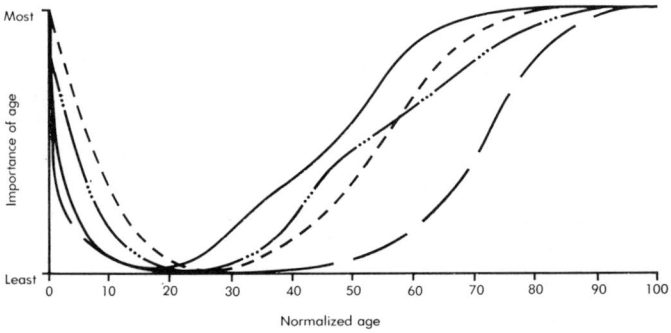

Development of Criteria Measures

Criteria measures were developed using nominal and interval scales. Size of burn was measured on an interval scale as a percentage of the body surface involved. Patient age was measured in single years rather than age categories. A list of 29 medical problems was developed for evaluating a patient's medical history; since it was considered that any of the problems on this list would significantly increase the severity of a burned patient's condition, the 29 problems were assigned equal weights. Nine primary burn sites were identified: face, chest and abdomen, perineum, back of head, neck, back, arms and hands, legs and thighs, and buttocks.

Development of Severity Functions

Of the available techniques for estimating utilities, the method of order has proved to be the most satisfactory for interval-scaled measues [4, 8, 9]. With this technique, subjects select the values of the criteria with which they would be most and least satisfied and then connect these two points with a curve that describes how satisfied they would be with values between these points. The four physicians on the panel used this approach for developing severity functions for full- and partial-thickness burn, age, and medical history. Results for size of full-thickness burn, results for size of partial-thickness burn, and results for age of patient are shown in Figs. 9.1-9.3. The similarity of the curves in these figures indicates that the judgments of the four physicians differed very little from each other.

The odds approach was used to estimate severity as a function of burn site. This method was chosen on the basis of work on the odds technique by Huber [4] and by Gustafson [2]; the work of Huber and Gustafson is consistent with the results of Phillips et al. [10] on subjective probability estimation. The four physicians on the panel selected the most important burn site in terms of severity and then estimated how much more severe a burn would be at this site than a burn at each remaining site. These estimates were made on a logarithmically calibrated scale of odds ranging from 1:1 to 1000:1. (This scale was chosen because the literature indicates that it tends to reduce estimation bias.) The results for the four physicians were averaged, and the aggregate odds estimates were then converted into weights on a 0-100 scale. A patient whose burns covered more than one site would thus be assigned a burn site severity function on the basis of the sum of the functions of the individual sites. The severity function for a patient burned at every site would be 100.

Weighting of Criteria

The five criteria (size of full- and partial-thickness burn, age, medical history, and burn site) were weighted by the four panel physicians using the odds technique described above, and the results were averaged. Table 9.5 shows the resulting scheme for weighting criteria, together with the severity functions for individual criteria.

TABLE 9.5

Criteria Used to Measure Burn Severity

Criterion	Criterion Weight	Criterion Severity Function
Percent of body covered by full-thickness burn	0.371	See Fig. 9.1
Age of patient	0.292	See Fig. 9.3
Number of past medical problems	0.218	Four or more = 100
		Three = 90
		Two = 75
		One = 55
		None = 0
Percent of body covered by partial-thickness burn	0.071	See Fig. 9.2
Burn site	0.048	Face = 32.5
		Chest and abdomen = 12.6
		Perineum = 12.6
		Back of head = 9.0
		Neck = 9.0
		Back = 8.1
		Arms and hands = 5.4
		Legs and thighs = 5.4
		Buttocks = 5.4

APPLICATION OF THE INDEX

The severity of a burn patient's condition is calculated on the basis of the five criteria described above. The severity associated with each measure is multiplied by the relative weight of the criterion, and the products are added. For instance, a 38-year-old patient with a history of one important medical problem who had full-thickness burns covering 40 percent of his body and partial-thickness burns covering 20 percent of his body and whose burns covered all of his body except his face, head, back, and arms would be assigned a severity index of 37, as shown in Table 9.6.

VALIDATION OF THE INDEX

Testing for Predictive Validity

Fifteen hypothetical patients were created, with different values across all five criteria, and the patients' conditions were described on cards in conventional terms. The same four physicians who determined relative weights and severity functions for the index rank-ordered the patient descriptions according to severity. The Spearman rank correlation coefficient between the average physician ranking and the index ranking was 0.89, indicating that the index is predictive.

Testing for Content Validity

Since the purpose of the burn severity index is to measure directly the severity of a burned patient's condition, and not merely to predict physician estimates of severity, further tests were required for validation.

Content validity testing [11] is often used for validation of models of this type, but since no one test can measure content validity, developers of such models must accumulate circumstantial evidence that indicates that their models behave as expected.

Comparison with Subjective Ratings by Physicians

The index ratings were first checked for content validity by comparing them with ratings of burn specialists unfamiliar with the index. Eight physicians at two other burn centers rated the 15 hypothetical patients according to perceived severity. Their ratings were compared to the index ratings and the ratings made by the four original physicians. The Spearman rank correlation coefficient between the

TABLE 9.6

Sample Calculation of Burn Severity

Criterion	Patient Information	Severity Function Value	×	Criterion Weight (from Table 1)	=	Index Weight
Percent of body covered by full-thickness burn	40	50		0.371		18.55
Age of patient	38	15		0.292		4.38
Number of past medical problems	1	55		0.218		11.99
Percent of body covered by partial-thickness burn	20	4		0.071		0.28
Burn site	Chest, abdomen, perineum, neck, legs, buttocks	45		0.048		2.16
				Severity index value		37.36

FIGURE 9.4

Relationship between Severity Index Scores and Percent Chance of Death According to Probit Analysis Model

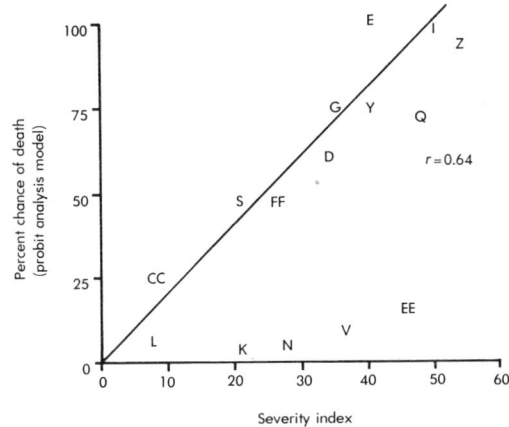

Note: Each letter indicates the position of an individual patient on the two scales.

index ratings and the ratings of six physicians at Burn Center 2 was 0.74. The correlation with the ratings of two physicians at Burn Center 3 was 0.87, which is comparable to the correlation of 0.89 registered by the physicians at Burn Center 1 who developed the index.

Comparison with Another Model

The performance of the index was also tested by comparing its ratings with the ratings of a probit analysis model developed at Burn Center 2 that is used to estimate probability of death from burns on the basis of age and percent of body surface affected (both variables are used as independent indexes) [12]. When the probit analysis model and the severity index model were applied to the 15 hypothetical patients, the correlation coefficient was 0.64. As shown in Fig. 9.4, this relatively low correlation is due in great part to the different ratings assigned to four of the patients (K, N, V, and EE) by the two models. The conditions of all four of these patients were more severe according to the severity index, in which the variables are not independent (for example, in applying the severity index model the relative effect of age cannot be estimated except as a function of size of burn).

TABLE 9.7

Comparison of Severity Index Model to Probit Analysis Model Using Selected Patients

Patient	Severity Index Rating	Percent Chance of Death According to Probit Analysis Model	Age of Patient	Percent of Body Burned	Number of Past Medical Problems
K	21.1	2	1	20	0
S	20.7	47	3	55	0
N	26.9	3	48	20	1
FF	26.3	47	8	55	1
V	36.8	8	53	25	3
G	36.2	72	29	70	0
EE	45.9	14	70	15	3
Q	46.8	70	70	40	0

It is conceivable that the severity index model would not work well in instances that required the independent weighting of criteria, but recent comparisons of additive and nonadditive models suggest that this problem may be overstated [13].

On the other hand, the severity index model considers other factors besides age and burn size. In this case the key additional factor seems to be past medical problems. If past problems influence severity, one would expect significant differences in results for the two models. In Table 9.7, probit analysis results and data on age and medical problems are given for the four patients for whom the severity index ratings did not correlate with chance of death as computed by probit analysis. Along with the data for these four patients are the comparable data for the four patients with the closest severity ratings (patients S, FF, G, and Q). Differences in ratings between K and S and between N and FF are seen to result from the treatment of age and burn size; differences between V and G and between EE and Q, however, result from differences in medical histories. Patients V and EE had significant past medical problems (myocardial infarction, hypertension, and marked obesity for EE; thrombophlebitis, peptic diathesis, and marked obesity for V), and patients G and Q had no record of significant medical problems. Results for these patients indicate that the severity index may be a more adequate measure of severity than the probit analysis model using only age and burn size.

It is interesting to note how much influence a model can have on physicians' thinking. Physicians at Burn Center 2 had been using the probit analysis model for several years to estimate percent change of death for all burn patients. The severity estimates made by physicians at Burn Center 2 correlated very well with probit analysis estimates ($r = 0.97$) but less well with the severity index ratings ($r = 0.74$). At Burn Centers 1 and 3, however, correlations between physicians' estimates and probit analysis were not nearly so high (0.56 and 0.65, respectively). Similarly, the correlation between physicians' estimates and severity index ratings was highest at Burn Center 1 ($r = 0.89$), where the index was developed.

Comparison with Survival Rates of Patients

A third test of content validity was the comparison of severity index ratings with actual outcome of care. For this test, data on 6243 burn patients from the National Burn Information Exchange [14] were used. Severity indexes were calculated and divided into eight severity ranges, and survival rates were then calculated for each patient group. Ranges for the higher severity ratings had to be very wide (for example, 40.0-99.9) in order to provide a sufficient number of observations per cell for each of five burn centers. Table 9.8

TABLE 9.8

Relationship between Survival Rates and Severity Index Ratings

Severity Index	Survival Rate (%) by Burn Center					All Centers
	A	B	C	D	E	
0– 3.9	100	99.4	99.5	97.5	100	98.4
4.0– 7.9	100	97.9	94.8	85.6	100	94.3
8.0–11.9	97.8	96.8	97.2	79.6	97.0	94.4
12.0–15.9	91.9	90.8	87.1	86.9	83.8	87.9
16.0–19.9	92.9	89.3	86.6	77.6	92.3	87.6
20.0–27.9	70.7	74.7	66.3	62.0	83.3	70.7
28.0–39.9	60.9	54.5	39.9	35.6	45.9	49.1
40.0–99.9	9.1	14.3	4.3	*	*	9.9

*There were not enough observations in these cells to develop reliable estimates.

shows the results. Except where noted, each cell represents at least 30 patients.

Survival rate is more or less monotonically related to the severity index in the column combining all five burn centers and approximates monotonicity in the five individual sites (see Table 9.8). Burn Center B shows a monotonic relationship. Burn Centers A and E have order reversals between categories four and five. Burn Center C shows an order reversal between the second and third categories. Burn Center D shows an order reversal between the third and fourth categories.

This analysis was performed in 1968, and the comparison with probit analysis was made in 1972. Testing the probit analysis model against the 6243 records would have been desirable. However, these records of actual cases were no longer available.

DISCUSSION

This study, completed in 1969, includes the first known use of a multiattribute utility model to measure health or health service needs. The results of the study suggest that such a model can predict the behavior of the persons who develop it and, very possibly, the behavior of other decision makers in similar situations. Its success in predicting behavior in settings other than the one in which it was developed suggests that there is a common wisdom among physicians around which decision models can be built.

The relatively low correlation (0.74) in one test setting occurred in a hospital in which another model using different severity criteria had been developed and was in operation. That model correlated better than the severity index model with decisions of physicians in that care setting. Does this suggest that the physicians involved use slightly different criteria in their decision making, or does it suggest that decision makers can be influenced by the very models built to aid them? If the latter is the case, it points to both the existing opportunities and the critical need for quality in models of this type.

Results of the present study suggest that it may be feasible to use models of this nature to ascertain medically underserved areas [15] and, possibly, to measure health status—an approach that would not require the major investments in data collection and processing that characterize other approaches to these problems. If the multi-attribute utility model works it can provide a quick and easy index to aid in a number of health service decisions.

REFERENCES

1. J. R. Miller, A Systematic Procedure for Assessing the Worth of Complex Alternatives. Report MTR-260, Defense Documentation Center #ESD-TR-67-90, 1967.

2. D. H. Gustafson, G. K. Pai, and G. C. Kramer, "A 'Weighted Aggregate' Approach to R&D Project Selection," IEEE Trans. 3 (March 1971).

3. R. Daneshgar, G. P. Huber, and D. L. Ford, "An Empirical Comparison of Five Utility Models for Predicting Job Preferences." Firm and Market Workshop Paper No. 6822, Social Systems Research Institute, University of Wisconsin, 1969.

4. G. P. Huber, V. K. Sahey, and D. L. Ford, "A Study of Subjective Evaluation Models." Firm and Market Workshop Paper No. 6817, Social Systems Research Institute, University of Wisconsin, 1968.

5. Kenneth MacCrimmon, "An Overview of Multiple Objective Decision Making." In J. Cochrane and M. Zeleny (eds.), Multiple Criteria Decision Making. Columbia, S.C.: University of South Carolina Press, 1973.

6. G. P. Huber, "Multi-attribute Utility Models: A Review of Field and Field-like Studies." Internal report, University of Wisconsin, 1972.

7. A. L. Delbecq, A. Van de Ven, and D. H. Gustafson, Group Techniques for Program Planning: A Guide to Nominal Groups and Delphi Process. Chicago: Scott, Foresman, 1975.

8. P. C. Fishburn, "Methods of Estimating Additive Utilities," Mgmt. Sci. 13 (March 1967):435.

9. G. K. Pai, "A Comparison of Three Methods of Determining a Utility Function for Money." Unpublished master's thesis, University of Wisconsin, 1970.

10. L. D. Phillips, W. L. Hays, and W. Edwards, "Conservatism in Complex Probability Inference," IEEE Trans. Hum. Fact. Electron. 7 (1966):7.

11. J. C. Nunnally, Psychometric Theory. New York: McGraw-Hill, 1967.

12. B. A. Waisbren, M. Stern, and G. E. Collentine, "Comparison of Methods of Burn Treatment by Probit Analysis." St. Mary's Hospital Burn Center, Milwaukee, Wis., 1974.

13. R. Keeny, "Multidimensional Utility Functions: Theory, Assessment and Application." Operations Research Center Technical Report No. 43, Cambridge, Mass., 1969.

14. I. Feller, "The National Burn Information Exchange, An Information System for Burns." Internal report, Burn Center, University of Michigan Medical School, Ann Arbor, 1966.

15. Bureau of Community Health Services, DHEW, "Report to Congress on the Criteria to Be Used for Designation of Medically Underserved Areas and Population Groups as Required by the Health Maintenance Organization Act of 1973." Unpublished report, Bureau of Community Health Services, 1974.

10

LINEAR PROGRAMMING

INTRODUCTION

This article is an example of a resource allocation problem in a hospital setting. The author utilized a linear programming model to solve the problem of finding the optimal way to use resources in accomplishing objectives. The objective function's purpose is to determine the maximum number of surgical patients that can be admitted and treated in a hospital, given the fixed capacities of resources to produce the service required. The constraints are the operating room hours, the recovery room hours, and the surgical service bed days. The author also cites many more applications of linear programming within the hospital setting.

Introduction to Technique

Of all management science techniques, linear programming is one of the most widely used. Linear programming was first introduced by George Dantzig in 1947 as a way of finding the optimal allocation of resources subject to constraints.

In general, linear programming deals with the maximization or minimization of a linear objective function of variables subject to one or more linear constraint functions of the variables.

The objective function is usually expressed as,

Maximize/minimize: $X_0 = C_1 X_1 + C_2 X_2 + C_3 X_3 + \cdots + C_n X_n$

subject to the following constraints:

$$A_{11}X_1 + A_{12}X_2 + \cdots + X_{1n}X_n \leq = \text{ or } \geq b_1$$

$$A_{21}X_1 + A_{22}X_2 + \cdots + A_{2n}X_n \leq = \text{ or } \geq b_2$$

$$A_{m1}X_1 + A_{m2}X_2 + \cdots + A_{mn}X_n \leq = \text{ or } \geq b_m$$

The X_j variables are the decision variables, whose values are determined when the linear programming model is solved. A_{ij}, C_j, and b_i are parameters. The objective function and constraints are linear representations of the decision to be made. The contributions of each activity are proportional to the level of the activity. The Simplex Method is commonly used to solve linear programs.

REFERENCES

Feldstein, M. S., Economic Analysis for Health Services Efficiency. Chicago: Markham, 1975.

Llewellyn, R. W., Linear Programming. New York: Holt, Rinehart and Winston, 1964.

Taha, H. A., Operations Research: An Introduction. New York: Macmillan, 1971.

Zionts, S., Linear Programming. Englewood Cliffs, N.J.: Prentice-Hall, 1973.

Baligh, H., and D. J. Laughhunn, "An Economic and Linear Model of the Hospital," Health Services Research 4 (Winter 1969):293-303.

Hulbert, F., "Minimizing the Hospital Patient Cost Through Linear Programming." Paper presented at the 31st National Meeting of the Operations Research Society of America, New York, May 1967.

Shuman, L., J. P. Young, and E. Naddar, "Manpower Mix for Health Services: A Prescriptive Regional Planning Model," Health Services Research 6 (Summer 1971): 103.

Wandel, S., "A Combined Linear Programming and Simulation Model for Aggregate Planning and Scheduling of Nurses in Hospitals," 41st National Meeting of the ORSA, April 1972.

THE APPLICATION OF LINEAR PROGRAMMING TO DECISION-MAKING IN HOSPITALS

William L. Dowling

Many of the decisions an administrator must make in managing his hospital involve the allocation or assignment of personnel and other resources to alternative ends or uses so as to accomplish certain objectives. The allocation of available operating room personnel and facilities to meet the demand for different surgical procedures, and the assignment of available RNs, LPNs, Aides, and Unit Managers to the different tasks which must be performed in caring for patients are examples of this type of decision.

Decisions of this type, called resource allocation decisions, deal with the problem of determining the most efficient way to use resources to accomplish objectives. All such decisions have three common elements. First, the decision-maker has an objective in mind. In the nursing example, the objective may be to determine the nursing staffing pattern that minimizes the cost of meeting the needs of patients on a given nursing unit. Second, there are alternative ways to accomplish the objective. RNs can be assigned to tasks requiring their level of skill or lesser levels of skill. LPNs and Aides can also be assigned in different ways. Unit Managers can be assigned some of the tasks usually performed by nurses. Third, there are constraints on the decision. All essential tasks must be performed. All personnel must be fully utilized. Certain tasks must be performed by RNs. Only so many nurses are available for each shift. When confronted with a problem of this type, the decision-maker seeks the optimal solution. That is, he seeks the solution that maximizes the results that can be produced with a given set of resources, or minimizes the resources that must be used to produce a given result.

Resource allocation decisions are made frequently in hospitals, often by department heads and supervisors guided by established criteria and policies. In many cases, good judgment is all that is required

---

Reprinted with permission from the quarterly journal of the American College of Hospital Administrators, Hospital Administration (now retitled, Hospital and Health Services Administration), Summer 1971, pp. 66-75.

to find a solution that is optimal or near-optimal. However, in more complex situations, where there are many resources, many tasks, many alternative ways of assigning resources to tasks, and many constraints on the acceptable assignments, it is difficult to make optimal decisions. In such situations, especially where non-optimal decisions result in a substantial waste of resources, more structured decision-making techniques should be considered.

One such decision-making technique is mathematical programming. Mathematical programming involves the formulation of a mathematical model to represent the resource allocation problem. The problem is then solved by a process (usually performed by a computer) of systematically searching for the optimal solution from among the alternative feasible solutions. Linear programming [1-6] is the simplest form of mathematical programming, but because many problems can be approximated by linear equations or functions, it is applicable in a great variety of situations. Linear programming has been used successfully in industry since the late 1940s, and in recent years it has been applied with increasing frequency to hospital problems.

THE ADMINISTRATOR'S ROLE

The administrator need not know the mathematics required to transform a problem into a set of equations or the computer technology required to obtain a solution. Industrial engineers and operations researchers have the required training. However, it is important that the administrator be able to recognize problems, such as those discussed above, which are amenable to solution by linear programming. Otherwise, opportunities to improve hospital efficiency may be missed. The administrator is also the person to specify the objectives of problems and to point out the institutional demands and policies that constrain their solution.

Specifying the objective function of a linear programming problem is often the most difficult aspect of applying this technique, and it is here that the expertise and judgment of the administrator are critical. If the specification of the objective of a problem does not reflect the real objectives of the hospital, the solution may impede or be irrelevant to the attainment of these objectives. The objective function must be expressed in terms of a set of decision variables (i.e., variables over which the hospital has control and to which the resources to be allocated can be related). For example, if a firm seeks to maximize profit, the objective function might express total profit (to be maximized) as a function of the unit profits of each of its products. The decision to be made is the amount of each product the firm should produce to maximize profit, given its fixed resources. Alternatively, the objective function might express total cost (to be minimized) as a function of the unit costs of producing a product by alternative processes. The decision to be made is the amount of each process the firm should use to minimize cost, given that it must produce so many units of the product.

A HYPOTHETICAL HOSPITAL PROBLEM

The concepts of linear programming can be illustrated by a hypothetical hospital problem. Note that in applying this technique it is necessary to

1. specify an objective function in terms of a set of decision variables,
2. specify the relationships between resources and decision variables,
3. specify the constraints that limit the acceptable values of the decision variables.

Suppose an administrator wishes to determine the maximum number of surgical patients that can be admitted and treated in his hospital during some period of time, given the fixed (in the short-run) capacities of hospital resources to produce the services required by these patients. Assume, for the sake of simplicity, that there are only three types of surgical patients, appendectomies, cholecystectomies, and tonsillectomies, and let x_1, x_2, and x_3 represent the number of each type of patient. Assume, again for simplicity, that there are only three resources that might constrain the number of surgical patients treated, operating rooms, recovery room beds, and surgical service beds, and let c_1, c_2, and c_3 represent the capacity of each resource expressed in terms of units of service (i.e., operating room hours, recovery room bed hours, and surgical service bed days). The decision that must be made is to determine the optimal number of each type of patient to be treated. Therefore, the xs are the decision variables. The relationships between resources and decision variables are the quantities of the different services required to treat the different types of patients. The constraints are the capacities of the different resources.

Since the hospital seeks to maximize the number of surgical patients treated, the objective function may be expressed as follows:

Maximize Surgical Patients = $x_1 + x_2 + x_3$

This equation simply states that total surgical patients is the sum of the number of each of the three types of surgical patients. The objective is to determine the combination of patients that maximizes total patients while at the same time taking into account the constraints imposed by the service requirements of the patients and the service capacities of the resources. More complex objective functions could be specified if different values are associated with different types of patients. For example, more value might be placed on patients who have the most serious illnesses, or who represent the best teaching cases, or who are admitted by certain physicians. In such cases, the objective would be to

$$\text{maximize } V = v_1 x_1 + v_2 x_2 + v_3 x_3$$

with the vs reflecting the benefit or value to the community or hospital associated with each type of patient.

PRODUCTION COEFFICIENTS

Let us assume that the quantities of the different services required to treat each type of patient are as follows:

	x_1	x_2	x_3
Operating room hours	1	2	1
Recovery room bed hours	3	5	1
Surgical service bed days	6	9	2

These values, called input-output or production coefficients, represent the average quantity of each service required by each type of patient.*They can be obtained from hospital records, reports (e.g., the last row of coefficients, which are simply average lengths of stay, can be obtained from PAS reports), or from special studies.

---

*The assumption of linearity, which is central to linear programming, simply means that these coefficients are fixed and independent. That is, (1) there are no economies in treating additional patients (e.g., if six patient days of care are consumed in treating one patient, twelve will be consumed in treating two) and (2) treating more or less of one type of patient does not affect the service requirements of the other types.

MATHEMATICAL EXPRESSION OF THE PROBLEM

Finally, the capacities of the resources for the period of time under consideration can be estimated from past output levels or special studies. Let us assume that

c_1 = 1000 operating room hours
c_2 = 2000 recovery room bed hours
c_3 = 3000 surgical service bed days

All of the information required to formulate the linear programming problem is now available, and the problem may be expressed as follows:

$$\text{Maximize Surgical Patients} = x_1 + x_2 + x_3 \qquad (1)$$
$$\text{subject to} \quad 1x_1 + 2x_2 + 1x_3 \leq 1000 \qquad (2)$$
$$3x_1 + 5x_2 + 1x_3 \leq 2000 \qquad (3)$$
$$6x_1 + 9x_2 + 2x_3 \leq 3000 \qquad (4)$$
$$x_1, x_2, x_3 \geq 0 \qquad (5)$$

Equation 1 is the objective function. Equations 2-4 are constraints that state that the total quantity of each service consumed by the three types of patients cannot exceed (must be equal to or less than) the service capacity of the corresponding resource. Equation 5 gives non-negativity constraints. Obviously, the hospital cannot treat negative numbers of patients, but since the computer does not know this without being instructed, non-negativity constraints must be included in any linear programming problem. The solution to this problem would indicate the combination of patients the hospital should admit and treat to maximize total surgical patients.

To make this problem realistic, many more types of patients and many more resources would be included in the model. In addition, constraints would be added to reflect institutional demands and policies. For example, the model could include constraints to prevent the hospital from exceeding its budget, or to prevent it from exceeding its desired occupancy level, or to require it to treat no less than some minimum number and no more than some maximum number of each type of patient.

The solution of linear programming problems yields two additional types of information which, for some problems, may be more important than the solution values of the decision variables. First, the imputed value or shadow price associated with each resource indicates the increase in the optimum value of the objective function (i.e., in the total number of patients treated) that could be obtained by increasing the capacity of the resource. For example, the shadow prices for this problem would indicate the number of additional surgical patients that could be treated with a one unit increase in the capacity of each of the resources. Positive shadow prices are given only for resources that are binding or constraining at the optimal solution. If, for example, the optimal number of patients fully used the capacity of the operating rooms but not that of the surgical service beds, the shadow price attached to the former would be positive, and that attached to the latter would be zero, since increasing the supply of beds would not enable the hospital to treat any more patients. This information could be useful in facility and personnel planning.

ANOTHER PRACTICAL APPLICATION

Second, the opportunity cost or tradeoff associated with each decision variable indicates the decrease in the optimal value of the objective function (i.e., in the total number of patients treated) that would be required by an increase in the decision variable. That is, starting from the optimal combination of surgical patients, how many patients would have to be discharged to make room for an additional patient of each type? This information could serve as the basis for scheduling admissions.

Finally, sensitivity analysis can be used to evaluate the effects of hypothetical or planned changes in hospital policies. This technique is applied after the optimal solution has been found to determine the impact on the optimum values of the objective function and decision variables of changes in individual input-output coefficients and constraints. Sensitivity analysis would allow the administrator to ask, "How many more surgical patients could be treated if another operating room was added, or if the average length of stay of appendectomy patients was reduced by one day, or if tonsillectomy patients were taken directly back to the nursing units after surgery?" Sensitivity analysis is also useful in determining the degree of accuracy required in specifying the input-output coefficients and constraints. If the optimal solution is sensitive to small changes in these values, sufficient data must be collected to determine them quite accurately, if not, estimates will give satisfactory results.

A VARIETY OF USES FOR LINEAR PROGRAMMING

Linear programming has been applied to a variety of hospital problems. Balintfy [7-9] has used linear programming in hospital menu planning. The problem is to minimize the cost of meals subject to constraints on the nutritional adequacy, balance, frequency, and portion size of the foods combined to make up meals. Gue [10] has conducted further work in this area. Wolfe [11] has applied linear programming to the assignment of nursing personnel to the activities that must be performed on a nursing unit. The problem is to determine the assignment pattern that minimizes personnel cost subject to a number of constraints reflecting the value of assigning different categories of personnel to different tasks and the requirement that every task be performed. Kant [12] has suggested the use of linear programming in planning the allocation and location of hospitals in one of the territories in Russia so as to provide optimal preventive medicine service for the population. Earickson [13] has demonstrated the potential usefulness of linear programming in selecting a location for a branch of Cook County Hospital in Chicago so as to minimize the aggregate cost of travel by users of the branch. He suggests that the same approach could be used to determine the optimal number and location of neighborhood health clinics. Holland [14] has worked on developing methods to evaluate the location of hospitals in rural areas. Park and Freeman [15] have used linear programming to determine the most effective allocation of community health resources.

Feldstein [16] has applied linear programming to the problem of determining the combination of cases that should be treated by hospitals in the British National Health Service. Hospital output is measured by the number of cases treated in each of nine medical specialties. Four inputs—bed days, doctors, nurses, and purchasables—are included in the model. The objective is to maximize the weighted sum of the number of cases treated, subject to the quantities of inputs available during the planning year. The solution indicates the number of cases of each type that should be treated, the excess quantity of each nonconstraining input, and the shadow price of each constraining input.

Hobbs and his associates [17] have applied linear programming to analyze the admission scheduling policy at Presbyterian-University hospital. The objective is to determine the number of patients in each of 24 elective surgery categories that should be admitted per month to maximize the total number of surgery patients treated. Bed capacity and operating room capacity constraints, as well as constraints reflecting hospital policies concerning occupancy levels, specialization requirements, and teaching requirements are included in the model. The problem is also solved for the objective of minimizing the cost of treating surgery patients. Dantzig [18] and Resh [19] have also applied linear programming to the admission scheduling problem.

THE BALIGH AND LAUGHHUNN STUDY

Baligh and Laughhunn [20] have developed a linear economic model for planning hospital admissions, although they make no attempt to operationalize the model. The model is based on the concept of "equivalence classes" of patients, each of which is defined by a set of requirements for hospital services and by a value or weight assigned by the hospital to treating the class of patients. The problem is to maximize the weighted sum of the number of patients treated, subject to available resources, budget, and hospital policy regarding the minimum number of patients in each class that are required for teaching purposes.

Dowling [21] has applied linear programming to model the production of patient care by a 275 bed community hospital. Hospital output is measured by the number of patients treated in each of 55 PAS diagnostic categories. The treatment of each category is viewed as a separate production process requiring a specific combination of diagnostic and therapeutic services. The constraints on output are the capacities of the hospital departments to produce these services. The problem is to determine the mix and volume of patients that maximize the total number of patients treated per year, subject to the capacities of the departments and to certain maximum and minimum patient requirements. Actual hospital output is compared to optimal output as a measure of hospital efficiency. Gurfield and Clayton [22] have demonstrated the value of linear programming in planning the expansion or reorganization of hospital facilities to meet changes in patient load or innovations in patient care by modeling the care of adult and pediatric cardiac patients at U.C.L.A. Hospital.

REFERENCES

(Citations with identifying numbers have appeared in Abstracts of Hospital Management Studies.)

1. Robert Dorfman, "Mathematical or 'Linear' Programming," American Economic Review 43 (December 1953).

2. A. Henderson and R. Schlaifer, "Mathematical Programming," Harvard Business Review 32 (May-June 1954).

3. William Baumol, Economic Theory and Operations Analysis (2nd ed.). Englewood Cliffs, N.J.: Prentice-Hall, 1965, pp. 70-128 and 270-94.

4. George Dantzig, Linear Programming and Extensions. Princeton, N. J.: Princeton University Press, 1963.

5. R. Dorfman, P. Samuelson, and R. Solow, Linear Programming and Economic Analysis. New York: McGraw-Hill, 1964.

6. Saul Gass, Linear Programming: Methods and Applications. New York: McGraw-Hill, 1964.

7. Joseph Balintfy, "Linear Programming Models for Menu Planning." In H. E. Smalley and J. R. Freeman (eds.), Hospital Industrial Engineering. New York: Reinhold, 1966, pp. 402-08.

8. J. Balintfy and E. Vetter, "Computer Writes Menus," Hospital Topics 42 (June 1964).

9. J. Balintfy and E. Nebell, "Experiments with Computer-Assisted Menu Planning," Hospitals 40 (June 16, 1966).

10. Ronald Gue, Mathematical Programming in Institutional Menu Planning. Southern Methodist University, Dallas, Texas, 1968 (DI2-5327).

11. Harvey Wolfe, A Multiple Assignment Model for Staffing Nursing Units. Operations Research Division, The Johns Hopkins Hospital, Baltimore, Md., 1964 (NU1-3694).

12. V. I. Kant, "The Use of Linear Programming in Perspective Planning of Preventive Medicine," Zdravookhranenie (Kishinev, USSR), No. 2, 1964.

13. Robert Earickson, "The Case for Decentralizing Cook County Hospital," Working Paper #111.4, Chicago Regional Hospital Study, January 1968 (AR-2102).

14. Max Holland, "An Efficient Allocation of General Hospital Facilities in Rural Areas: A Computer Algorithm Methodology," Ph.D. dissertation, Clemson University, Clemson, S.C., 1970 (AR0-5617).

15. K. Park and J. Freeman, Community Health Resource Allocation with Linear Programming Methods. Health Systems Research Division, University of Florida, Gainesville, 1969 (MN-2040).

16. Martin Feldstein, Economic Analysis for Health Services Efficiency. Chicago: Markham, 1962. Pp. 168-82.

17. Terrance Hobbs et al., "Linear Programming as Applied to the Admissions of Elective Surgery Patients at Presbyterian-University Hospital," Department of Industrial Engineering, University of Pittsburgh, Pittsburgh, Pa., 1963; and "Some Mathematical Techniques Applicable to Presbyterian-University Hospital," Department of Industrial Engineering, University of Pittsburgh, Pittsburgh, Pa., 1963 (MN-1004).

18. George Dantzig, A Hospital Admission Problem. Operations Research House, Stanford University, Palo Alto, Calif., 1970 (AM1-5533).

19. Michael Resh, "Mathematical Programming of Admissions Scheduling in Hospitals," Ph.D. dissertation, Johns Hopkins University, Baltimore, Md., 1967 (AM-2011).

20. H. Baligh and H. Laughhunn, "An Economic and Linear Model of the Hospital," Health Services Research 4 (Winter 1969).

21. William Dowling, "A Linear Programming Approach to the Analysis of Hospital Production," Ph.D. dissertation, University of Michigan, Ann Arbor, 1970 (MN2-6294).

22. R. Gurfield and J. Clayton, Analytic Hospital Planning: A Pilot Study of Resource Allocation Using Mathematical Programming in a Cardiac Unit. Rand Corporation, Memorandum RM-5893-RC, April 1969 (SC1-6837).

Bibliographic citations for this commentary were compiled through the resources of the Cooperation Information Center for Hospital Management Studies at the University of Michigan. Subscriptions to Abstracts of Hospital Management Studies, the quarterly publication of the Information Center, are available at $25 per year from the Center at Room 420, City Center Building, 220 East Huron Street, Ann Arbor, Mich. 48108.

11

INTEGER PROGRAMMING

INTRODUCTION

This paper describes an integer programming model which determines an optimal mix of staff for a large psychiatric hospital. Staff activities are classified into interchangeable and noninterchangeable activities. Psychiatrists, psychologists, social workers, mental health associates, RNs, and LPNs were asked to rank the staff categories according to the appropriateness for the performance of the interchangeable therapeutic activities. The ranking formed the basis for index scores, which together with the time each staff member spent on performing therapeutic activities served as the objective function of the model. Constraints were imposed on the model to limit expenses, numbers of staff categories, and the time spent on performing administrative, supervisory, and therapeutic activities.

Introduction to Technique

The general structure of integer programming differs from that of linear programming in only one conceptual respect: some or all of the variables in the model are restricted to discrete or integer values. If all the variables concerned have integer values, the algorithms are known as pure-integer programs. If only some of the variables in the models have discrete values, while the rest have continuous values, such algorithms are known as mixed-integer programs.

Integer programming methods can be divided into: a) cutting methods, and b) search methods. Techniques such as fractional algorithm, applicable to pure integer problems, and mixed algorithm, applicable to mixed-integer problems, are categorized under cutting methods. "Branch and bound" algorithm is classified under search methods.

REFERENCES

Connor, P. J., "A Hospital Inpatient Classification System," Ph.D. dissertation, Industrial Engineering Department, Johns Hopkins University, 1960.

Hillier, F., and G. Lieberman, Operations Research (2nd ed.). San Francisco: Holden-Day, 1974.

Shuman, L. J., P. Hardwick, and G. A. Huber, "Location of Ambulatory Care Centers in a Metropolitan Area," Health Services Research 8 (Summer 1973):121-38.

Zionts, S., Linear and Integer Programming. Englewood Cliffs, N.J.: Prentice-Hall, 1974.

A STAFF ALLOCATION MODEL FOR
MENTAL HEALTH FACILITIES

Joseph P. Lyons
and
John P. Young

This article describes a model for allocating staff within a large psychiatric hospital. The model provides an objective framework within which one can test alternative staff operating policies before making critical decisions concerning the employment of one category of personnel as opposed to another. It is based on objective data describing patient needs and staff functioning patterns, rather than subjective opinions concerning staff deployment. Besides being useful for the short-term deployment of staff

---

Research supported by training grant no. 5T 31MH 12813 from the Alcoholism, Drug Addiction, and Mental Health Administration, DHEW. Reprinted with permission from Health Services Research 11, No. 1 (Spring 1976). Copyright 1976 by the Hospital Research and Educational Trust, 840 North Lakeshore Drive, Chicago, Ill. 60611.

and budgetary resources, it can also be used as a long-
range planning tool for testing modifications in policy
decisions and budget proposals. The algorithm employed,
mixed-integer linear programming, is readily available;
computer costs and running time are relatively minimal.

The setting for this research was Springfield Hospital Center, a state psychiatric hospital of approximately 2,000 beds that serves seven counties of central Maryland in addition to parts of northern Baltimore City. At the time the research was initiated, during the early part of 1974, the hospital was involved in a massive reorganization aimed at implementing the concept of "unitization," defined by Abrams [1] as "the process of administrative reorganization of a large hospital into several separate units; usually, each has its own chief, a separate staff and responsibilities, each unit is autonomous; together the several units form a confederation that is supervised by the hospital director or superintendent."

Initial plans called for reorganization into six units, each providing inpatient psychiatric services for a specific geographic area. Each unit would be semiautonomous in that it would admit and discharge its own patients. The units were to be similar in organization, administrative structure, and treatment processes.

A hospital unitization committee, while planning for the anticipated reorganization, was faced with the problem of reallocating staff to meet the aggregate needs of both present and future patients in each unit. This is, of course, a perplexing problem that repeatedly confronts many mental health administrators: the determination, within a fixed budget, of an optimal mix of personnel to be employed in a facility that provides psychiatric services to a defined population and that operates under a set of clinical and administrative constraints. The research discussed here represents the response to a request from the unitization committee for assistance in solving this problem.

The objectives of the study reported here were (1) to structure a descriptive model of the present use of staff that, when combined with professional psychiatric opinions, could become the basis for the development of a normative model for allocation of staff, (2) to develop a staffing model that could be used for staff reallocation by the unitization committee, and (3) to test the use of the model for long-term planning of staff requirements on the unit level. This model would then be modified as necessary to fit each unit and each new setting in which the model was to be applied.

In setting up the study it was assumed (1) that some personnel types are more appropriate than others for the provision of particular therapeutic activities, (2) that the staff can adequately perceive each patient's problems and prescribe therapies to positively affect these problems, (3) that treatment of these problems has a positive (or at least nonnegative) effect on the patient, and (4) that the needs of patients for both custodial and behavioral care can be estimated in terms of hours of care required.

RELATED STUDIES

Initially it was thought that methods developed by Connor [2] and by Wolfe and Young [3, 4] would be suitable for staffing daily care activities on a unit. Connor's methodology was to be used for classifying patients according to identifiable care needs and for determining the total hours of nursing time required to respond to these needs. Wolfe and Young's methodology, based on Connor's classification procedures and using an integer programming format, would then be used to determine the appropriate manpower mix and specific staffing allocations for a basic unit staff, with additional staff drawn from a pool or other units as required.

Although Wolfe and Young's use of integer programming techniques provided a basis for the design of the preliminary model in this research, two difficulties with this approach emerged. First, since Wolfe and Young's model was developed for the allocation of nursing staff in a short-term general hospital, it did not consider the variety of additional personnel types involved in longer-term mental health care or the appropriateness of a particular care assignment. Second, as a result of unitization, each unit was to be administratively semiautonomous, thereby restricting the flow of personnel between units. Personnel assigned to one unit would be required to remain on that unit and provide services for the patients from the unit's geographic area.

Some elements of a staffing methodology for mental hospitals had been developed by others, and these proved to be of great help at Springfield. Staff times required to provide purely custodial care could be estimated using Naleway's SCOPE methodology [5]. This method entails an analysis of each patient's custodial needs for care in several defined areas: medical, social, development, behavioral, and activities of daily living. However, the method cannot be utilized to predict staffing needs for planned therapeutic activities. Certain planned therapeutic activities are defined as being interchangeable between different levels of professionals with varying degrees of effectiveness. Accordingly, in addition to assessing the custodial needs of the patient, the professional must specify the type of personnel required for each hour of planned therapeutic activity. In a parallel work, Binner and Nassimbene [6] developed a classification system for use in the analysis of time utilization for personnel employed on a ward or unit of a psychiatric hospital. This classification system divides professional time into eight functional areas. Although both methods were useful in the present work, neither directly fitted the requirements at Springfield because the staffing models produced by both methods are primarily descriptive, relying on only one individual's judgment concerning staff assignments; neither Naleway nor Binner and Nassimbene attempted to develop a normative model using a composite of professional judgments and constraints reflecting institutional policy decisions.

The normative mathematical programming model of Liebman [7, 8] seemed to fill the methodological gap. This model, developed in 1970, had as its objective to maximize the effective utilization of nursing personnel in a long-term-care setting and used a psychometric Q-sort technique [9] to quantitatively measure existing nursing conceptions of effective utilization of personnel, according to educational level, training, and experience. Although this model, like that of Wolfe and Young, could not be directly applied in a psychiatric hospital because it considered only the utilization of nursing personnel, it provided an additional ingredient for the methodology finally developed at Springfield.

CLASSIFICATION OF STAFF ACTIVITIES

Using the results of Naleway [5] and Binner and Nassimbene [6], a classification system was developed that categorizes activities of staff as either interchangeable or noninterchangeable. Interchangeable activities were those that could be performed by more than one type of personnel, whereas noninterchangeable activities were those that were considered to be within the domain of only one specific personnel type. Naleway considered individually planned program activities to be interchangeable and defined them as "treatment or growth and development activities which are specifically planned for each patient, directed toward his goals and objectives, and documented in written plans" [5]. The following were considered interchangeable activities at Springfield Hospital Center: individual counseling, individual therapy, group therapy, resocialization group, occupational therapy, patient education, poetry therapy, family counseling, addiction counseling, marital counseling, good grooming group, and vocational counseling. Admissions, discharges, behavioral and daily living care activities, reports, records and community liaison activities, administrative time, off-ward activities, clinical supervision, and staff meetings on the unit were considered noninterchangeable activities.

CRITERION FOR OPTIMIZATION

Use of this classification scheme, in conjunction with data obtained through a patient needs survey based on the SCOPE methodology and statistics on admissions and discharges, made it possible to develop a descriptive model of one unit. In this model staff members were assigned to interchangeable activities on the basis of existing staff complement and availability, but the principal contention was that by relaxing this restriction and allowing the manpower complement to vary according to some criterion the descriptive model could be transformed into a normative one.

A psychometric Q-sort technique similar to that employed by Liebman was used to quantify professional judgments concerning alternatives in deployment of staff. A stratified random sample of 30 professionals was chosen from the staff of Springfield Hospital Center. The sample consisted of five groups, each of which included a psychiatrist, psychologist, social worker, mental health associate, registered nurse, and licensed practical nurse. Each member of the sample was asked to rank types of personnel according to appropriateness for the performance of the planned therapeutic activities considered to be interchangeable. Each participating professional was given a scaling board divided into 12 consecutively numbered slots and a deck of 12 cards, with a personnel type listed on each card. The personnel types were: psychiatrist; psychologist; master's level social worker; social worker assistant; recreation therapist; mental health associate; registered nurse; licensed practical nurse 1,2; licensed practical nurse 3,4; health aide 1,2; health aide 3,4; and recreation aide. Next the professional was instructed to shuffle through the cards and choose the card he felt represented the most appropriate personnel type for performing the therapy in question. That card was then placed on the board in slot no. 1. He was then asked to select the least appropriate personnel type, and that card was placed in slot no. 12. In a similar manner the second most appropriate personnel type would be placed in slot no. 2 and the second least appropriate would be placed in slot no. 11, and so on.

The rankings were converted into normal deviate scores [10], on the assumption that they were normally distributed, and were subsequently adjusted to an intuitively realistic base of 100. For example, if all 30 professionals ranked one personnel type as most appropriate for the performance of a therapy, then that personnel type would receive a score of 100, that is, 30×1.63 (a normal deviate score) = 48.90×2.045 (multiplier) = 100.

The professionals were also asked to judge which personnel types should not be allowed to provide each therapy. If more than 10 of the professionals indicated that a particular personnel type should

TABLE 11.1

Normalized Appropriateness Indexes, by Personnel Type and Therapeutic Activity (highest possible score = 100, lowest possible score = -999)

Therapeutic Activity	Personnel Type										
	Psychiatrist	Psychologist	MSW	SWA	Rec. Ther.	MHA	RN	LPN 1,2	LPN 3,4	HA 1,2	HA 3,4	Rec. Aide
Individual counseling	24	21	38	25	-999	38	19	1	14	-999	-24	-999
Group therapy	57	78	45	3	-999	15	31	-999	-5	-999	-999	-999
Individual therapy	91	74	46	-999	-999	22	23	-999	-999	-999	-999	-999
Resocialization group	-999	-999	-999	-999	18	30	10	8	26	-19	2	-999
Occupational therapy	-999	-999	-999	-999	92	-999	-999	12	10	21	24	61
Recreational therapy	-999	-999	-999	-999	97	-999	-999	14	11	26	36	69
Patient education	17	4	0	2	-999	29	73	12	38	-999	-10	-999
Poetry therapy	20	37	23	13	-999	40	19	-999	-999	-999	-999	-999
Family counseling	58	61	75	27	-999	35	18	-999	-999	-999	-999	-999
Addiction counseling	61	68	51	12	-999	29	31	-999	-2	-999	-999	-999
Marital counseling	76	75	59	20	-999	24	-999	-999	-999	-999	-999	-999
Good grooming group	-999	-999	-999	-999	-13	20	34	35	47	17	-19	-19
Vocational counseling	-20	24	67	54	-999	55	22	-999	-5	-999	-999	-999

TABLE 11.2

Analysis of Variance Comparing Raters, Therapists, and Therapies

Therapeutic Activity	F Ratio*		Residual Mean Square Error
	Therapist Rating/ Error Score	Rater Type/ Error Score	
Individual counseling	12.02	0.513	0.1814
Group therapy	27.26	0.0132	0.1324
Individual therapy	105.33	0.0703	0.0444
Resocialization group	3.34	0.0212	0.2210
Occupational therapy	50.47	3.41×10^{-13}	0.0712
Recreational therapy	52.09	1.02×10^{-13}	0.0716
Patient education	29.75	8.53×10^{-14}	0.0814
Poetry therapy	10.62	0.0011	0.1439
Family counseling	106.78	0.0034	0.0430
Addiction counseling	70.65	0.0025	0.0518
Marital counseling	94.99	0.0030	0.0480
Good grooming group	20.32	0.0014	0.1165
Vocational counseling	43.16	3.84×10^{-13}	0.0717

*All of the ratios for therapist rating/error score were significant at the 0.01 level for 11, 55 degrees of freedom (1-percent level 2.59). None of the ratios for rater/type error score was significant at the 0.01 level with 5, 55 degrees of freedom (i.e., the 1-percent level of significance is 3.37).

not be allowed to perform a task, then that personnel type would receive a score of -999. Ten was chosen as a logical cutoff point since the tallied data tended to cluster above or below 10. Table 11.1 shows the resultant normal deviate and negative valuation scores and illustrates the perceived appropriateness levels of the 12 personnel types for the performance of the 13 planned therapeutic activities. Selection of an equal number of raters in each professional category was based on the assumption that the biases exhibited would cancel each other out. In order to estimate the magnitude of the biases of each professional type and to examine the degree of consensus of all raters, an analysis of variance was performed on the ratings. The results of the analysis of variance indicated (0.01 confidence level with 11, 55 d.f.) that there was no significant difference between professional types; that is, the 30 professionals from Springfield Hospital Center could have been chosen at random without regard to the numbers of each professional category represented and the data would not have been significantly different. Also, the professional opinions concerning the appropriateness of a therapist for the performance of a therapy were significantly different from those that could have been generated randomly.

F scores for each therapy were also examined. These scores are shown in Table 11.2. All of the therapist rating/error score F ratios were significant at the 0.01 confidence level, although some were much larger than others. None of the rater type/error score F ratios was significant at the 0.01 confidence level. These F ratios were interpreted as representing the degree of consensus among the raters concerning the appropriateness of all personnel types for the performance of therapies, that is, an appropriateness index that approaches 100 represents a high degree of consensus. Consequently, each appropriateness index not only reflects the suitability of each personnel type for a therapy, but also illustrates the consensus level of all types of raters.

MATHEMATICAL FORMULATION OF AN ALLOCATION MODEL

The above classification and appropriateness criteria were used in developing a mathematical formulation of an allocation model. The allocation model included current operating constraints relating to the utilization of staff time for custodial and planned therapeutic activities, together with a variety of other clinical and budgetary restrictions. The formulation used a mixed-integer linear programming format consisting of mathematical statements of constraint equations as well as an objective function; the branch and bound algorithm for mixed problems [11, 12] was used as a solution technique.

Objective Function

The objective of this allocation model is to maximize the aggregate appropriateness score of all personnel performing interchangeable planned therapeutic activities. This score is represented by the dependent variable Z. Mathematically, the objective function can be stated as follows:

$$\text{MAX } Z = \sum_{i=1}^{I} \sum_{k=1}^{K} b_{ik} X_{ik}$$

where b_{ik} = appropriateness index score of personnel type i performing therapeutic activity k (i = 1, ..., I; k = 1, ..., K)

X_{ik} = number of hours personnel type i spends performing therapeutic activity k per time period

Constraints

The objective function is subject to the constraints shown in Eqs. 1-5 below:

$$\sum_{k=1}^{K} X_{ik} + V_i - [U_i - (C_i + M_i)] A_i F_i \leq 0 \qquad (1)$$

with $X_{ik} \geq 0$ and continuous and $F_i \geq 0$ and integer and

where V_i = amount of time per time period required of personnel type i to perform the following noninterchangeable activities: admissions, discharges, behavioral and daily living care activities, reports, records and community liaison, and additional administrative activities

U_i = percentage of time that personnel type i will normally spend in unit activities

C_i = percentage of time that personnel type i will normally spend in giving or receiving clinical supervision

M_i = percentage of time that personnel type i will normally spend attending staff meetings on the unit

A_i = average number of hours worked per time period by personnel type i

F_i = total number of personnel type i to be employed on the unit

$$F_i \leq T_i \qquad (2)$$

where T_i = upper limit of the number of personnel i that are available

$$\sum_{i=1}^{I} X_{ik} = D_k \qquad (3)$$

where D_k = number of hours of therapy k demanded per time period being considered

$$\sum_{i \in P} C_i A_i F_i - \sum_{i \notin P} C_i A_i F_i \geq 0 \qquad (4)$$

where $\sum_{i \in P} C_i A_i F_i$ = number of therapy hours per time period allocated for the provision of clinical supervision by those personnel types belonging to a set P of providers of clinical supervision, for example, psychiatrists, psychologists, and master's level social workers

$\sum_{i \notin P} C_i A_i F_i$ = number of therapy hours per time period required by those not in set P who need clinical supervision, such as RNs, LPNs, mental health associates, social worker assistants, and health aides

$$\sum_{i=1}^{I} S_i (1 + Y_i) F_i \leq B \qquad (5)$$

where S_i = salary per time period of personnel type i

B = total personnel budget available per time period

Y_i = fringe benefits received by personnel type i (a percentage)

The above model is a mixed-integer linear programming problem with IK continuous variables (X_{ik}S) as well as I integer variables (F_iS); in addition, there are 2I + K + 2 constraints.

A PILOT STUDY

The above notions were illustrated by considering the problem of planning for the allocation of staff within the Springfield Tricounty Unit, a 55-bed unit that was to provide inpatient psychiatric services for the citizens of three central Maryland counties: Howard, Carroll,

TABLE 11.3

Distribution of Time Spent in Noninterchangeable Activities, by Personnel Type

Personnel Type	Total Hours per Month Required for Noninterch. Activities* (V_i)	Percent of Time Spent in Off-Ward Activities ($100 - U_i$)	Percent of Time Spent in Clinical Supervision (C_i)	Percent of Time Spent in Staff Meetings (M_i)
Psychiatrist	93	15	16	15
Psychologist	0	25	16	0
MSW	0	15	16	0
SWA	112.5	15	2	15
Rec. ther.	0	20	2	0
MHA	136	15	2	15
RN	251	5	2	15
LPN 1,2	692	0	0	0
LPN 3,4	0	0	2	0
HA 1,2	1038	0	0	0
HA 3,4	692	0	0	0
Rec. aide	0	0	0	0

*Admissions and discharges; behavioral and daily living care activities; reports, records, and community liaison; and additional administrative activities.

TABLE 11.4

Total Number of Hours of Planned
Therapeutic Activities per Month

Therapeutic Activity	Number of Hours per Month (D_k)
All	631
Individual counseling	476
Group therapy	21
Individual therapy	9
Resocialization group	22
Occupational therapy	17
Recreational therapy	42
Patient education	8
Poetry therapy	1
Family counseling	17
Addiction counseling	0
Marital counseling	0
Good grooming group	13
Vocational counseling	5

and Frederick. In 1974 its average admission rate (and its discharge rate) was 30 patients per month, or approximately one per day. Staff activities were classified as either interchangeable or noninterchangeable according to the previously mentioned classification system. Table 11.3 shows the distribution of time spent in noninterchangeable activities for each personnel type. The estimated times for behavioral and living care activities were determined by applying the SCOPE methodology directly. Estimated times for the remaining noninterchangeable activities were obtained through observation and activity analysis of staff. (Since the figures in Table 11.3 reflect the existing treatment and administration philosophy, applications to different settings must depend on data that reflect the philosophies of those settings.)

While the needs of patients for behavioral intervention and daily living care were being inventoried, the required number of hours of planned therapeutic activities (interchangeable) was determined by the unit staff. Table 11.4 is a listing of the number of hours to be provided per month.

Since the allocation model is a macro model to be used by the administrator or director in planning for the hiring and deployment of staff, it may be based on expected values for the parameters involved. Accordingly, average monthly salary levels, as shown in Table 11.5, were taken from State of Maryland salary structures as of July 1972. The figures in this table represent the third level in the average pay schedule for each personnel type and include a 15-percent adjustment for fringe benefits.

The allocation model has as its objective the maximization of the appropriate use of staff for interchangeable therapeutic activities, given noninterchangeable clinical and administrative activity constraints. Table 11.6 illustrates the results of applying the allocation model to the Tricounty Unit setting as it existed in 1974. In this application the number of personnel was constrained at the 1974 level and mix. In addition to the personnel listed in Table 11.6, the staff included 13 health aides and one recreation aide, but no interchangeable therapeutic activities were assigned to them. The resultant appropriateness score was 14,935 units. This score represents an optimal value of the objective function for the Tricounty Unit under prevailing conditions. Given the 1974 staff level and mix, all of the planned therapeutic activities could be performed without resorting to the use of overtime by any personnel type.

However, at the time of the pilot study, four personnel types (psychiatrist, social worker assistant, MHA, and RN) regularly spent a total of 38 hours per month per person more than the standard

TABLE 11.5

Average Monthly Salary, by Personnel Type

Personnel Type	Monthly Salary in dollars $[S_i(1 + Y_i)]$
Psychiatrist	2360
Psychologist	1573
MSW	1376
SWA	983
Recreational therapist	983
MHA	915
RN	1130
LPN 1,2	806
LPN 3,4	838
HA 1,2	620
HA 3,4	746
Recreational aide	668

TABLE 11.6

Allocation of Planned Therapeutic Activities among Personnel Types on the Basis of 1974 Personnel Mix and Total Hours of Planned Therapeutic Activities Listed in Table 11.4 (total appropriateness score = 14 935 units; monthly budget = $23 400)

Therapeutic Activity	Personnel Type (Number)						Total Hours
	Psychi- atrist (1)	SWA (1)	Rec. Ther. (1)	MHA (3)	RN (2)	LPN 1,2 (6)	
Individual counseling				159		317	476
Group therapy				20	1		21
Individual therapy	1			8			9
Resocialization group			22				22
Occupational therapy			17				17
Recreational therapy			42				42
Patient education					8		8
Poetry therapy				1			1
Family counseling				17			17
Addiction counseling							0
Marital counseling							0
Good grooming group						13	13
Vocational counseling		5					5

258

requirement of 173 hours per month. Application of the model on the basis of this staff deployment yielded a total appropriateness score of 23,837, but this was obviously achieved under unacceptable working conditions.

The administrative interpretation of these results is that, given the current staff mix and without eliminating noninterchangeable activities or working overtime, the best deployment of personnel time can be obtained by combining the fixed amounts of time given in Table 11.3 and the hours of planned therapeutic activities as depicted in Table 11.4. In this application the hours of staff time were sufficient to perform the noninterchangeable as well as interchangeable planned therapeutic activities. This may not be the case in all applications. The budget, although not a binding constraint in this application, was fixed at $23,400 per month.

In order to take advantage of the prescriptive potential of the model, the constraints were modified by allowing the number of personnel in each category to vary, and the data were reprocessed using the branch and bound mixed-integer programming algorithm and computer program. In this second application the operating budget was again restricted to $23,400 per month and the level of activity in clinical supervision and noninterchangeable activities remained the same.

As a byproduct of the process of applying the SCOPE standards and performing the necessary activity analysis, a surplus number of personnel in the less highly trained categories was identified. Application of the model made it possible to determine the number of these surplus positions that should be converted into more highly trained professionals in order to provide the highest possible level of planned therapeutic activities.

The reallocation of planned therapeutic activities is detailed in Table 11.7. Allowing the number of personnel in each category to vary distinctly modified the therapeutic assignments for the various personnel types and increased the aggregate appropriateness score from 14,935 units to 28,060 units. By comparing Table 11.7 with Table 11.6 one can note the change in staff mix: one psychologist, one master's level social worker, and one mental health associate were added and two LPNs were dropped. The recommended changes also made it possible to reduce the number of health aides from 13 to 10 and to eliminate the one recreational aide. It should be noted that the recommended changes resulted in a more appropriate allocation of highly trained personnel to provide the planned therapeutic activities without sacrificing the hours and manpower needed to provide daily living care.

TABLE 11.7

Allocation of Planned Therapeutic Activities among Personnel Types on the Basis of Modified Staff Mix and Total Hours of Planned Therapeutic Activities Listed in Table 11.4 (total appropriateness score = 28 060 units; monthly budget = $23 400)

Therapeutic Activity	Psychiatrist (1)	Psychologist (1)	MSW (1)	SWA (1)	Rec. Ther. (1)	MHA (4)	RN (2)	Total Hours
Individual counseling		33	116	5		322		476
Group therapy		21						21
Individual therapy	1	8						9
Resocialization group					22			22
Occupational therapy					17			17
Recreational therapy					42			42
Patient education							8	8
Poetry therapy		1						1
Family counseling		17						17
Addiction counseling								0
Marital counseling								0
Good grooming group						12	1	13
Vocational counseling			5					5

APPLICATION OF THE MODEL TO NEW TRICOUNTY UNIT

Further reorganization at Springfield Hospital Center led to the expansion of the Tricounty Unit to three buildings with a total inpatient census of 125 patients in 1974. This expansion was based on recommendations made by the unitization committee in an attempt to accommodate clients from the three counties housed in the past in other units because of a shortage of beds. Staffing of the new Tricounty Unit was also based on committee recommendations and occurred while the allocation model discussed here was still being developed and validated using earlier Tricounty Unit data. Therefore, although there was no opportunity to prescribe staff allocation in advance, it became clear that the model should be applied to the expanded setting, so that the hospital administrator would be able to make changes in staff mix where appropriate.

This application of the staff allocation model once again included a patient needs survey and an activity analysis of staff functions. The aggregate appropriateness score for the expanded Tricounty Unit, based on existing staff mix, was 61,836 units; this score reflected an increase in patient load from 55 to 125 and an increase in operating budget from $23,400 to $44,840 per month. The distribution of interchangeable therapeutic activities among personnel types is shown in Table 11.8. In addition to the personnel listed in the table, the staff included nine LPNs and 24 health aides, none of whom were assigned interchangeable therapeutic activities.

Application of the SCOPE standards to this new setting and translation of these standards into the numbers of full-time personnel needed to provide behavioral and daily living care revealed a deficit of less-trained personnel (Table 11.8). The recommended number of hours of planned therapeutic activities shown in the right-hand column of Table 11.8 reflects a change in program direction from that of the original Tricounty Unit in that more hours of therapy per patient were requested. Only 85 percent of the requested behavioral and daily living care could be provided on the reorganized unit given the current staff. In addition, a check of the number of hours available among the more highly trained professionals revealed that only 85 percent of the recommended hours of planned therapeutic activities could be provided. The latter determination was based on the patient needs survey and the total available hours of all the more highly trained professionals and was not dependent on the specific allocation of personnel types to planned therapeutic activities.

These results suggested that some of the more highly trained positions should be converted into less highly trained positions in order to make up the deficit in hours of behavioral and daily living care. In addition, the number of middle-range professionals (MHAs,

TABLE 11.8

Allocation of Planned Therapeutic Activities among Personnel Types in Expanded Tricounty Unit on the Basis of Available Staff
(total appropriateness score = 61 836; monthly budget = $44 840)

Therapeutic Activity	Psychiatrist (2)	Psychologist (1)	MSW (2)	SWA (3)	Rec. Ther. (1)	MHA (3)	RN (4)	Rec. Aide (1)	Total Hours
Individual counseling			28	342		156			526[a]
Group therapy		33							33
Individual therapy	70	71	53						194
Resocialization group						77			77[b]
Occupational therapy					126				126
Recreational therapy					26			110	136
Patient education						16	4		20[c]
Poetry therapy						5			5
Family counseling			39						39
Addiction counseling									0
Marital counseling			17						17
Good grooming group						38			38[d]
Vocational counseling									0

[a]539 hours were requested.
[b]90 hours were requested.
[c]23 hours were requested.
[d]46 hours were requested.

TABLE 11.9

Allocation of Planned Therapeutic Activities among Personnel Types in Expanded Tricounty Unit on the Basis of "Ideal" Staff Mix (total appropriateness score = 69 078 units; monthly budget = $44 840

Therapeutic Activity	Personnel Type (Number)							Total Hours
	Psychiatrist (2)	Psychologist (1)	MSW (1)	SWA (1)	Rec. Ther. (2)	MHA (5)	RN (5)	
Individual counseling						539		539
Group therapy							33	33
Individual therapy	70	87					37	194
Resocialization group					30	51	9	90
Occupational therapy					126			126
Recreational therapy					136			136
Patient education							23	23
Poetry therapy						5		5
Family counseling			25	14				39
Addiction counseling								0
Marital counseling		17						17
Good grooming group							46	46
Vocational counseling								0

RNs, and SWAs) would have to be increased in order to provide more of the planned therapeutic activities and pick up the slack created by the shifting of positions from more highly trained to less highly trained categories.

In order to determine the staff levels necessary to provide the additional services, the model was reapplied, this time allowing the number of personnel to vary (clinical and budgetary constraints were kept at the same levels). The appropriateness score increased from 61,836 units to 69,078. In addition, the new staff mix allowed for the provision of 100 percent of the needed hours of behavioral and daily living care (provided by less-trained professionals) as well as 100 percent of the requested hours of planned therapeutic activities. The distribution of interchangeable activities is shown in Table 11.9. With this distribution, the nine LPNs and 24 health aides were retained but the recreation aide position was eliminated.

UTILIZATION OF RESULTS

As noted earlier, the Tricounty Unit was expanded into three buildings before the allocation model could be validated; as a result, there was no opportunity to prescribe and implement an optimal staff mix before the expanded unit became operational. However, by applying the model to the expanded Tricounty Unit, once it was operational and the appropriate data were obtained, the unit director, who was also chairman of the unitization committee, was able to use the results to obtain supplementary funding to hire the extra personnel recommended to implement the model. The number of personnel in the less-trained categories, such as health aides, LPNs, and recreational aides, was increased as recommended. The additional personnel made it possible for the more highly trained professionals to provide more planned therapy, since they no longer had to contribute to the behavioral care activities or the daily living care activities. Recommended reductions of staff were left to normal personnel attrition.

The unitization committee was asked to plan for and reorganize five other units at Springfield Hospital Center. Since the allocation model had proven to be useful for evaluating staffing requirements on the expanded Tricounty Unit, it was felt that it would be of considerable value as a conceptual framework for discussion of budgets, patient needs, staff activities, clinical supervision, and the appropriateness of assigning various personnel types in the provision of specific kinds of care. Staffing of the five units was proposed with increased insight as to constraints that applied and the manner in which staff could be allocated so as to maximize the appropriateness of the services delivered. Since then, many of the concepts underlying the structure of the model have been used in numerous clinical and administrative meetings at all levels within the institution to help professionals define their roles for patient care and administrative supervision.

GENERALIZATION OF THE MODEL

The mathematics of the staff allocation model follows a generalized programming format; as a result, it can be applied in many similar settings. However, the clinical and administrative requirements built into the definitions of the variables, constraints, and coefficients will restrict its use to those facilities that meet the following criteria: (1) the facility, unit, or ward is a defined entity whose director has fiscal responsibility for evaluating the trade-off between appropriateness and cost of personnel types; (2) the personnel working within the facility must be accountable to the administrator for a specified percentage of their time—loose arrangements for personnel types to "get the work done" cannot be built into the model; (3) classification of staff activities into mutually exclusive categories (interchangeable and noninterchangeable) must be realistic in the setting being considered; (4) the operating policies of the particular setting must be accurately reflected in the constraint equations; (5) if the setting also includes an outpatient component, verification of the SCOPE standards will have to be performed and the appropriate variables and constraints must be inserted into the model; and (6) the design of the model requires that an appropriateness score be developed for each new setting, using the same procedure as described above, since the index must reflect the peculiarities of the institution in which it is being implemented.

Further experience with the model [13] suggests the following strategy for implementation of the model in a large psychiatric hospital: (1) Apply the model using overall budget as an upper limit and determine the optimum appropriateness score and allocation of activities among personnel. (2) Reapply the model disregarding the budget constraint but using the present number of personnel in each category as an upper limit to determine the number of personnel in each category to be transferred from unit to unit. (3) Transfer the designated personnel to meet the estimated levels of patient care on each unit. Since the model is designed to allocate activities among only the required number of personnel in order to maximize the aggregate appropriateness score, it is possible that surplus positions will be identified. These surplus positions can then be distributed at the discretion of the hospital director. (4) After personnel have been transferred (or at any strategic point in time, such as the end of the fiscal year or just before the submission of a new budget proposal), take an inventory of the total staff complement and note any reduction in staff as a result of attrition. (5) If a reduction has occurred, reapply the data collection instruments and obtain new values for V_i, U_i, C_i, M_i, and D_k. Using the recalculated data base as lower limits, rerun the model using the original budget (or proposed budget) as an upper limit; as a result of this application, employ additional personnel in specific categories if an increase in aggregate appropriateness is noted. As time passes and personnel turnover occurs, reapply steps 4 and 5 as needed. In this way, staffing mix can be varied to approach the optimum.

REFERENCES

1. A. Abrams, "Geographical Unitization in Large State Hospitals," Hosp. Community Psychiatr. 22 (1971):285.

2. R. J. Connor, "A Hospital Inpatient Classification System," doctoral dissertation, Industrial Engineering Department, Johns Hopkins University, 1960.

3. H. Wolfe and J. P. Young, "Staffing the Nursing Unit, Part I: Controlled Variable Staffing," Nurs. Res. 14 (Summer 1965):236.

4. H. Wolfe and J. P. Young, "Staffing the Nursing Unit, Part II: The Multiple Assignment Technique," Nurs. Res. 14 (Fall 1965):299.

5. M. Naleway, Staffing Care of Patients Effectively, SCOPE: A Study of Pennsylvania Mental Hospitals. Harrisburg, Pa.: Pennsylvania Department of Public Welfare, 1970.

6. P. Binner and R. Nassimbene, "An Approach to Workforce Estimating," Research paper, Fort Logan Mental Health Center, Denver, 1972.

7. J. S. Liebman, "The Development and Application of a Mathematical Programming Model of Personnel Allocation in an Extended Care Unit," doctoral dissertation, Department of Operations Research, Johns Hopkins University, 1971.

8. J. S. Liebman, J. P. Young, and M. Bellmore, "Allocation of Nursing Personnel in an Extended Care Facility," Health Serv. Res. 7 (Fall 1972):209.

9. J. C. Nunnally, Psychometric Theory. New York: McGraw-Hill, 1967. P. 55.

10. F. Yates and R. A. Fisher, Statistical Tables for Biological Research. London: Oliver and Boyd, 1963.

11. A. H. Land and R. Dirg, "An Automatic Method of Solving Discrete Programming Problems," Econometrica 28 (July 1960): 497.

12. R. Sharestein, BBMIP Branch and Bound Mixed Integer Programs. IBM Share Users' Library No. 260, D-15.2.005. IBM, 1969.

13. J. P. Lyons, "Staffing Models for a Unitized Mental Hospital," doctoral dissertation, School of Hygiene and Public Health, Johns Hopkins University, 1975.

12

QUEUEING THEORY

INTRODUCTION

This paper illustrates a practical application of queueing theory to the problem of determining the staff size for providing adequate service by a hospital messenger unit.

Messenger service is provided on a first-come, first-served basis by an available messenger, with each messenger viewed as a separate service facility. If no messenger is available, service calls must wait, thus forming a queue. In addition, the messenger unit provides routine service scheduled at specified times. Staffing level is constrained by a) the budget, and b) the desire to provide service with minimum waiting times.

Messenger service is characterized by a Poisson arrival process, an exponential distribution of service times, a first-come, first-served queue discipline, and a service arrangement of multiple messengers acting in parallel.

The central problem is concerned with the expected queue length and the probability that a call will have to wait longer than a specified desired time limit. After determination of these two values, a ratio consisting of the cost of waiting per unit time to the cost of service per unit time is determined. The derived ratio is used to study the effect on the system.

Introduction to Technique

Queueing theory was first developed to telephone traffic congestion with the aim of finding a solution to randomly arising demands placed upon the services supplied by an automatic telephone system. The basic feature of a queueing system is that elements to be served are provided with a service by a service channel. Queues develop by the elements to be served while waiting for the service channels to service them.

The rate of arrival of the elements to be served and the service times are usually specified by frequency distributions. The distributions may be approximations of the observed distributions. The two most common distributions are the Poisson for arrival rates and the exponential for service times.

The behavior of the elements to be served within the system is defined as the queue discipline. Among the components of queue discipline is the order in which the elements to be served enter the system.

Service systems are designed so that average servicing capacity is greater than average arrivals for service, but problems arise because arrivals are random. The object behind queueing theory is to minimize the time spent in the system by both the service channel and the element to be served and also to minimize the costs of the waiting time involved. The output of a queueing problem, therefore, consists of the average length of the queue, the average number of elements waiting in the queue, and average utilization rates of the service channels.

Queueing problems can be solved by use of a mathematical approach or a simulation approach. Among the mathematical approaches available are: a) the use of differential difference equations, b) exponential distribution, c) Erlang distributions, d) integral equations, and e) Markov chains. Simulation involves experimentation on a proposed model using different combinations of arrival and service times.

REFERENCES

Di Roccaferrera, G., Operations Research Models. Cincinnati, Ohio: Southwestern, 1964.

Griffith, J. R., Quantitative Techniques for Hospital Planning and Control. Lexington, Mass.: D. C. Heath, 1972.

Kabak, I., "On Scheduling and Delivery of Babies," Operations Research 20 (January-February 1972):19-23.

McClain, J. O., "Bed Planning Using Queueing Theory Models of Hospital Occupany: A Sensitivity Analysis," Inquiry 13 (June 1976):167-76.

Panico, J. A., Queueing Theory. Englewood Cliffs, N.J.: Prentice-Hall, 1969.

Shonick, W., and J. Jackson, "An Improved Stochastic Model for Occupancy-Related Random Variables in General-Acute Hospitals," Operations Research 21 (July-August 1973):952-65.

HOSPITAL MANPOWER PLANNING
BY USE OF QUEUEING THEORY

Ishwar Gupta
Juan Zoreda
Nathan Kramer

Queueing theory dates back to the work of A. K. Erlang in 1908 [1]; in Erlang's and subsequent work up to approximately 1945, its applications were restricted mainly to operations of telephone systems [2, 3]. Since then it has been extended and applied to a wide variety of phenomena [4-7]. Welch and Bailey [8, 9] pioneered its use in the health field in evaluating appointment systems for an outpatient department, and the study of scheduling systems and waiting times remained its main application in the health field [10] until Haussmann [11] took a different perspective in using it to establish an index of quality of care based on waiting times for service.

The present study illustrates the practical application of queueing theory to a simple problem in manpower planning: how large a staff is required to give adequate service from a hospital messenger unit? The problem is simple enough to be amenable to an analytic solution, and the optimal solution arrived at by the use of queueing theory resulted in a considerable saving to the hospital studied.

Reprinted with permission from Health Services Research 6, No. 1 (Spring 1971). Copyright 1971 by the Hospital Research and Educational Trust, 840 North Lakeshore Drive, Chicago, Ill. 60611.

THE PROBLEM

The function of the messenger unit at Presbyterian-St. Luke's Hospital is to transport patients, specimens and reports, and miscellaneous objects in response to requests from any section of the hospital. Whenever a call is received the dispatcher sends a messenger, if one is available, to provide service. The service facility is arranged in parallel, as shown in Fig. 12.1: messengers M_1, M_2, etc., may be viewed as separate service facilities, and incoming calls are served by any free messenger. If no messenger is free calls must wait and may thus accumulate, forming a queue. Requests are usually all given the same priority, so that service is on a first-come first-served basis.

In addition to these nonroutine services, the unit provides routine services scheduled at definite times. It is easy to estimate the man-hours required to provide this routine service, but it is not a simple task to estimate man-hours to be allocated to nonroutine activities: calls arrive at random, and the time required to complete the service is also random, depending on the type of request. Hiring an unlimited number of messengers would allow immediate service for calls at any time but is obviously not economically sound. On the

FIGURE 12.1

The Queueing System: One Line, Multiple Servers in Parallel

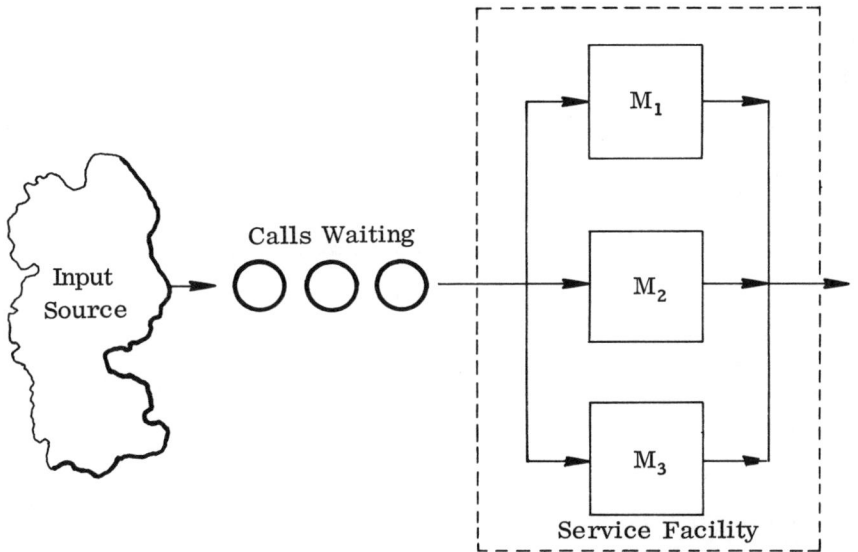

other hand, significant understaffing of the unit would result in poor service. The choice of staffing level must be consistent with acceptable labor costs and with acceptable waiting times for service on calls.

DATA COLLECTION AND ANALYSIS

To apply queueing theory to the problem, it is necessary to know the distributions of arrival time and of service time and the queue discipline (in this case first-come first-served, as indicated). To determine arrival-time and service-time distributions, data were collected from 8 a.m. to 3 p.m.—the busiest part of the day—over a two-week period; the time was noted as each request for service arrived, and also when the messenger departed and returned. The difference between the latter two times was defined as the service time.

Data were obtained for 375 calls for service; these were grouped by time required to perform the service, as shown in Table 12.1. The mean service time was calculated as 11.9 min.; for convenience, 12 min. was taken as an approximation. The distribution of service times is compared in Fig. 12.2 with an exponential distribution calculated from

$$T(>t) = Ne^{-t/m}$$

TABLE 12.1

Distribution of Calls Grouped by Service Time Required

Service Time, Minutes	Number of Calls
0–5	92
>5–10	103
>10–15	82
>15–20	39
>20–25	26
>25–30	8
>30–35	9
>35–40	16

FIGURE 12.2

Distribution of Service Times

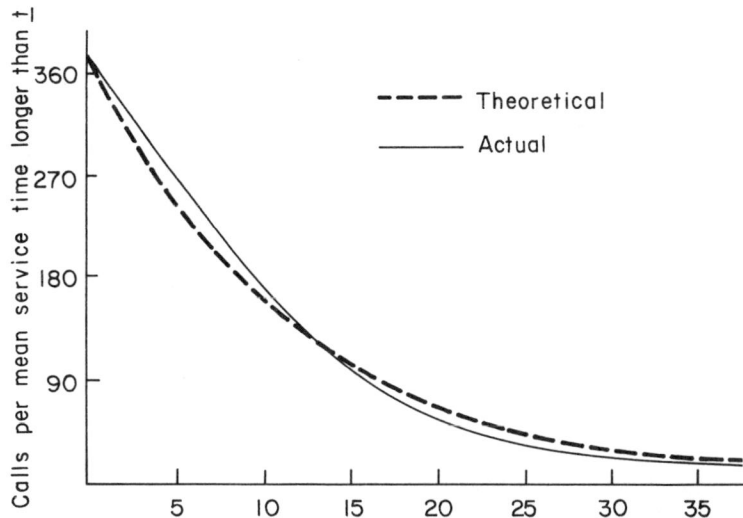

where t is the time in minutes, N is the number of calls observed (375), and m is the mean service time. A goodness-of-fit test gave a χ^2 value of 12.4, while the critical value of χ^2 ($\alpha = .05$, d.f. = 7) is 14.07, indicating that the observed service times conform to the theoretical exponential distribution.

The data were then tabulated by number of calls arriving during each consecutive 12-min. interval of the data-collection period, and the mean number of arrivals per 12-min. interval (that is, per mean service-time interval) was determined to be 1.16. On the assumption of a Poisson arrival process, the theoretical frequency distribution of arrivals per mean service time was calculated as

$$T(x) = \frac{1.16 M e^{-1.16}}{x!}$$

where x = calls per mean service time and M = 315, the number of service-time intervals observed. The observed and the calculated frequency distributions are shown in Table 12.2; a goodness-of-fit test of these distributions gave a χ^2 value of 1.7, comparing well with the critical value for χ^2 of 11.07 ($\alpha = .05$, d.f. = 5) and justifying the assumption of a Poisson process for the arrival of calls.

TABLE 12.2

Observed and Theoretical Frequency Distributions of Calls per Mean Service Time

Number of Calls	Frequency	
	Observed	Theoretical
0	96	98
1	112	113
2	74	69
3	20	24
4	10	9
5	3	2

APPLICATION OF THE QUEUEING MODEL

It has been established that the messenger service possesses the characteristics of a Poisson arrival process, an exponential distribution of service times, a first-come first-served queue discipline, and a service arrangement of multiple servers acting in parallel. It is assumed that the system operates in a steady-state condition, that is, that the current state is independent of the initial conditions. Under these circumstances it may be assumed that a simple queueing model will describe the service adequately. No attempt is made here to develop the mathematical model in detail. The interested reader will find detailed discussions of the formulas in the works of Hillier and Lieberman [12], Morse [13], and Saaty [14].

Staffing Level and Service Delay

For the present problem, the parts of the model that are of interest are those which express, as functions of the number of messengers, L_q, the expected queue length, and $P(>t)$, the probability that a call will have to wait some time longer than t. Let λ denote the mean number of arrivals per unit time, μ the mean number of calls serviced by one messenger per unit time, and s the number of messengers. If the mean arrival rate is less than the mean service rate, $\lambda < \mu s$; for convenience, let $\rho = \lambda/\mu s$, and note that $\rho < 1$. The probability that no calls are waiting can be defined as

$$P_0 = 1 \bigg/ \left[\sum_{n=0}^{s-1} \frac{(\lambda/\mu)^n}{n!} + \frac{(\lambda/\mu)^s}{s!(1-\rho)} \right]$$

where n is the number of calls in the queueing system. Then the waiting-time probability may be calculated as

$$P(>t) = \frac{P_0 (\lambda/\mu)^s}{s!(1-\rho)} e^{-s\mu t(1-\rho)} \tag{1}$$

and the expected queue length may be obtained from

$$L_q = \frac{P_0 (\lambda/\mu)^s \rho}{s!(1-\rho)^2} \tag{2}$$

Curves were drawn from Eq. 1 for the probability of delays of service with different staffing levels (Fig. 12.3). Expected queue length (L_q) was calculated from Eq. 2 for various staffing levels; the results are given in Table 12.3.

Staffing Level and Cost

The cost of waiting is intangible in most cases and is difficult to estimate. One can, however, get an insight into the problem by arbitrarily varying the ratio of cost of waiting per unit time to cost of service per unit time and studying its effect on the system. To construct an example, let unit time be one hour; C_1 is service cost per messenger per hour and C_2 is waiting cost per call per hour.

At any time $[s - (\lambda/\mu)]$ messengers are idle; the cost of idleness is $C_1[s - (\lambda/\mu)]$. Also, L_q calls are waiting to be served, with an additional cost of $C_2 L_q$, so that the equation describing the total hourly cost is

$$F(s) = C_1 \left(s - \frac{\lambda}{\mu} \right) + C_2 L_q$$

The objective is to minimize F, which is a function of s. The equation can be solved by trial and error: let $C_1 = \$2/\text{hr}$, and assign

FIGURE 12.3

Probability of Waiting Times Longer Than t at Different Staffing Levels

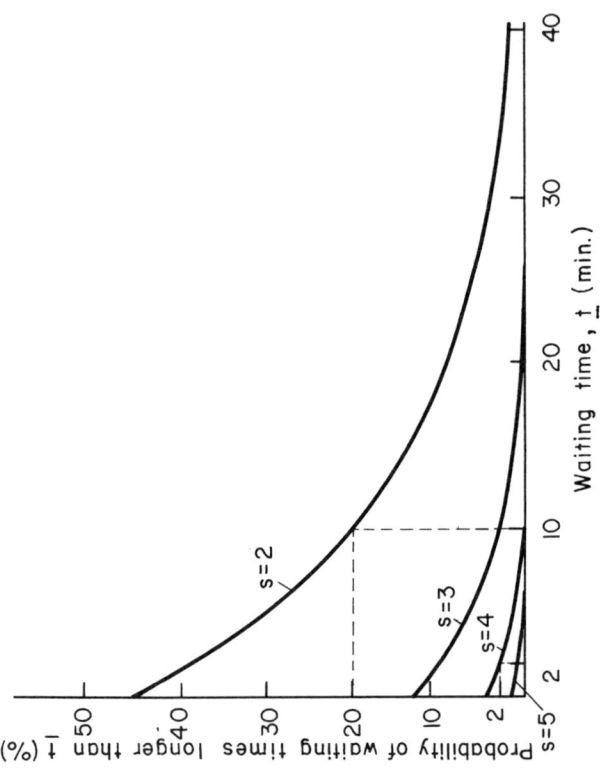

TABLE 12.3

Expected Queue Length with Various Numbers of Messengers

Number of Messengers	Calls Waiting for Service
2	0.675
3	0.094
4	0.016
5	0.003

TABLE 12.4

Hourly Cost of Various Staffing Levels at Two Different Ratios of Waiting Cost (C_2) to Service Cost (C_1)

| Number of Messengers | Cost per Hour | |
	$C_2/C_1 = 5$	$C_2/C_1 = 15$
2	$8.35	$21.82
3	4.54	6.42
4	5.76	6.08
5	7.63	7.68

alternative values 5 and 15 to the ratio C_2/C_1. The resulting values for hourly cost are shown in Table 12.4.

DISCUSSION

The administrator must decide which one of several criteria is the most relevant as the basis for choosing a staffing level. He may decide that a given percentage of calls may not be allowed to wait for service longer than a certain time or that no more than a certain percentage of calls may be waiting in the queue for service at any time, or he may choose to minimize the total cost of the operation, balancing the cost of waiting against the cost of providing additional messengers.

As shown in Fig. 12.3, with two messengers 20 percent of the calls would wait longer than 10 minutes, while with three messengers only 2 percent of the calls would wait longer than 10 minutes. The choice of criteria must dictate which of these values is to be regarded as optimal.

By inspecting Table 12.3, one can also decide on a tolerable limit for calls waiting to be serviced at any time. It is obvious from the results that increasing the number of messengers from two to three has a marked effect on the queue length, while a further increase to four or more has relatively little effect. Adding an additional person is not always an effective solution.

With regard to the cost values shown in Table 12.4, it can be seen that when waiting cost (C_2) is excessively high, it is economical to have four messengers instead of three. This sort of result was expected intuitively. In emergency units, therefore, a higher level of service should be provided. Such calculations can provide estimates of staffing costs for emergency service.

In this particular application, it was found that the data on service times and arrival rates were adequately represented by the theoretical distributions. In more complex cases these distributions may not approximate the real-life situation: for example, in an emergency department there may be priorities of service dependent on the condition of each newly arrived patient. The analysis of such a situation is involved and may sometimes be impossible, so that computer simulation would be necessary to provide an objective basis for decisions on staffing. The messenger service problem, however, proved to be simple enough that the analytic approach of queueing theory was both feasible and effective; as a consequence of this analysis, it was decided that three messengers would be the optimal on-duty staff for the first (day) shift. With this staffing level, about 86 percent of the requests would be satisfied immediately, while 14 percent would wait an average of four minutes to be served. After making allowance for absenteeism, turnover, and 7-day-week scheduling, six messengers were assigned to the first shift.

After the desired staffing level was achieved, departmental records showed that the messenger unit was providing adequate service and that waiting times were within the desired limits. The recommended reduction in manpower from 11 to 6 resulted in a saving of close to $25,000 per year.

REFERENCES

1. E. Brockmeyer, H. L. Halstrom, and A. Jensen, "The Life and Works of A. K. Erlang," Trans. of the Danish Acad. of Tech. Sci. 2 (1948):9.

2. T. C. Fry, Probability and Its Engineering Uses. New York: Van Nostrand, 1928.

3. E. C. Molina, "Application of the Theory of Probability to Telephone Trunking Problems," Bell Systems Tech. J. 6 (1927):461.

4. J. A. Bather, "Optimal Relation Policies for Finite Dams," J. Soc. Ind. App. Math. 10 (1962):395.

5. F. Benson and D. R. Cox, "The Productivity of Machines Requiring Attention at Random Intervals," J. Roy. Stat. Soc. (Ser. B) 13 (1951):65 and 14 (1952):200.

6. L. C. Edie, "Traffic Delays at Toll Booths," Op. Res. 4 (1956):107.

7. G. Brigham, "On a Congestion Problem in an Aircraft Factory," Op. Res. 3 (1955):412.

8. N. T. J. Bailey and J. D. Welch, "Appointment Systems in Hospital Outpatient Departments," Lancet 262 (1952):1105.

9. N. T. J. Bailey, "A Study of Queues and Appointment Systems in Hospital Outpatient Departments with Special Reference to Waiting Time," J. Roy. Stat. Soc. (Ser. B) 14 (1952):185.

10. M. J. B. White and M. C. Pike, "Appointment Systems in Outpatient Clinics and the Effect of Patients' Unpunctuality," Med. Care 2 (1964):133.

11. R. K. D. Haussmann, "Waiting Time as an Index of Quality of Nursing Care," Health Serv. Res. 5 (Summer 1970):92.

12. E. S. Hillier and G. J. Lieberman, Introduction to Operations Research. San Francisco: Holden-Day, 1967.

13. P. M. Morse, Queues, Inventories and Maintenance. New York: Wiley, 1958.

14. T. L. Saaty, Elements of Queueing Theory. New York: McGraw-Hill, 1961.

13

MARKOV CHAIN APPLICATION

INTRODUCTION

An absorbing Markov chain model is used to evaluate two blood bank crossmatch policies. Before any patient is infused with the blood of another human, the two bloods must be mixed (crossmatched) to determine if there will be an adverse reaction. The crossmatching process usually takes place the day before the blood infusion may be required. Since the period during which a patient may need the blood may extend over two or three days, the crossmatched blood remains usually reserved for that period of time. This study compares the common policy of using the oldest blood first with the policy of using the oldest blood available for those patients with the highest probability of actually needing the blood and using fresher (younger) blood for those patients with a lower probability of needing the blood. It was found that the latter policy results in more efficient utilization of blood.

Introduction to Technique

A Markov model is often applicable to a decision problem. The basic assumptions of a Markov process are:
1. There is a finite number of states of the system.
2. Moves from one state to the next are made in discrete steps, thus ruling out the continuous-flow type of movement or transition.
3. The probability of moving from one state to another is constant, and it is dependent only on the current state and not on the manner in which the current state is reached.
4. The steady-state probabilities are the long-run probabilities of being in a particular state after the process has been operating long enough to "washout" the initial conditions.

REFERENCES

Bhat, N., Elements of Applied Stochastic Processes. New York: Wiley, 1972.

Bush, J. W., M. B. S. Chen, and J. Zaremba, "Estimating Health Program Outcomes Using a Markov Equilibrium Analysis of Disease Development," American Journal of Public Health 61 (December 1971):2362-74.

Bush, J. W., and S. Fansnel, "A Health Status Index," Operations Research 18 (November-December 1970):1021-66.

Harris, R., M. Maggard, and W. Lasso, Computer Models in Operations Research, Operations Research. New York: Harper & Row, 1974.

A COMPARISON OF TWO BLOOD BANK
CROSSMATCH POLICIES

C. Carl Pegels
and
Andrew E. Jelmert

The process of crossmatching blood is an integral part of blood bank operations. Human blood is specialized in the sense that one person's donated blood cannot be used randomly for another person. Before blood is infused to a patient, a test is performed to determine if the patient's blood matches the blood to be infused. Only blood that

---

The research contained in this article was performed pursuant to Contract No. PH-43-68-1281 with the National Institutes of Health, Department of Health, Education, and Welfare. Findings and conclusions do not necessarily represent views of the Public Health Service. Reprinted with permission from AIIE Transactions 3, No. 1, pp. 69-75. Copyright 1971 by the American Institute of Industrial Engineers, Inc. All rights reserved.

matches the patient's blood is acceptable. Two blood crossmatch policies are compared. The commonly used policy is compared to a modified policy and it is found that the latter can produce considerable savings in blood and concomitant costs. The absorbing Markov chain model is used to evaluate the two crossmatch policies.

Human blood is a perishable commodity with a limited life. Its only source is the healthy human being, and its major demand originates from the injured or ailing human being. The fact that one person's donated blood cannot be used randomly on another person makes it extremely specialized. Human blood is divided into four main blood groups: O, A, B, and AB. It is broken down into two types, those with the Rh factor, called Rh positive, and those without the Rh factor, called Rh negative, yielding a total of eight major blood types.

Almost the entire supply of human blood for noncommercial blood bank inventories is obtained from voluntary donors. The demand for human blood originates in the hospital from sick or injured human beings. Surgeons estimate the amount of blood they think adequate for each particular operation. Whenever blood needs are anticipated for injuries or medical needs, the attending physician estimates the maximum normal blood requirement. Occasionally this maximum is exceeded and additional blood is requested.

All anticipated blood needs are forwarded to the hospital blood bank. Normally this demand is supplied by the shelf inventory of the hospital bank. If there is insufficient inventory to meet these needs, the blood bank must obtain blood from its suppliers.

Before any patient is infused with the blood of another human, the two bloods must be mixed (crossmatched) to determine if there will be an adverse reaction. Generally, blood of the same type is acceptable but occasionally even blood of the same type will not crossmatch. If the two bloods are compatible, the unit is considered crossmatched for the particular patient. It is generally reserved for that patient 24-48 hours following the expected blood need.

If the blood is not used in the prescribed period, it is removed from crossmatch and is once again available for the blood needs of other patients. This procedure continues until the blood is either infused or until it expires. Blood is a perishable commodity and can only be transfused within 21 days of the time it is drawn. Although it may still be used for other purposes, it has a 21 day life as whole blood. Blood which exceeds this age is considered outdated.

When blood is requested for a patient, it is the common practice in blood banks to crossmatch the oldest blood first. This practice is followed because it is generally assumed that it results in a more efficient utilization of available blood. The above policy of course is not followed when fresh blood is specifically requested and required.

This article will demonstrate that a modified policy of assigning the oldest blood to those with the highest probability of transfusion and fresher blood to those with a lower probability of transfusion will result in a more efficient utilization of blood.

The technique used to study the difference between the two crossmatch policies is the absorbing Markov chain. For a more extended treatment the reader is referred to any of several operations research textbooks currently in use.

THEORY OF MARKOV CHAINS

A Markov chain is a process that moves successively through a set of states $s_1, s_2, \ldots, s_n$. With each state s_i a vector of probabilities is associated p_{ij}, $j = 1, 2, \ldots, n$, which indicate the probabilities that the process will move from state s_i to s_j. The n^2 probabilities, p_{ij}, $i, j = 1, 2, \ldots, n$ are assumed to remain unchanged throughout the process. Collectively, the probabilities can be written in the form of a transition matrix, P.

$$P = \begin{array}{c} \\ s_1 \\ s_2 \\ \vdots \\ s_n \end{array} \begin{array}{c} s_1 \quad s_2 \quad \cdots \quad s_n \\ \begin{bmatrix} p_{11} & p_{12} & \cdots & p_{1n} \\ p_{21} & p_{22} & \cdots & p_{2n} \\ \vdots & \vdots & & \vdots \\ p_{n1} & p_{n2} & \cdots & p_{nn} \end{bmatrix} \end{array} \quad (1)$$

For each state s_i, the probabilities p_{ij}, $j = 1, 2, \ldots, n$ describe a probability distribution, and according to the postulates of probability

$$\sum_{j=1}^{n} p_{ij} = 1$$

A regular transition matrix has the property that all elements are positive for some power of P. If the matrix P is multiplied successively by itself, and if the resultant matrix eventually turns out to be a matrix with positive elements, then P is called a regular transition matrix. A regular matrix has the interesting, and often useful, property of tending to a matrix of which all rows are identical as the power, n, of the matrix P, grows larger.

The Markov chains to be used in this paper are called absorbing Markov chains. An absorbing Markov chain is identified as such because once in an absorbing state it becomes impossible to leave that state. The states are thus called absorbing states. Although it is impossible to leave these absorbing states, it is possible to eventually reach each absorbing state starting at any nonabsorbing state. The matrix below is a typical example of an absorbing Markov chain.

$$M = \begin{array}{c} \\ 1 \\ 2 \\ 3 \\ 4 \end{array} \begin{array}{cccc} 1 & 2 & 3 & 4 \\ \left[\begin{array}{cccc} 1 & 0 & 0 & 0 \\ 0 & 1 & 0 & 0 \\ .2 & .3 & 0 & .5 \\ .1 & .8 & .1 & 0 \end{array}\right] \end{array} \qquad (2)$$

The absorbing states are states 1 and 2. Note that the 2 × 2 matrix for 1 and 2 is an identity matrix with ones on its main diagonal and zeros elsewhere. Absorbing matrices are most conveniently written in the so-called "canonical form." The matrix M is written in canonical form as

$$M = \begin{bmatrix} I & O \\ S & Q \end{bmatrix} \qquad (3)$$

where I is the 2 × 2 identity matrix, O is the 2 × 2 matrix with nothing but zeros and S and Q are regular 2 × 2 matrices.

For the application of Markov chains to evaluate the two policies, one should mainly be concerned with the matrices S and Q. If the matrix I - Q is inverted, and if the inverse $[I - Q]^{-1}$ is identified as the matrix T, then two interesting properties can be obtained from T postmultiplied by the vector of ones, e. The first case, TS, provides the probabilities of ending up in either absorbing state 1 or 2, if the process originates from the two nonabsorbing states 3 and 4. The second case, Te, provides the expected number of steps required to move from the nonabsorbing states 3 and 4 to either one of the two absorbing states, 1 and 2.

Application of Model to a Typical Common Policy

In a typical blood crossmatch policy the oldest blood is assigned first. This policy is followed regardless of what the probability of transfusion is for the assigned unit of blood. As stated previously, this policy is generally assumed to reduce outdating to a minimum while maintaining the largest possible available inventory.

The above policy can be represented by the absorbing Markov chain input matrix in Table 13.1. The first two states (represented by the first two columns) are the transfusion and outdating states, respectively. The third state represents blood which is in the process of being crossmatched for a particular patient. All blood must be crossmatched, and therefore enter this state, before it can be transfused. The next five states are assigned states and are called states A, B, C, D, and E. They are the probability of transfusion states with each state representing one-fifth of the probability range between zero and one. The last state is the unassigned state.

Blood can pass from the assigned states to the transfusion state, the outdating state or the crossmatch state, where it is crossmatched again for another patient.* The last state, the unassigned, is reserved for blood from the time it enters the system until it is crossmatched for the first time. The numbers in the body of the table represent the probability of moving from one state to another.

Blood from the unassigned state is crossmatched to meet demand. The probability that blood outdates without ever being assigned is estimated to be 1 percent for this application. From the crossmatch state the blood is assigned to any one of the five probability transfusion states which have equal probabilities of 0.20.

The assumption of equal probabilities of blood being assigned to each of the five probability transfusion categories is reasonable because the demand for each category is approximately uniform. The effect of relaxing this assumption is examined later in the article.

The probability figures (4th to and including 8th row) in the transfusion column represent the midpoints of the probability of transfusion ranges, for example, the .40 to .60 range is represented by the midpoint probability of .50. If a unit of blood is not transfused, it must enter one of two possible states, the outdated state or the crossmatch state. If it does not become outdated, it will be cross-

---

*In actual blood banking practice, blood may also become unassigned after it has been crossmatched. From the unassigned state it moves to either the crossmatch state or it may outdate. In our model this state change has been skipped without affecting the results in any way. Blood which outdates before reassignment is represented as moving directly to the outdate state; and blood which is eventually reassigned proceeds directly to the crossmatched state.

TABLE 13.1

Input Probability Matrix—Common Policy

State	Transfusion	Outdating	Crossmatch	A	B	C	D	E	Unassigned
				\multicolumn{6}{c}{Probability of a given state in state column moving to any other state}
Transfusion	1	0	0	0	0	0	0	0	0
Outdating	0	1	0	0	0	0	0	0	0
Crossmatch	0	0	0	.2	.2	.2	.2	.2	0
A (0–.2)	.1	.18	.72	0	0	0	0	0	0
B (.2–.4)	.3	.14	.56	0	0	0	0	0	0
C (.4–.6)	.5	.10	.40	0	0	0	0	0	0
D (.6–.8)	.7	.06	.24	0	0	0	0	0	0
E (.8–1.)	.9	.02	.08	0	0	0	0	0	0
Unassigned	0	.01	.99	0	0	0	0	0	0

TABLE 13.2

Output Matrix—Common Policy

	Probability of transfusion given the state	Probability of outdating given the state	Probability of transfusion	Probability of outdating	Expected number of assignments
Crossmatch	0	0	.833	.167	3.33
A (0–.2)	.10	.18	.700	.300	3.40
B (.2–.4)	.30	.14	.767	.233	2.87
C (.4–.6)	.50	.10	.833	.167	2.33
D (.6–.8)	.70	.06	.900	.100	1.80
E (.8–1.)	.90	.02	.967	.033	1.27
Unassigned	0	.01	.825	.175	4.30

matched for reassignment; it is impossible to proceed directly from one assigned state to another assigned state without first being crossmatched. Blood in the crossmatched state must enter one of the assigned states. It cannot move from the crossmatched state to the outdated state.

The matrix in Table 13.1 represents a policy which assigns the oldest blood to the first request. As a result, the probability of outdating, given that a unit was not transfused, will be independent of the particular assigned state of a unit of blood. In this model, the probability of blood outdating after having been in one of the assigned states is 0.20. This is empirically based on the fact that blood which becomes outdated has been crossmatched an average of five times.

The probability of outdating, r, is then found by the equation,

$$r = s(1 - p) \qquad (4)$$

where p is the probability in each respective transfusion column entry and s is a constant (0.20) estimated from historical data. Since the probabilities in each row must add up to one, the probability values, q, in each respective entry in the third column are found by the equation,

$$q = 1 - p - r \qquad (5)$$

Applying the absorbing Markov chain solution technique to the common policy represented by the matrix in Table 13.1 results in the output matrix shown in Table 13.2. The essential information contained in Table 13.2 can be summarized by the percentage of 82.5 of blood transfused and a concomitant outdating percentage of 17.5 (last line in 3rd and 4th columns). The average age of the blood leaving the system is 15.05 days if 3.50 days are assumed to elapse between each assignment.* However, the average age calculation also includes blood that outdates at the age of 21 days. A recalculation† results in an average age at transfusion of 13.76 days.

---

*The elapsed time between assignments of 3.50 days is used only for illustrative purposes. The elapsed time of 3.50 days times 4.3 assignment results in an average age of 15.05 days.

†Calculated by the formula .825(x) + .175(21) = 15.05; x is found to be 13.76 days.

Application of Model to a Modified Policy

The modified policy follows the policy of crossmatching older blood to patients with a high probability of transfusion and fresher blood to patients with a low probability of transfusion. If more than one unit of blood is requested to be crossmatched, different probabilities of transfusion are estimated for each unit of blood even though all units are assigned to the same patient. Hence, a given patient for whom three units are requested to be crossmatched will have assigned to him a certain amount of old and fresh blood.

The modified policy does put certain demands on a blood bank manager. He must estimate the probability of transfusion ranges for each unit of blood requested, and he must have some advance knowledge or estimates of blood demand over a one day horizon to make the modified policy effective. A typical blood demand schedule is shown in Table 13.3 for a given day. The probabilities of transfusion are assumed to have been estimated by the blood bank manager. Most blood bank personnel have a great deal of historical information on the blood needs of each surgical procedure and the ordering policies of individual physicians. Based on the demand schedule in Table 13.3, the older blood will be assigned to the .8-1 probability of transfusion categories, the next older blood to the .6-.8 probability categories, and so forth.

The input probability matrix is shown in Table 13.4, which is the same as the input matrix for the common policy as far as the unassigned column is concerned. The transfusion column is also the same for both matrices, but the remainder is different. The outdating column is once again found by Equation 4. However, under the modified policy, s is no longer a constant but is a function of the assigned

TABLE 13.3

A Typical Blood Demand Schedule

Type of surgery or therapy	Units requested	Probability that x units will be transfused		
		$x=1$	$x=2$	$x=3$
i	1	.4–.6	—	—
ii	3	.8–.1	.4–.6	0–.2
iii	2	.6–.8	0–.2	—
iv	1	.2–.4	—	—
v	3	.8–1	.6–.8	.2–.4

TABLE 13.4

Input Probability Matrix—Modified Policy

State	Transfusion	Outdating	Crossmatch	A	B	C	D	E	Unassigned
Transfusion	1	0	0	0	0	0	0	0	0
Outdating	0	1	0	0	0	0	0	0	0
Crossmatch	0	0	0	.2	.2	.2	.2	.2	0
A (0–.2)	.1	0	.90	0	0	0	0	0	0
B (.2–.4)	.3	.07	.63	0	0	0	0	0	0
C (.4–.6)	.5	.10	.40	0	0	0	0	0	0
D (.6–.8)	.7	.09	.21	0	0	0	0	0	0
E (.8–1.)	.9	.04	.06	0	0	0	0	0	0
Unassigned	0	.01	.99	0	0	0	0	0	0

Probability of a given state in state column moving to any other state

TABLE 13.5

Output Matrix—Modified Policy

State	Probability of transfusion given the state	Probability of outdating given the state	Probability of transfusion	Probability of outdating	Expected number of assignments
Crossmatch	0	0	.893	.107	3.57
A (0–.2)	.10	0	.904	.096	4.21
B (.2–.4)	.30	.07	.863	.137	3.25
C (.4–.6)	.50	.10	.857	.143	2.43
D (.6–.8)	.70	.09	.888	.112	1.75
E (.8–1.)	.90	.04	.934	.046	1.21
Unassigned	0	.01	.884	.116	4.54

state. Since older units of blood are assigned to patients for which the probability of transfusion is high, the units are more likely to become outdated if they are not transfused. Conversely, only fresh blood is assigned to patients with a low probability of transfusion and none becomes outdated. Under this policy $s = 0$ for the 0–.2 probability range, $s = .10$ for the .2–.4 range, $s = .20$ for the .4–.6 range, $s = .30$ for the .6–.8 range, and $s = .40$ for the .8–1.0 probability range. Since each probability interval occurs with equal relative frequency, the average value of s is 0.20, which is the same as the value used for the common policy. The probability values in the last column are determined by using Equation 5.

Application of the absorbing Markov chain model results in the output matrix shown in Table 13.5. The percentage of blood transfused under the modified policy is 88.4 with a concomitant outdating percentage of 11.6. The average age at which blood leaves the system is 15.89 days under the assumption of a 3.50 day elapsed time between assignments. Recalculation to eliminate outdated blood results in an average age of 15.22 days at transfusion.

A Comparison of the Two Policies

The two policies are compared in Table 13.6. Under the modified policy, the percentage transfused has increased by 5.9 percentage points which represents a much better utilization of blood.* The

---

*Percentage of blood transfused is also a function of the amount of blood in inventory. Large inventories result in lower percentage of blood utilization; small inventories result in higher blood utilization. In this study inventory level is assumed to be a constant and

TABLE 13.6

Comparison of the Two Policies

	Common policy	Modified policy
Percentage transfused	82.5	88.4
Percentage outdated	17.5	11.6
Average age at transfusion in days	13.76	15.22

average age at transfusion is 1.46 days more under the modified policy. The result is not surprising because older blood is assigned to those patients having a high probability of transfusion. However, the increase in average age is not significant enough to warrant concern.

SENSITIVITY ANALYSIS

Although the parameter estimates were based primarily on empirical data, the actual values will vary between hospitals and even within a given hospital as the ratio between demand rate and inventory level fluctuates. As blood inventory increases, the probability that blood will become outdated without being assigned will also increase. The model representing the common policy was used to determine the effect this will have on outdating. Table 13.7 shows

TABLE 13.7

Transfusion as a Function of Outdating before First Assignment

Probability of outdating before first assignment	Probability of transfusion	Probability of outdating
$\frac{1}{2}\%$	82.9	17.1
1%	82.5	17.5
3%	80.8	19.2

the degree of improvement should be attainable under other inventory levels as well.

TABLE 13.8

Probability of Outdating as a Function of Demand Distribution and the Ability of Blood Bank Managers to Estimate the Probability of Transfusion

Policies	Historical constant s for given p	Probability of transfusion for five assignment probability distributions				
		$P(A) = .3$ $B = .3$ $C = .2$ $D = .1$ $E = .1$ (1)	$P(A) = .25$ $B = .25$ $C = .2$ $D = .15$ $E = .15$ (2)	$P(A) = .2$ $B = .2$ $C = .2$ $D = .2$ $E = .2$ (3)	$P(A) = .15$ $B = .15$ $C = .2$ $D = .25$ $E = .25$ (4)	$P(A) = .1$ $B = .1$ $C = .2$ $D = .3$ $E = .3$ (5)
I (Common) A	.2	25.4	21.1	17.5*	14.4	11.8
B	.2					
C	.2					
D	.2					
E	.2					
II (Modified) A	.1	19.8	16.9	14.7	12.8	11.2
B	.15					
C	.2					
D	.25					
E	.3					
III (Modified) A	.05	15.9	14.3	13.0	12.0	11.1
B	.1					
C	.2					
D	.3					
E	.4					
IV (Modified) A	.0	13.3	12.4	11.6**	11.0	10.5
B	.1					
C	.2					
D	.3					
E	.4					

Note: Each column represents a different probability distribution of blood being transfused given that it is crossmatched. Columns 1 and 2 indicate that low probabilities of transfusion are more common than high probabilities; column 3 indicates that low, medium, and high probabilities of transfusion are equally likely; columns 3 and 4 indicate that high probabilities of transfusions are more common than low probabilities.
*Common and **modified policies were previously discussed.

293

TABLE 13.9

Sensitivity of Reduction in Outdating of Modifield Policy over Common Policy in Percentage Points

Policies	(1)	(2)	(3)	(4)	(5)
II	5.6	4.2	2.8	1.6	.4
III	9.5	6.8	4.5	2.4	.7
IV	12.1	8.7	5.9	3.4	1.3

Note: For more detailed headings see Table 13.8.

the effect of varying the probability of outdating before the first assignment on the probability of transfusion and outdating.

In the previous discussion both the common and modified policies assumed that the demand distribution for blood with different proba-

TABLE 13.10

Percentage Outdating as a Function of the Mean Value of s

State	s/p	Mean value of s		
		$\bar{s} = .25$	$\bar{s} = .20$	$\bar{s} = .15$
A	$s = \bar{s}$			
B	$s = \bar{s}$			
C	$s = \bar{s}$	20.8	17.5	13.9
D	$s = \bar{s}$			
E	$s = \bar{s}$			
A	$s = \bar{s} - .15$			
B	$s = \bar{s} - .075$			
C	$s = \bar{s}$	16.4	13.2	9.2
D	$s = \bar{s} + .075$			
E	$s = \bar{s} + .15$			
Improvement in percentage points of modified policy over common policy		4.4	4.3	4.7

bilities of transfusion was uniform. In practice, the average probability that a crossmatched unit will be transfused is somewhat less than 0.5. Hence, assignments with lower probabilities of transfusion are more common.

An accurate evaluation of the modified policy depends upon the ability of the blood bank director to estimate the probability of transfusion. The effect of a nonuniform probability distribution and errors in classifying demand by these categories are demonstrated in Tables 13.8 and 13.9. As the relative frequency of crossmatches with a low probability of transfusion increases, the percentage of blood outdating naturally increases. The expected savings from using the modified policy also increases.

Table 13.10 investigates the effect of varying the mean value of s. As the mean value of s increases, the associated improvement decreases if the variance of s is constant. In practice, increasing s will probably also increase the variance associated with s under the modified policy, thereby increasing the advantages of this policy.

ECONOMIC IMPLICATIONS

Implementation of the modified assignment policy can be expected to result in a reduction in the percentage of blood outdating of approximately 5 or 6 percent. For example, a typical, large hospital with approximately 700 beds could be expected to use at least 4000 units of blood per year. Let us assume that 5 percent of blood requests are for fresh blood and that the remaining 3800 units of blood are currently transfused by the first, common policy of using oldest blood first. If 18 percent of the blood drawn for shelf inventory becomes outdated—a typical figure—the hospital must then acquire 4630 units during a one-year period. (The units are calculated by 3800/ 1.00 - 0.18.) Implementation of the modified policy could thus potentially reduce the outdated number by 230 to 250 units per year.

Although many hospitals do not pay for the blood they receive, they do pay processing fees. Typically, these fees are approximately $20 per unit. Use of the modified policy could thus result in the hospital saving $4600-$5000 annually. In addition, better use of donated blood is made. There are few benefits from the use of outdated blood.

Perennial blood shortages point to a need for better utilization of the existing blood supply. If adopted, the proposed modified policy can make a substantial contribution in that direction.

14

SIMULATION

INTRODUCTION

This paper presents a partially deterministic and a partially probabilistic simulation model to reproduce a pattern of hospital utilization in the Chicago area. The model has two additional useful features: a mechanism to achieve replication of the system, and an ability to explore reallocation of hospital capacity in order to improve on the present system. The model applied to the metropolitan Chicago hospital system indicates that relocation of hospital beds could decrease patient travel, but the same improvement could be achieved by relaxing existing constraints of income and race.

Introduction to Technique

The term "simulation" refers to a set of techniques for manipulating a model of some complicated process for the purpose of finding numeric solutions which might be impossible or too costly to obtain mathematically. Simulation deals with the study of dynamic systems over time. Inventory, queueing, scheduling, and forecasting are some examples. Simulation models are designed to sample the characteristics of the system they represent by observing the system over time and subsequently gathering pertinent information.

There are three general types of simulation:
1. Analogous model
2. Continuous model
3. Discrete model

Continuous and discrete models are mathematical models, while the analogous model replaces the original system by an analogy which is easier to manipulate. Continuous models represent the system experiencing smooth changes in characteristics over time. In discrete models, a system is simulated by observing it only at selected points in time. All the models could be either deterministic or stochastic in nature. The most common type of simulation is the discrete model.

There are several types of simulating procedures that are commonly used:
1. Monte Carlo methods
2. Tactical simulation
3. Strategic simulation
4. Business gaming
5. Experimental gaming
6. Heuristic programming

REFERENCES

April, J., "Simulation as an Aid in Community Planning: A Case Study of a Community to be Built Around a Health Center in Guadalajara, Jalisco, Mexico," Socio-Economic Planning Science 8 (October 1974):301-07.

Charba, R. W., and J. L. Sanders, "Planning Models for Tuberculosis Control Programs," Health Services Research 6 (Summer 1971):144-64.

Griffith, J. R., Quantitative Techniques for Hospital Planning and Control. Lexington, Mass.: D. C. Heath, 1972.

Maisel, H., and G. Guiliano, Simulation of Discrete Stochastic System. Chicago, Ill.: Science Research Associates, 1972.

Rabinowitz, M., "Blood Bank Inventory Policies: A Computer Simulation," Health Services Research 8 (Winter 1973):271-82.

Thompson, D. A., "Financial Planning for an HMO," Health Services Research 9 (Spring 1974):68-73.

Yett, D. E., L. Drabek, M. D. Intriligator, and L. J. Kimbell, "Health Manpower Planning: An Econometric Approach," Health Services Research 7 (Summer 1972):134-47.

LOCATIONAL EFFICIENCY OF CHICAGO HOSPITALS: AN EXPERIMENTAL MODEL

Richard L. Morrill
and
Robert Earickson

An experimental simulation model is described by which imbalances in the distribution of hospitals may be evaluated and location shifts suggested to meet future needs. The model, partly deterministic and partly probabilistic, is here used to project the effects on patient travel of shifting capacity and of shifting demand. Applied to the metropolitan Chicago hospital system, the model results indicate that relocation of hospital beds would considerably decrease patient travel, but that the same improvement in patient travel and in hospital utilization could be achieved, with a far less radical and costly shift of beds, by relaxing existing constraints of income and race.

Hospitals are costly institutions to construct and maintain, and physician and hospital care are costly items for most families. The federal government spends large sums through the Hill-Burton Act to aid in the financing of hospital construction, through Medicare and Medicaid to aid the aged and the indigent, and in other programs. It is to the advantage of all concerned, therefore, that these monies be wisely spent; specifically, that the character and location of hospitals be such as to assure a viable operation while meeting the needs of the patient population [1].

From the Chicago Regional Hospital Study, supported by National Institutes of Health Research Grant HM 00452. The Study is cosponsored by the Hospital Planning Council for Metropolitan Chicago and the Illinois Department of Public Health, with the participation of the Center for Urban Studies and the Center for Health Administration Studies of the University of Chicago. Reprinted with permission from Health Services Research 4, No. 2 (Summer 1969). Copyright 1969 by the Hospital Research and Educational Trust, 840 North Lakeshore Drive, Chicago, Ill. 60611.

The present study was designed to find ways for cities and regions to evaluate the adequacy of the present distribution of hospitals and to locate or relocate facilities to meet future needs. This required, first, identification of pertinent variables, that is, the variability in patients, in hospitals, and in policies that must be taken into account in any realistic appraisal; and second, derivation of a model that would adequately reproduce existing patient use of the hospital system [2]. Only then could a normative model be created—one that could measure imbalances in the present distribution and suggest location shifts that would better meet the needs of both patients and hospitals. This article reports on the development of such a model and its application to the metropolitan Chicago hospital system.

The traditional approach to evaluation has been to take the population of given administrative units (cities, counties, etc.) and find the ratio of population to beds, comparing this to national standards. The inadequacy of this approach has long been recognized. Studies of hospital utilization [3, 4] and of hospital service areas [5] have provided a more satisfactory basis for estimating needs and for measurement and planning.

Patient variables identified in earlier stages of the study as affecting the demand for hospital care were: level and type of care needed [6-8], ability to pay [9-13], race [13, 14], and religion [15]. Variables related to physicians and hospitals and therefore influencing the supply of medical care were: for physicians, location and differentiation [16-19]; and for hospitals, location [16, 17, 20, 21], level and type of care provided [22, 23], and policies and type of control [13, 14, 24]. Survey data on patient travel to hospitals served to distinguish the separate influences of the physician [19, 25], of the pattern of hospital service areas [20], of distance [25-27], of level and type of care, and of economic [9-11, 28, 29], racial [14, 28, 30], and religious [15, 28] variables.

These relations and influences were summarized by a factor analysis of the characteristics of hospitals and their utilization, and regression analysis revealed that flows between communities and hospitals were about equally influenced by size of demand and opportunities and by amount of intervening demand and opportunities, with the flow modified upward when there was religious or racial similarity between hospital and community. Reduced volume was found to accompany increased hospital quality, since hospitals of high quality tended to treat smaller numbers of more difficult cases from a wide area [22].

APPROACHES TO MODELING THE PATIENT-PHYSICIAN-HOSPITAL INTERACTION

The first requirement of an adequate model is that it be able to replicate use of the system [2]. This involves the recognition of a degree of irrationality or uncertainty, and especially indeterminacy; that is, patients being confronted with a decision between approximately equally good choices. The model must accommodate experiment in order first to discern what modes of behavior better characterize actual decision making and then to test the effects of possible changes in behavior or outside constraints. Finally, the model must be able to evaluate the adequacy of the system and to prescribe changes that will raise the level of satisfaction of patients, physicians, and hospitals. Since patients desire easier access in space and time to physicians and hospitals with desired characteristics, physicians desire both access to hospitals and full use of their capacities, and hospitals desire a high rate of occupancy without congestion and excessive waiting, evaluation of the system should identify groups of patients and physicians who are required to travel unusually far or suffer unusually long waits and hospitals with excessive or deficient demand. The model should then be able to prescribe shifts in physician and hospital capacity that will bring all patients within maximum travel times (to be specified by society ultimately) and all hospitals to a viable level of operation.

Very simple models incorporating optimizing principles of spatial, social, and economic behavior were found able to account for much of the variation in behavior, but they fell short of satisfying the above requirements [31]. Specifically, interactance models fairly well described use of the system and, to a degree, indicated imbalances in it. Distance-minimizing transport models failed to allow sufficient flexibility in behavior, but they proved valuable in identifying groups of patients who were poorly served and hospitals that were poorly located. In this study, therefore, a simulation approach is used that attempts to combine the descriptive advantages of the interactance model and the prescriptive values of the transport model, in order to allow the necessary experimentation, capture actual variation in behavior, and at the same time retain the ability to evaluate the efficiency of the system [32, 33].

Distance-Minimizing Models

The transport model of linear programming embodies a simple hypothesis of spatial behavior: that distance is minimized within the constraints of demand and supply; or, here, that patients go to the nearest available hospital that competition permits. The model typically has an objective function of minimizing aggregate distance traveled or costs of travel; but this goal is constrained by the necessity that all demand be met (here, all patients treated) and all supplies (here, all hospital treatment capacity) be utilized. The optimal solution is found by an iterative search. While the results are economically highly efficient, they are behaviorally unrealistic. The main problem is that, mathematically, the number of routes taken (as between communities and hospitals) must be less than $3n - 4$, even though other destinations may be only marginally less satisfying or even equally good [34]. In reality, many times more paths are taken.

Despite descriptive shortcomings, the transport model has prescriptive utility. An optimal solution indicates which sets of patients have to travel farthest for care and which hospitals must reach farthest for patients, thus suggesting mutually profitable shifts in capacity. Another evaluative benefit comes from comparison of highly disaggregated solutions (as by race, religion, or income of patients) with more aggregate ones. For example, the model can first permit Negroes to visit only those hospitals known to accept them and then permit them to seek the nearest available hospital. The difference in distances traveled constitutes a measure of the cost of existing constraints [30].

Gravity-Interactance Models

As indicated above, an interactance model did rather well in reproducing the structure of flows. While distance is not strictly minimized, the model is behaviorally rational. A set of patients viewing the opportunities around them cannot be expected to think alike; some may consider a closer hospital "best," while others may view a farther one as better because it is larger. From the aggregate point of view, with people varyingly substituting size for distance, various destinations may be equally good. This decision-making hypothesis is really a rather good one [27]. But the individual or group evaluation of opportunities may also represent differences in perceived attractiveness of destination due to religion, race, or ability to pay; and with uncertainty as to what goals people have in fact pursued, mathematical difficulties give rise to misgivings about evaluative use of interactance model results.

A SIMULATION MODEL OF PHYSICIAN AND HOSPITAL USE AND EVALUATION

The simulation model that has been developed is an interactance model to the extent that probabilities of patients from an area visiting various hospitals are estimated from such a construct, though modified. But this stage provides only an initial estimate of hospital use. The model has two additional useful features: a mechanism to achieve replication of the system and one to reallocate hospital capacity in order to improve on the present system (Fig. 14.1).

Data on communities, physician clusters, and hospitals are presumed available. Numbers of patients with various characteristics and demands are known or can be estimated. There is obviously little or no substitution possible among obstetric, pediatric, and medical-surgical units of hospitals; similarly, the higher level hospitals have a "monopoly" on the care of many kinds of cases [22, 23]. Thus if data permit division of patients by types and levels of demand, the simulation model must be run separately for significant combinations of type and level of care.

The first stage allocates patients to physicians. For each community, studies of trips to services show that white patients seem to view the attractiveness of physician clusters as a simple function of the number and variety of physicians (white only). But the likelihood of patients visiting the clusters is influenced by the cost of reaching them, the existence of closer intervening physicians, and the lack of information about farther opportunities. Patient reaction to distance, determined from actual behavior, is one of indifference up to about two miles, after which attractiveness falls rapidly—that is, a physician twice as far away is viewed as something less than half as attractive [19]. If there are large numbers of patients and not too many potential destinations, the probabilities derived from such a modified interactance approach can become deterministic proportions; otherwise a Monte Carlo random number routine allocates the patients in accordance with the probabilities. Negro patients are similarly allocated, visiting either white or Negro physicians, with a moderate preference for the latter.

The computer program used (in Fortran IV) provides a deterministic or probabilistic option. Because the first is faster and less costly on common computers (IBM 7094, CDC, etc.), most of the experiments were deterministic, and solutions were found in from three to five iterations of a fairly simple allocative formula. The main technical problem was lack of storage memory for very large problems.

SIMULATION / 303

FIGURE 14.1

Flow Chart of Model Process

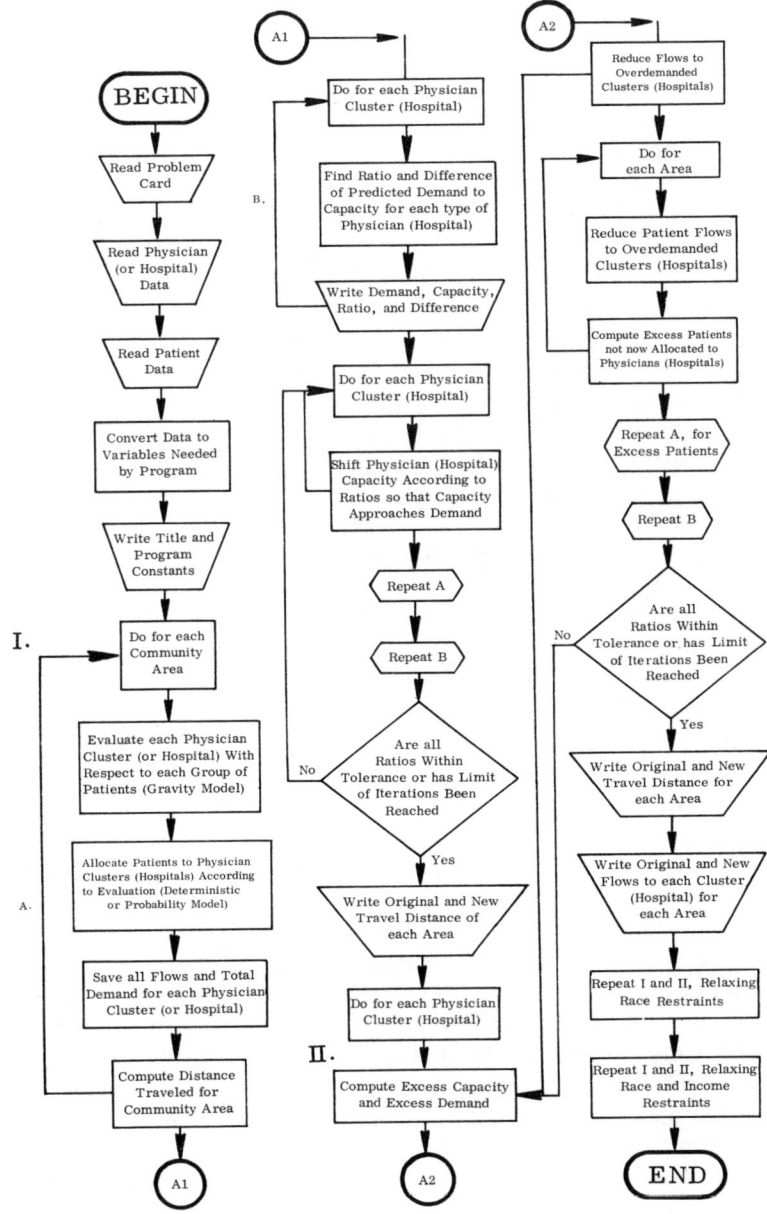

This initial allocation may be interpreted as where patients would like to go, given the present distribution of physicians. Since, however, physicians are not evenly distributed among all people, the demand for physician care at some locations will exceed their capacity and at others fall short. For example, too many patients will be allocated to a small isolated physician cluster in a heavily populated area. According to the mathematical operation of the modified interactance prediction of flows, a large cluster of physicians with nearby competing clusters will not attract enough. Since a consistent basis for choice is applied, the differences can be interpreted as a measure of the imbalance or inefficiency of the location of capacity.

The first option shifts physician capacity until the demand on each physician cluster comes within some acceptable range of divergence. For example, assume that the initial demand on one physician cluster is twice its normal capacity and that on another cluster half. Presumably there are too few physicians in the first and too many in the second. As a guess, the model doubles the number of physicians in the first and halves the number in the second. The allocation is repeated with the altered capacities, and the divergence between normal and predicted demand is rechecked until the demand comes within an acceptable level of divergence.

The second option conversely shifts patients from overdemanded physician clusters to underdemanded ones, in order to replicate, as closely as possible, the actual pattern of travel. After the initial allocation, flows to overdemanded clusters are proportionally reduced to actual capacity. The residual demand is then reallocated to underdemanded clusters only, a procedure that also requires iterative allocation. The greater aggregate travel distance that is required will be a direct measure of the inefficiency of capacity location: that is, an estimate of the extra effort patients in fact must exert to get care. Comparison with the shifted-capacity solution measures the savings possible from such relocation.

The second stage allocates patients to hospitals. The replications of actual patient-to-physician flows are taken as inputs. Using the already identified patient variables of race, religion, and ability to pay, the patient population is divided into six subgroups: paying Negro patients (as above); charity patients (those who did not visit a physician at all but will visit hospitals directly); and four white paying subgroups—Jews, Protestants, Catholics, and the religiously indifferent. Since the capacity of hospitals to care for Negro and charity patients is known, each of these allocations is done separately. All white paying patients are allocated in the same model run, but the religion of the patients is recorded. Within the white paying group, allocation to hospitals reflects a balance among the factors of distance, size, and religious character of hospital. Within the Negro group and the charity group the balance is between distance and size only.

Charity patients are allocated to hospitals in the same manner as patients were allocated to physicians above—as a simple function of distance to hospitals and their capacity to treat charity patients. For Negro patients, allocation is as before, except that the probability of visiting a particular hospital is a function of both the patient's and the physician's evaluation of size and distance. The working hypothesis here, that the choice is a function equally of distance from patient and of distance from physician, seems more reasonable than that the desires of one or the other should be controlling (in effect, the mean of the hospital distance from physician and from patient is substituted for distance from patient).

White subgroups evaluate distance "religiously" as well as geographically—that is, a mental barrier is erected against a hospital operated under the auspices of a different religion that increases the effective distance to it [20, 28]. Analyses of actual flows and experimental operation of the model suggest that on the average Jews evaluate distance to non-Jewish hospitals as about three times farther; Catholics evaluate distance to non-Catholic hospitals as about twice as far; Protestants evaluate Catholic and Jewish hospitals as about twice as far but evaluate nonreligiously oriented hospitals about the same as Protestant hospitals. These factors, applied to the distances to hospitals, affect the probabilities of visiting various hospitals; otherwise the allocation method is the same as before.

Again, the first option shifts hospital capacity until the demand on each hospital comes within some acceptable range of divergence (for paying Negroes, for charity patients, and for white paying patients separately). The same iterative procedure as before shifts beds from underdemanded to overdemanded hospitals. This substage of the model has the capability, if desired, of creating new hospitals and estimating their ideal size. Plausible locations are given a "token" hospital of but one bed; if these locations are superior, beds will be shifted from poorer existing locations. Some present hospitals may in fact be eliminated by the model, although it is also possible to prevent an uneconomic reduction in size of existing hospitals.

The second option shifts patients, again for paying Negro, charity, and white paying patients separately, from initially overdemanded hospitals to underdemanded ones. Again, the greater aggregate distance traveled measures the extra effort patients must exert, given the present distribution of capacity. Comparison with the shifted-capacity solution measures the savings attributable to relocation.

Since all the disaggregated flows will have been allocated, it is then possible to summarize all flows and demands on hospitals and to make summary comparisons. Addition of initially predicted demands on hospitals by the three subgroups will yield net measures of capacity imbalance. Summing of the suggested capacity shifts will indicate net shifts as between both locations and subgroups—for example, from white paying to charity patients.

The final stage of the model is experimental. The substages of initial allocation, shifting of capacity, and shifting of patients are repeated for any desired "external" changes. For example, several new hospitals or expansions may be approved or anticipated. The effects of such planned relocations on aggregate travel of patients and on the demand for existing hospitals may be measured. Estimated populations as of some future date may provide the basis for estimates of patient demand by area. The resultant imbalances and suggested shifts become a valuable indication of where new hospitals or expansions are needed.

A particularly valuable experiment, given present demands and capacities, measures the effects of relaxation of constraints. It may not be necessary to carry out all the shifts suggested in the model in an attempt to meet the separate demands of the many subgroups. Certainly it would be so costly that only some portion of suggested relocation or new capacity would be justified. Thus it is important to discover whether it would in the end be cheaper and easier to relax some of the present restrictions on entry to hospitals. Some or much of the apparent imbalance might disappear if patients and physicians had freer access to the system. This can be tested by appropriate aggregation of subgroups. The most feasible changes are in regard to race and ability to pay, since legal and financial arrangements can be made to permit entry to hospitals irrespective of color and income. Since preference on the basis of religion is personal, relaxation here is somewhat academic, so long as hospitals under religious control exist. Aggregations to be tested, then, are (1) all patients irrespective of race, (2) all patients irrespective of income, and (3) all patients irrespective of both race and income. These tests of relaxation of constraints may be applied to both the patient-physician and the patient-hospital stages of the model.

RESULTS

For purposes of clarity, map presentation of model results is limited to a sample set of communities across Chicago's south side, extending to the suburb of Evergreen Park. These communities are characterized by wide variations in race, income, and religion.

FIGURE 14.2

Changes in Cluster Size and Patient Travel Resulting from Shifting Physicians

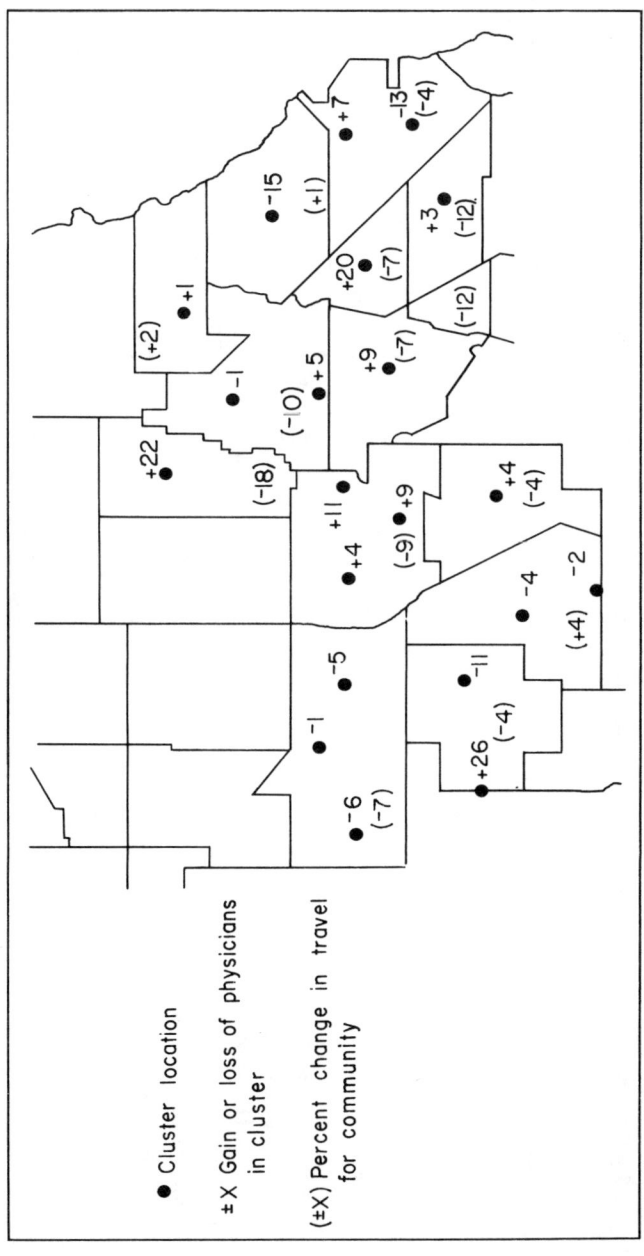

FIGURE 14.3

Changes in Patient Load and Patient Travel Resulting from Shifting Demand on Physicians

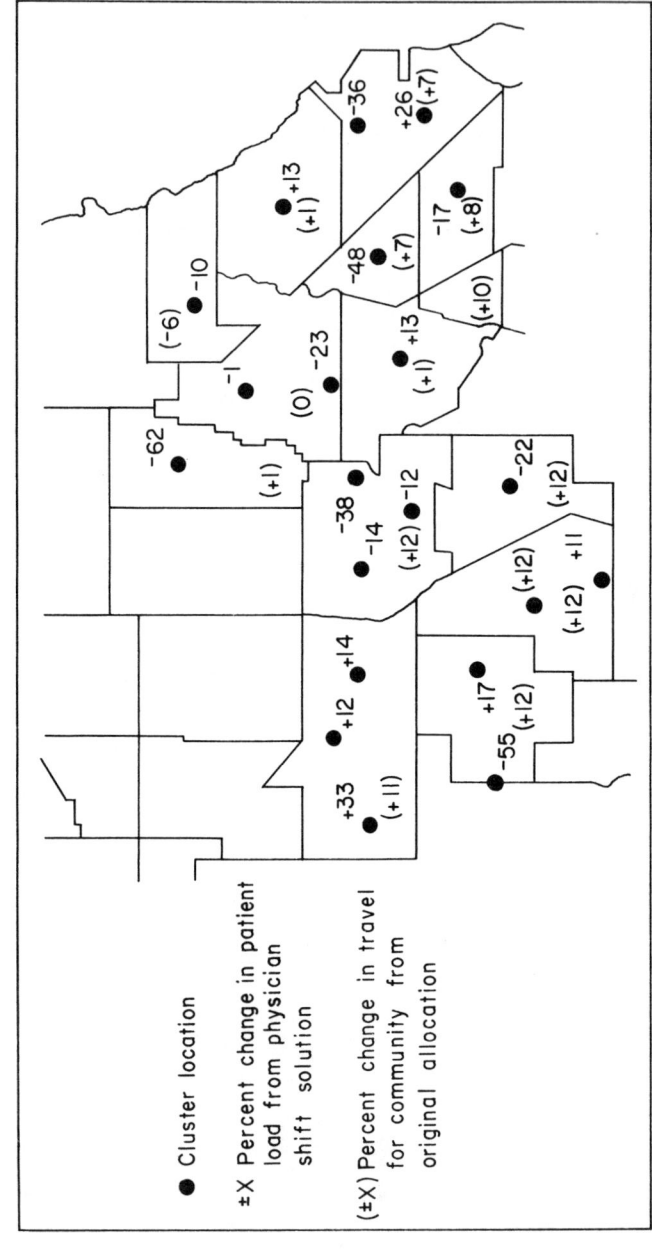

Allocation to Physicians

<u>Shifts of Capacity</u>. As expected, the initial allocation resulted in excess demand on physician clusters in newer and poorer areas and insufficient demand on older and larger clusters. Almost all demands were brought to ±10 percent of the mean demand (11 patients per physician) within five iterations. Some 1500 physicians (about 15 percent) were shifted, mainly from the Loop (central business district) and other very large clusters to smaller clusters closer to the population (Fig. 14.2). Although this shift greatly reduces aggregate patient travel, it is recognized that this breakup of agglomerations may be uneconomic. Inefficient reduction of clusters can be avoided in the model, however, by disaggregation of patients and physicians by major specialty groups.

<u>Shifts of Patients</u>. When patients are forced to use the existing system, total travel reasonably approximates that actually observed. Aggregate travel exceeds that for the physician-capacity-shift solution by 90,000 patient-miles, or about 20 percent (Fig. 14.3). These model results are particularly useful in pinpointing which specific groups and areas presently incur the greatest excess travel. Not surprisingly, these are paying patients in poor communities and patients in rapidly growing newer communities.

<u>Race and Income Barriers Removed</u>. If patients, irrespective of race and ability to pay, are able to visit all physicians, an even greater shift of physicians is forecast by the model, mainly from the Loop and from wealthy areas specifically to Chicago's poverty areas. This physician shift is a measure of the great latent demand for physicians in low income areas—in other words, of the unmet need.

Allocation to Hospitals

For the hospital trip, patients modify the distance according to religious preference. The model worked rather well in this respect, requiring, for example, greater average travel for Jewish patients, owing to the limited number of Jewish-affiliated hospitals. The capacity-shift portion of the model also differentiated by religion. For example, in heavily Catholic southwest Chicago, bed complements of Catholic hospitals were increased and those of Protestant hospitals reduced, reflecting demand shifts in the postwar period.

<u>Shifts of Capacity</u>. The initial allocation resulted in excess demand on hospitals in Negro areas and in many suburban areas and

FIGURE 14.4

Changes in Bed Complement of Selected Chicago Area Hospitals Resulting from Shifting Capacity to Charity, Negro, and Other Patients

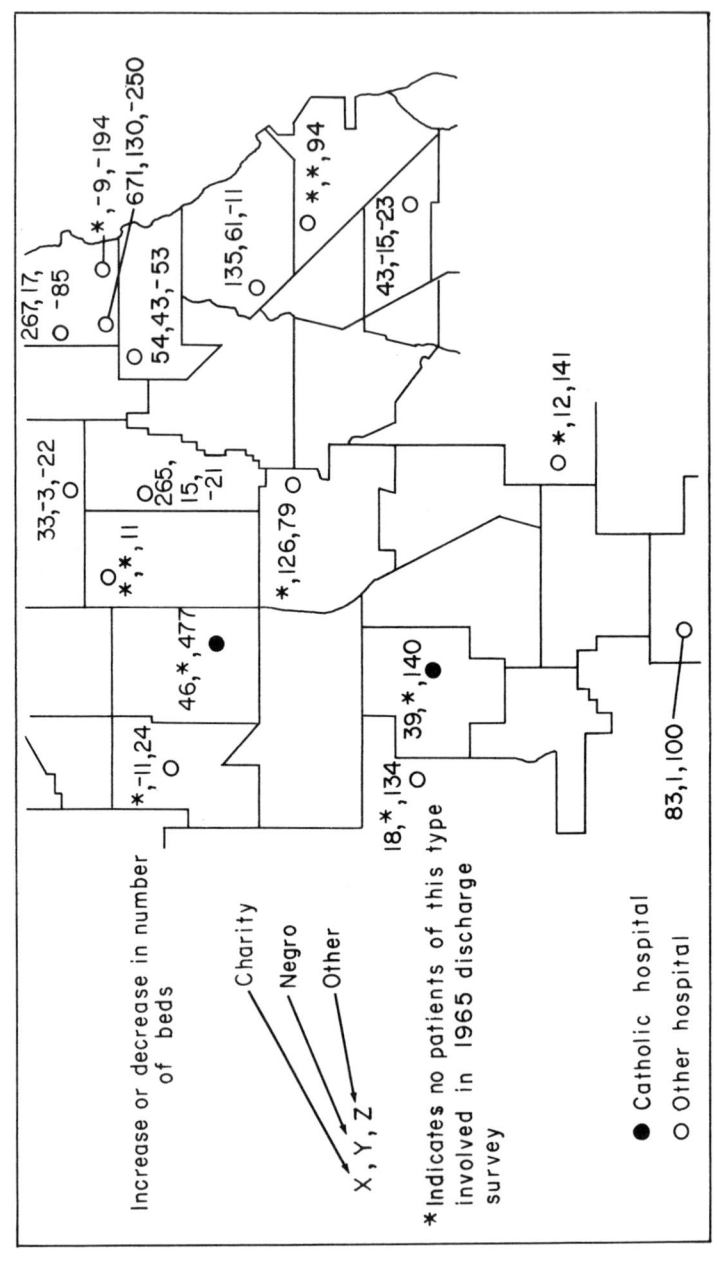

FIGURE 14.5

Changes in Charity, Negro, and Other Patient Travel in Selected Chicago Areas Resulting from Shifting Hospital Capacity

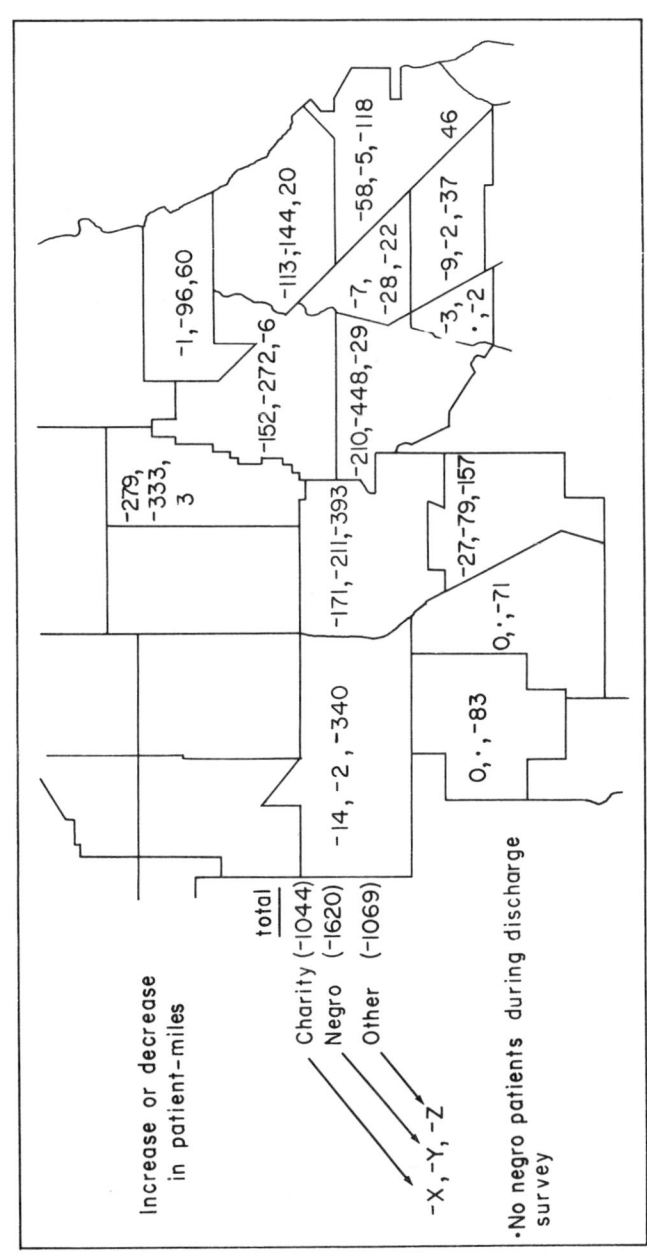

FIGURE 14.6

Changes in Patient Travel with Existing Distribution of Hospital Capacity when Race and Income Barriers are Removed

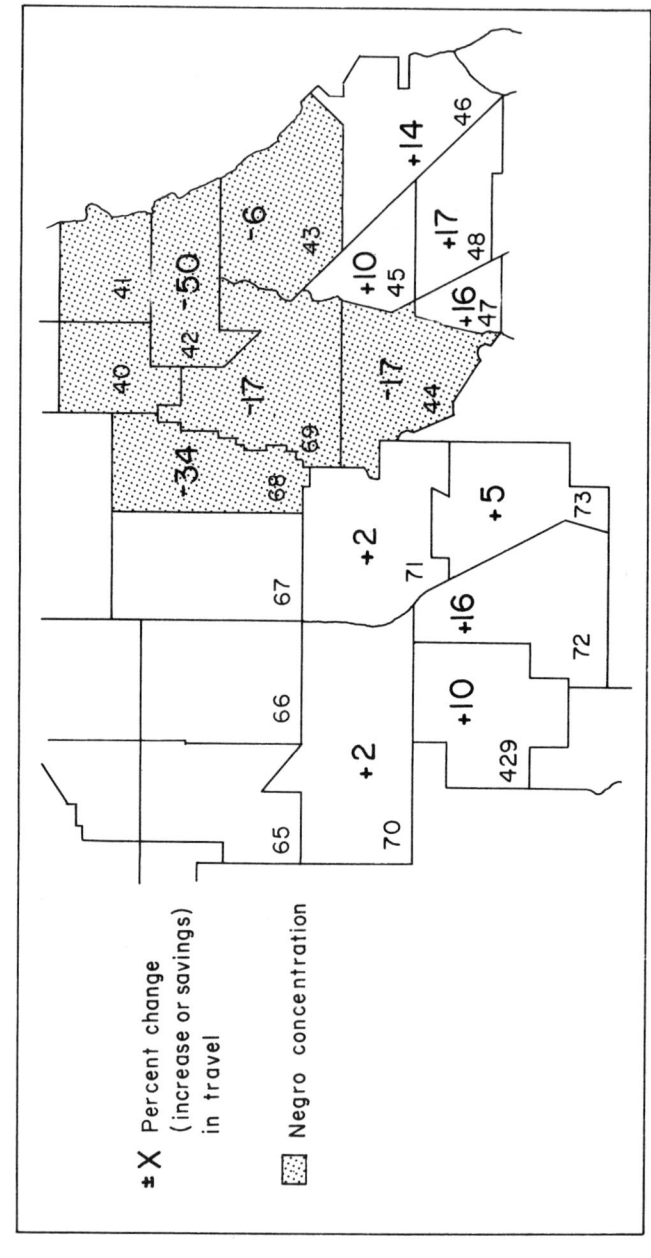

insufficient demand for inner city hospitals and for charity and veterans' institutions. The model results suggest a shift of over 12,000 beds, or about 16 percent (Fig. 14.4). Beds for both paying and charity Negro patients are shifted to ghetto area hospitals at the expense of close-in hospitals and especially Cook County Hospital (charity), with resultant savings in patient travel (Fig. 14.5). Beds are added to many suburban hospitals in rapidly growing areas. Many hospitals on the Chicago north side are reduced in size, reflecting long-term population shifts.

As with trips to physicians, level of hospital care was not explicitly treated in these first runs. Thus Chicago's best and largest hospitals are slashed in size, since they are indeed too large and central with respect to general levels of care. In later model runs, a separate solution will be obtained for cases that could be handled only by larger hospitals enjoying scale and agglomerative advantages.

Shifts of Patients. If patients are again forced to use the existing system, travel exceeds that for the capacity-shift solution by 116,000 patient-miles (about 20 percent). Most of the excess travel is incurred by black and poor patients generally, since they are presently restricted to so few hospitals.

Race and Income Barriers Removed. When the barriers against unrestricted use of hospitals by paying Negro patients are removed, patients' demands are ideally met through the shifting of only 1380 rather than 1700 beds to ghetto area hospitals. Likewise, patients are forced to travel less far, given the present distribution of capacity. If the barriers against free entry to hospitals by charity patients are also removed, patients using the existing system enjoy great savings in travel, and a far less radical and therefore less costly shift of beds is required to achieve the same improvement in patient travel and hospital utilization. For example, Cook County Hospital is reduced from 2700 only to 1590 rather than to 800 beds, and altogether 8650 rather than 12,167 beds are shifted, for an almost identical travel saving (Fig. 14.6).

CONCLUSIONS: EVALUATION OF THE MODEL

The simulation model outlined above is intended both to reproduce an actual pattern of use satisfactorily, on the basis of properly understood and formulated decision-making criteria, and, by extension, to evaluate present imbalances of capacity and estimate the shifts necessary for desired improvement. A fair degree of complexity was required in order to depict the system realistically. A partly deterministic and partly probabilistic simulation model resulted, since the range of choice confronting the residents of an area seems too great for deterministic assignment.

The model works moderately well at replicating use of the system and at evaluating locational efficiency and suggesting shifts in location and policies that would raise the general level of satisfaction with the least dislocation. On the other hand, certain problems must be noted: (1) The model results are quite sensitive to the particular parameters of the equation (patient interpretation of distance, size, and religion), hence it cannot be claimed that the results are "right" until more evidence of patient perception and behavior is obtained, including personal interviews; (2) the authors are not fully satisfied with the specific mathematical operations of the model; (3) the value of the present results is limited by lack of breakdown by physician specialty and by level of hospital care; and (4) the model may place too much stress on reducing patient travel and not enough on institutional viability and quality.

Anticipated experiments in the near future include some breakdown by type and level of care; prediction of the effects of estimated 1980 population distribution and of planned new hospitals and expansions; use of the model to suggest new hospitals and their optimal size; and extension to data for Seattle and Honolulu.

Although the model was developed for the hospital use context, the programming is flexible enough to permit a much broader application, at least to problems involving movements of persons, differential location of demand and supply, and evaluation of the efficiency of travel patterns and supply patterns. The authors believe the evaluative portion to be the most important contribution. If it proves useful, then further application to movements to shopping centers, schools, churches, recreation sites, and other destinations would be appropriate and necessary to demonstrate true generality.

REFERENCES

1. R. Earickson, "Spatial Interaction of Patients, Physicians, and Hospitals: A Behavioral Approach," Ph.D. dissertation, University of Washington, 1968.

2. P. de Visé, "Methods and Concepts of an Interdisciplinary Regional Hospital Study," Health Serv. Res. 3 (Fall 1968):166.

3. P. J. Feldstein, "Research on the Demand for Health Services," Millbank Mem. Fund Quart. 44, Part 2 (July 1966):128.

4. G. D. Rosenthal, The Demand for General Hospital Facilities. Chicago: American Hospital Association, 1964.

5. P. de Visé, Hospital Study Districts for Metropolitan Chicago. Technical Report No. 2. Chicago: Hospital Planning Council for Metropolitan Chicago, 1966.

6. R. E. Coughlin, "Hospital Complex Analysis: An Approach to Analysis for Planning a Metropolitan System of Service Facilities," Ph.D. dissertation, University of Pennsylvania, 1965.

7. J. P. Schneider, "Planning the Growth of a Metropolitan System of Public-service Facilities: The Short-term General Hospital," Ph.D. dissertation, University of Pennsylvania, 1966.

8. P. de Visé, Predicting Pediatric and Geriatric Population Needs of New Life Communities. Working Paper III.6, Chicago Regional Hospital Study, 1968.

9. Charlotte Muller, "Income and the Receipt of Medical Care," Am. J. Pub. Health 55 (April 1965):510.

10. G. Bugbee, "Medical Care for Low Income Families," Inquiry 5 (March 1968):5.

11. M. E. Odoroff and L. M. Abbe, "Use of General Hospitals: Variations with Methods of Payment," Pub. Health Rep. 74 (April 1959):316.

12. G. Pyle, "The Geography of Disease in Large Cities," M.A. dissertation, University of Chicago, 1968.

13. P. de Visé, Slum Medicine, Chicago Style: How the Medical Needs of the City's Negro Poor Are Met. Working Paper IV.8, Chicago Regional Hospital Study, 1968.

14. Chicago Commission on Human Relations, Negro Physicians and Medical Students Affiliated with Chicago Hospitals and Medical Schools. Chicago: The Commission, 1966.

15. S. Kaplan, Report on Jewish Births and Jewish Population in Cook County, Illinois, 1963. Chicago: Jewish Federation of Metropolitan Chicago, 1966.

16. R. L. Morrill and R. Earickson, Hospital, Physician and Commercial Location. Working Paper I.7, Chicago Regional Hospital Study, 1966.

17. J. Schneider, "The Spatial Structure of the Medical Care Process," Discussion Paper 14, Regional Science Research Institute, Philadelphia, 1967.

18. P. Rees, Numbers and Movement of Physicians in Southeast Chicago: 1953-1965. Working Paper I.13, Chicago Regional Hospital Study, 1967.

19. R. L. Morrill and P. Rees, Influence of the Physician on Patient to Hospital Distance. Working Paper I.16, Chicago Regional Hospital Study, 1968.

20. R. L. Morrill and R. Earickson, Hospital Service Areas, Parts I-IV. Working Papers I.3, I.4, I.5, and I.6, Chicago Regional Hospital Study, 1967.

21. R. L. Morrill, Historical Development of the Chicago Hospital System. Working Paper I.2, Chicago Regional Hospital Study, 1966.

22. R. L. Morrill and R. Earickson, "Variation in the Character and Use of Chicago Hospitals," Health Serv. Res. 3 (Fall 1968): 224.

23. W. J. Carr and P. Feldstein, "The Relationship of Cost to Hospital Size," Inquiry 4 (June 1967):45.

24. M. F. Long and P. Feldstein, "Economics of Hospital Systems, Peak Loads and Regional Coordination," Proc. Am. Econ. Assoc. 1967, p. 119.

25. R. L. Morrill and R. Earickson, "Hospital Variation and Patient Travel Distance," Inquiry 5 (December 1968):26.

26. D. L. Drossness and J. W. Lubin, "Planning Can Be Based on Patient Travel," Mod. Hosp. 106 (April 1966):92.

27. R. L. Morrill, "Relationship between Transportation and Hospital Location and Utilization," Proc. ASME 1967, p. 117.

28. R. L. Morrill and R. Earickson, Influence of Race, Religion and Ability to Pay on Patient to Hospital Distance. Working Paper I.17, Chicago Regional Hospital Study, 1968.

29. R. Earickson, The Case for Decentralizing Cook County Hospital. Working Paper III.4, Chicago Regional Hospital Study, 1968.

30. R. Earickson, Simulation Model of Nonwhite Hospital Use in Chicago. Working Paper III.3, Chicago Regional Hospital Study, 1967.

31. R. L. Morrill and R. Earickson, Problems in Modelling Interactance: The Case of Patient Travel for Hospital Care. Working Paper III.5, Chicago Regional Hospital Study, 1968.

32. Gunnar Olsson, "Central Place Systems, Spatial Interaction and Stochastic Processes," Papers, Regional Sci. Assoc. (European) 18 (1967):13.

33. H. S. Guetzkow (ed.), Simulation in Social Science. Englewood Cliffs, N.J.: Prentice-Hall, 1962.

34. B. H. Stevens, "A Review of the Literature on Linear Methods and Models for Spatial Analysis," J. Am. Inst. Plan. 26 (August 1960):253.

PART III
OTHER SYSTEMS ANALYSIS TECHNIQUES

15

DELPHI METHOD

INTRODUCTION

Delphi forecasting was used for determining the major trends of health care organization and delivery in a large San Francisco hospital prior to the implementation of physical plant changes. Twenty-four panel members were selected from different professions of health care providers. Questions were asked concerning the trends in organizational patterns of health care delivery, the patterns of reimbursement, the foreseeable changes, and the resultant impact on hospitals. The results of the study convinced the hospital to drop its plan for a traditional medical practices building expansion. An alternative plan, which included the sponsorship of an ambulatory clinic and a health maintenance organization, was considered.

Introduction to Technique

The Delphi Method is a group consensus method that was originally developed to forecast technically oriented phenomena. Several other uses of Delphi have been developed, such as the gathering of data, examining the significance of historical events, exploring urban and regional planning options, and exposing priorities of personal values and social goals.
In the Delphi Method, a group or panel responds to questions regarding possible future events without coming into face-to-face contact. By this process each panelist is forced to compare his descriptions and predictions of the future with those of his colleagues. There are two main forms of the Delphi processes. They are:

1 Delphi-Exercise (Conventional Delphi)—a monitor team develops a questionnaire, elicits responses, develops a new questionnaire

(with prior responses paraphrased and summarized), elicits new responses, and continues this process until a satisfactory forecast has been made.
2 Delphi-Conference (Real-Time Delphi)—a computer replaces the monitor team in the data compilation. This approach is faster but it requires that the characteristics of the communication are well defined.

REFERENCES

Linstone, H. A., and M. Turoff, The Delphi Method Techniques and Applications, Reading, Mass.: Addison-Wesley, 1975.

Schoeman, M., and V. Mahajan, "Using the Delphi Method to Assess Community Health Needs," Technological Forecasting and Social Change 10 (1977):203-10.

DELPHI FORECASTING OF
HEALTH CARE ORGANIZATION

David B. Starkweather
Louis Gelwicks
Robert Newcomer

The research described in this paper originated as part of a master plan for redevelopment and expansion of the services and

---

David B. Starkweather, Dr. P. H. is Associate Professor of Public Health, and Director, Graduate Curriculum in Hospital Administration, School of Public Health, University of California at Berkeley.

Louis Gelwicks, A. I. A., is Research Associate, Gerontology Center, University of Southern California, and President of Gerontological Planning Associates, Santa Monica.

Robert Newcomer, Ph. D. is Lecturer, Graduate Program in Urban and Regional Planning, University of Southern California, and Director of Planning, Gerontological Planning Associates.

Reprinted with permission of the Blue Cross Association, from Inquiry 12, no. 1, pp. 37-46. Copyright 1975 by the Blue Cross Association. All rights reserved.

facilities of an urban hospital in the western United States. Hospital officials asserted, appropriately, that no major changes in the institution should be made without first obtaining as clear a picture as possible of the nature of health care organization 10 years hence; only in this context should changes be contemplated. Efforts to obtain such a forecast relied primarily on the Delphi process, a technique designed to obtain consensus from a panel of experts on future events and conditions.

Results from four realms of prediction are reported here, for their general interest and as an illustration and critique of a useful planning technique which has wide potential application. The four realms are 1) predominant organization patterns of health care delivery, 2) methods of financing health care, 3) modes of reimbursement, and 4) the nature and role of hospitals.

The Delphi technique [1] arose out of a recognized need to eliminate the interpersonal dynamics that exist in face-to-face group meetings. It has been found that in such groups agreement is likely to represent the views of member(s) with greatest status, despite other valid views, and that people in such groups are often reluctant to change their publicly expressed opinions even in the face of substantial contrary evidence or argument [2].

In the Delphi method, a group, or panel, responds to questions regarding possible future events without coming into face-to-face contact. Panel participants are not identified to each other during the course of the study, although background information and specific comments of the panelists are anonymously included in subsequent stages of inquiry.

A Delphi survey is conducted over several rounds, typically three or four [3], in order to permit interactive but impersonal feedback and re-evaluation. The question, response, and evaluation process is carried out by mail, with contributions of each panelist processed by one or a few persons conducting the study. By this process, each panelist is forced to compare and contrast his descriptions and predictions of the future with those of his colleagues. This leads to juxtaposition, re-evaluation, refinement, and clarification of predictions, resulting in either strong convergence or lack of consensus—with outcomes based on a thoughtful weighing of alternatives and counter views rather than on ignorance or unchallenged speculation.

In short, the Delphi process is characterized by 1) relative efficiency in the use of experts' time, 2) anonymity of response, 3) multiple iterations, 4) convergence of the distribution of answers, and 5) a statistical group response which preserves a distribution that may remain wide.

APPLICATIONS OF THE DELPHI PROCESS

Since it is likely that Delphi surveying will become, in the near future, a popular planning tool in the health field, it would seem worthwhile to identify some of its inherent strengths and weaknesses. Delphi was originally designed by the Rand Corporation for technologic forecasting. It has been used in this way in the health field to predict different stages and types of breakthroughs in medical instrumentation [4]. However, the application reported in this paper—and presumably most others that will follow—deals with forecasting of social and organizational variables. In comparing the two types of applications, we are struck by the differences and difficulties in dealing with high-articulation versus low-articulation subjects. In technologic forecasting, experts are chosen for their in-depth knowledge of some narrow field, whereas in social forecasting, experts must clearly possess knowledge of a broad range of factors to be able to assess the strength and direction of their interaction and to be capable of ferreting out crucial determinants from a confusing array of possibilities. Thus, the qualifications of panelists for social forecasting run more toward breadth and balance than to depth and mastery of facts.

There is an increasing tendency to stretch the Delphi to entirely different uses, notably 1) searching for goals and objectives, 2) planning, and 3) developing evaluation criteria [5, 6]. While these are worthwhile possibilities, important differences should be recognized. In particular as regards the first and third use, the emphasis shifts from description and prediction, i.e., what is and what is likely, to normative questions of values, i.e., what should be. In the former instance, experts should be capable of objective analysis, and in the latter, they should be "experts" in the strength of their own subjective opinions. Further, the content and style of both questions and response evaluation are changed.

COMPOSITION OF THE PANEL

The selection of panelists is crucial, as it is, of course, in conventional techniques where persons are appointed to a task force, asked to participate in a series of group meetings, or chosen by sampling technique to be representative of some large group. Heterogeneity among panelists, rather than homogeneity, is important, since the Delphi process purposely emphasizes confrontation of predicted futures or contrast of different values. Without different vantage points represented on a panel, there is a danger of false consensus derived from persons "inbred" by virtue of common background or setting. As an example, in the study reported herein we sought heterogeneity by first identifying four categories of experts to be included: health services administrators, physicians, health care consumer advocates, and health economists.

Another important feature of Delphi panels—particularly important in forecasting as compared to the alternative applications mentioned—is that they be composed of seasoned experts. Making sense out of the future of health care organization is obviously difficult business; misleading conclusions can result from panelists who do not possess sufficient scope or experience. Without these attributes, individual panelists are likely to be either "oversold" by fellow panelists who hold differing views, or "undersold" for lack of judgment applied to logically developed counterviews [7].

Panel fatigue is a problem in the Delphi technique; it bears on whether conclusions are valid or whether they have resulted from over or under consensus. Panelists usually become fascinated by the Delphi process at rounds 2 and 3; but just as typically, they may "agree to anything" to avoid recycling the survey beyond round 3 or 4. Thus false consensus or divergence is possible. This phenomenon varies widely among different Delphis, and is not well understood by students of Delphi methodology [8]. However, an analyst can usually tell when closure is premature or overdue by examining the amount of change in responses between rounds 2 and 3 or 3 and 4. If each individual panelist's responses are identified (only to the analyst) and the Delphi is processed by computer, this monitoring is easily performed.

USE OF THE DELPHI IN HOSPITAL STUDY

The Delphi was used as a forecasting technique in a study conducted by the authors for a large hospital in San Francisco [9]. Hospital officials had decided that no major changes should be made in the physical plant without knowing more clearly the major trends in health care organization and delivery. The Delphi process was chosen as one primary means of obtaining this view.

Twenty-four panel members were selected for participation in this study. They were drawn from four general backgrounds in order to give a broad base of judgment: 1) hospital and health services administrators and planners, 2) physicians with experience in different modes of practice, 3) health care consumer advocates and voluntary health and welfare agency executives, and 4) health care financing officials, both private and government. These 24 persons were selected from an original list of 33 experts, the reduction in number being due to nonavailability of some experts coupled with a wish to keep the four types of panelists in equal proportion. By agreement, the panelists' names are not published herein; however, they are recognized experts in their fields.

This study was conducted in three rounds. The questions for round 1 were purposely general and open-ended, serving primarily to identify and delimit the scope of forecasting. Four realms were identified by the following set of questions [10]:

1 What general organizational pattern(s) for the delivery of health services do you see predominating within five to 10 years?
2 What do you see as the methods of reimbursement for providers for the patterns indicated by you in your answer to question 1?
3 What major changes do you project for the next five to 10 years as regards ways in which consumers will finance medical care? Please be specific as to: a) the role of prepayment and insurance plans, b) the role of government financial programs, and c) sources of any new financing.
4 How will hospitals be affected by the predominant organization patterns indicated by you in your answer to question 1 in respect to a) sponsorship, b) public accountability, c) relationships between hospitals, and d) medical staff organization?

Subsequent rounds were developed from the initial responses given to round 1 questions; thus, panelists were responding to issues they had collectively raised. This was done by 1) abstracting round 1 responses to eliminate redundancies and restating long answers in cryptic phrases; 2) distributing results to all panel members for their individual reconsideration; 3) further summarizing round 2 responses and representing them in a format that juxtaposes contrasting views; 4) redistributing results once again to all panelists; and 5) performing statistical analysis and final presentation of round 3 results.

Only round 3 results are fully reported here, consisting of the final index of consensus obtained in this Delphi [11]. However, as an example of the iteration process, the details of response and analysis of the first question—"What general organization patterns . . . do you see predominating . . . ?"—are briefly presented in the sequence outlined in the preceding paragraph.

1 Round 1 responses indicated widely divergent assessments of future organization patterns, including a variety of new formal ties between previously independent providers, new physician-hospital relationships, and new forms of ambulatory care delivery. Some panelists predicted marked increase in group practice, while others saw continuation of present pluralism in modes of medical practice.

The full array of responses was restated in the general phraseology shown in the narrative portion of Table 15.1 (excluding the numerical predictions of likelihood). At this point, however, the phraseology was not as specific as shown in the table. For instance, item (a) of Table 15.1 simply asked the panelists to indicate the nature of specific organizational ties, without indicating which providers would be involved, the likelihood of hospital consolidations, or reference to either health care corporations, item (b), or health maintenance organizations, item (c).

2 Round 2 was distributed to all panelists approximately six weeks after round 1 [12], the intervening time having been used by panelists to develop round 1 responses (three weeks) and by Delphi analysts to restate their responses (three weeks).

3 Round 2 responses were again restated in order to articulate important details and contrasting views. Where different meanings and uses of words had been revealed, common definitions were provided. For instance, concerning items (a), (b), and (c) of Table 15.1, parties to specific collaboration were indicated, as well as both clarification of and distinction between health care corporations and HMOs. Concerning item (e), group practice, the phrase "at least 50%" was added in order to provide a uniform basis for panelist forecasting.

4 The round 3 survey was more abbreviated than round 2, one wide array of initial responses having been reduced both by restatements of analysts and reconsiderations of panelists [12]. A format for predicting likelihoods was added to this distribution.

5 Round 3 responses were analyzed to identify the predictions upon which there was consensus and those upon which there remained a divergence of views. Results are shown in Table 15.1.

For the study as a whole, Tables 15.1-15.4 contain final responses to all initial questions. These tables show the proportion of panelists, rounded to the nearest 5 percent, who estimated with .90, .50, and .10 probability, respectively, that the conditions paraphrased by each statement will occur in the next five to 10 years.

Rectangles and squares are used to graphically indicate the degree of consensus for each statement. We define consensus as 75 percent or more of the panel having reached agreement on one or two probability choices. If that proportion of the panel agreed on two probability choices (i.e., .10 and .50 or .50 and .90), we believe "general consensus" was achieved. If the 75 percent proportion converged on a single probability choice (i.e., .10 or .50 or .90), we believe "strong consensus" was evidenced. General consensus is indicated by rectangles, and strong consensus by larger squares. A smaller square within a rectangle denotes a future circumstance in which 50 percent or more but not 75 percent of the panel converged on one probability estimate.

The results reported here are undifferentiated by respondent background. Each panel member's assessment was equally weighted. Since the panel used in this study was made up of persons with widely divergent expertises and approaches to medical care, the futures upon which consensus was reached would seem to have general significance.

FINDINGS

Organizational Patterns

Table 15.1 presents forecasts with respect to the broad dimensions of future health services organization. All but two forecasts received general consensus for .50 or higher probability, including several where approximately half of the experts who provided .50 assessments were joined by additional panelists whose assessments of likelihoods were very high.

Clearly, the panelists anticipate important changes in health services organizational patterns. There was strong consensus that specific functional and organizational ties between providers would increase. This is seen more as a hospital-based development than as one arranged by health care corporations or health maintenance organizations. Since the three approaches are by no means mutually exclusive, the experts were probably reflecting the fact that hospitals currently exist and are, therefore, clearly available for this role, whereas the other two mechanisms are less extant. The assessments concerning marked increase in group practice are significant; and the specifications of particular affiliation of many such groups with hospitals is both consistent with the general forecast of new organizational ties between many providers (item (a)) and details identified in subsequent tables as regards financial reimbursement (Table 15.2, item (i)) and medical staff-hospital relationships (Table 15.4, items (x), (y), (z)).

While panelists agreed on certain fundamental changes, they also indicated considerable uncertainty as to specific forms of future health care organization. This is revealed by the general consensus on continuation of pluralism. However, several experts commented in the narrative response of round 2 that while pluralism would undoubtedly prevail, there will likely be a substantially different mix of specific delivery forms. Thus, the probability assessments as regards pluralism (item (d)) are seen as consistent with the responses to other items of Table 15.1 and subsequent tables.

TABLE 15.1

Predominating Health Service Organization Patterns

Futures	Percent of Panelists Indicating Likelihood of Occurrence in Next 10 Years of:		
	90%	50%	10%
(a) More specific organizational ties between medical groups, hospitals, ambulatory care, and specialized facilities as a result of hospital consolidations	75	10	5
(b) Same as (a) except as a result of health care corporations*	15	45	40
(c) Same as (a) except as a result of health maintenance organizations*	15	60	25
(d) Continuation of today's pluralistic pattern of the organization of medical practice (solo, small partnership or group), large group as with Kaiser, salaried or contract practice at some hospital	30	65	5
(e) Marked increase in medical group practice to the point of incorporating at least 50% of all practicing physicians	45	55	0
(f) Affiliation of group practices with specific hospitals with most larger sized groups so linked	35	60	5
(g) Neighborhood-oriented ambulatory care clinics featuring practice of physicians in primary care teams	25	60	15

*Definitions provided panelists:

Health care corporations have the following characteristics: 1) a corporate structure with capacity to deliver health maintenance on a primary, specialty, restorative, and custodial care basis; 2) cover health needs of defined geographic area; 3) every practicing physician would have opportunity to affiliate with HCC; 4) various forms of medical practice, including group practice would be permitted; 5) evaluation of the quality of health care would be conducted by corporation; 6) identification and responsibility by the corporation for its own manpower needs; 7) operating under new regulatory controls established by state legislation (utility type commission); 8) reimbursement to providers by mutually agreeable means.

Health maintenance organizations are based on the following principles: 1) organized system of health care which accepts responsibility of providing an agreed upon set of comprehensive health maintenance and treatment services for a voluntarily enrolled group of persons in a geographic area; and 2) reimbursed through a prenegotiated and fixed prepayment based on each enrolled person or family unit.

329

TABLE 15.2

Predominating Methods of Medical Care Reimbursement

Futures	Percent of Panelists Indicating Likelihood of Occurrence in Next 10 Years of:		
	90%	50%	10%
Predominating Reimbursement Mode to Doctors			
(a) Continuation of fee-for-service	30	55	15
(b) Capitation payment (i.e., based on an agreed number of persons rather than for services rendered) by both government and private insurance	25	55	20
(c) Salary	0	40	60
Predominating Reimbursement Mode to Hospitals			
(d) Incentive reimbursement (payment arranged so that if the provider economizes relative to some previously agreed standard he is paid a portion of the difference as a "bonus")	35	60	5
(e) Negotiated rates rather than costs or charges	45	45	10
(f) Regulated prices (as in the case of public utilities)	35	35	30
(g) Reimbursement based on budget submission and review	30	40	30

Predominating Reimbursement Mode to Both Doctors and Hospitals

(h) Continuation of fee-for-service for physicians and cost-based reimbursement for hospitals	20	50	30
(i) Capitation payments which would cover both physician, hospital and other services, inspiring providers to cooperate for mutual financial gain (as is the case with Kaiser)	30	45	15
(j) Return to more of a free market approach with rates determined by forces of competition, supply and demand	10	35	55

Predominating Method of Payment to Doctors and Hospitals

(k) Continuation of current pattern, i.e., use of private (indemnity, Blue Cross) plans for those persons able to purchase premiums, and use of same plans as fiscal intermediaries for patients who are financially sponsored by government	45	45	10
(l) Same as above, except assumption of actuariy risk by fiscal intermediaries instead of by government	10	45	45
(m) Elimination of private plans as fiscal intermediaries for government–sponsored patients, with direct payment by government in its place	0	40	60
(n) Elimination of private plans for all types of patients with virtually all payments coming from government through national health insurance	5	20	75

Medical Care Reimbursement

Three distinct categories of medical care reimbursement—to doctors, to hospitals, and to both doctors and hospitals—were investigated, as well as methods of payment to each. Results are shown in Table 15.2. The Delphi panelists identify no single predominating mode of reimbursement for the next 10 years. Several alternatives received approximately equal likelihoods of occurrence, indicating lack of consensus. However, several major shifts from current practices were predicted, including use of capitation payments to physicians and physician-hospital combinations, and incentive reimbursements to hospitals, probably based on negotiated rates. Again, closer relationships between physicians and hospitals seem implied. It is interesting that the panel rejected utility-type rate regulation as a predominating mode for hospitals, as it did reimbursement based on budget submission and review (as is the case in Canada). The forecast for private insurance companies was approximate to their present role: fiscal intermediaries for government, without assuming actuarial risk, and continued underwriting of private coverage. The panel clearly rejected the extremes of socialized medicine in respect to salaried physicians, as well as unfettered free-market medicine.

Methods of Financing

Likelihood of prior existing, current, and nationalized methods of medical care financing were predicted, and are shown in Table 15.3.

National health insurance was given a .50 or better chance of implementation within a period of five to 10 years by almost 90 percent of the Delphi panel. Within the same probability range, fewer experts (60 percent), still a majority, forecasted its implementation within five years. National health insurance is expected to evolve in two stages—catastrophic coverage followed by comprehensive benefits. The scope of benefits of this insurance is not clearly perceived at this time, although relatively comprehensive benefits are predicted as the 10-year eventuality. Panelists agreed that national health insurance will be financed by a combination of general tax revenues, employer contributions, and individual payments. As previously noted, national health insurance is not expected to occur to the exclusion of existing private plans (an observation that has held true in virtually all nations that have moved to nationalized forms).

TABLE 15.3

Predominating Methods of Consumer Medical Care Financing

Futures	Percent of Panelists Indicating Likelihood Of Occurrence in Next 10 Years of:		
	90%	50%	10%
(a) Return to previous patterns of private financing, i.e., private, individual and employer	10	10	80
(b) Continuation of present patterns of financing, i.e., approximately 50% from private sources (private payments and insurance) and approximately 50% from the government (federal, state and local)	10	20	70
As Regards National Health Insurance:			
(c) Catastrophic or excessive costs only	30	40	20
(d) Relatively comprehensive or full benefits (including catastrophic/excessive coverage)	25	70	5
(e) No implementation within next 10 years	5	30	65
(f) Implementation within next 10 years, not within next five years	30	60	10
(g) Implementation within next five years	30	30	40
(h) Implemented within one stage, catastrophic/excessive coverage only	10	45	45
(i) Implemented within one stage, comprehensive benefits (including catastrophic/excessive coverage)	10	30	60
(j) Implemented within 10 years, in two stages, catastrophic/excessive first followed by comprehensive benefits	45	40	15
(k) Financed by general tax revenues	5	30	65
(l) Financed primarily by specific employer/employee contributions (as in Medicare)	10	60	30
(m) Financed by a combination of general tax revenues, employer contributions and individual payment (made either as wage deductions or direct payments)	65	35	0

TABLE 15.4

Medical Service Organizational Patterns and Their Effect on Hospitals

Futures	Percent of Panelists Indicating Likelihood of Occurrence in Next 10 Years of:		
	90%	50%	10%
Hospitals in Respect to Sponsorship			
(a) Little or no change	20	20	60
(b) More profit-oriented ownership	0	35	65
(c) Government run hospitals will convert to private nonprofit status	15	45	40
(d) Hospitals will assume status of quasi-public utilities	45	50	5
(e) Federation of hospitals into central sponsorship/ownership	20	45	35
Hospitals in Respect to Public Accountability			
(f) Little or no change	5	5	90
(g) More voluntary public responsiveness in terms of types of services, financial accounting, expansion, etc.	35	55	10
(h) More representation of the underserved public on hospital boards	55	45	0
(i) Public disclosure of hospital income, expenses and plans	95	5	0
(j) Officially authorized agency review of performance in fiscal management and of service quality	55	45	0
(k) Greater commission-type regulation of services, expansion, and rates	80	20	0

Hospitals in Respect to Relationship with Other Hospitals

(l) Little or no change	5	20	75	
(m) Continued voluntary development of shared services not involving patient contact	35	55	10	
(n) Greater voluntary coordination, cooperation and functional specialization among hospitals regarding all services, research, and education	65	30	5	
(o) Stronger management alliances	55	35	10	
(p) Formation of consortia of hospitals which will jointly assume financial risk	35	40	25	
(q) Physical consolidations and complete organizational merger	15	40	45	

Hospitals in Respect to Medical Staff Organization

(r) Physicians will be required to admit all of their cases to one hospital rather than several	0	35	65	
(s) Hospitals will continue to have their own medical staff and will continue to be closed to non-staff physicians	50	25	25	
(t) Hospitals will no longer have their own medical staff, physicians will become members of a common staff which is sponsored by a federated organization such as a health care corporation	10	20	70	
(u) Staff privileges among hospitals will be interchangeable	20	40	40	
(v) Hospitals will contract with medical care foundation for medical staff	5	55	40	
(w) One medical staff for two or more hospitals	45	40	15	
(x) Greater physician participation in hospital affairs, including direct operating responsibilities	40	45	15	
(y) Doctors will be closer to their principal hospital, having an interlocking incentive and penalty system linked to the hospital	10	80	10	
(z) Medical staff will be more oriented into health teams coordinated with neighborhood clinics in addition to hospitals	30	50	20	

Impact of Medical Care Organization Patterns on Hospitals

Four general areas were examined under this heading: hospital sponsorship, public accountability, relationships with other hospitals, and medical staff organization. Results are shown in Table 15.4

With the exception of the fourth subcategory, the Delphi panel predicted definite changes from the status quo. Hospitals are given a .50 or better likelihood by most respondents of assuming the status of "quasi-public utilities" and of becoming federated into varying forms of consolidated sponsorship. One-third of the panel predicted an increase in profit-oriented ownership, a circumstance that is not inconsistent with utility status. Additionally, there was strong consensus among panelists that public accountability in terms of broader hospital board membership, public disclosure, agency review, and commission regulation will occur. Concerning utility regulation, the combination of the panel's strong consensus of high likelihood as regards item (k) in Table 15.4, and its lack of consensus on item (f) in Table 15.2 suggests that commission regulation may fall short of rate control, although it will most certainly apply to other forms of supervision.

Consensus was somewhat lower in the prediction of relationships among hospitals, partly because the panelists were not required to regard their several options as mutually exclusive. Four alternatives each received majority support for probability assessments of .50 and higher. One—greater voluntary coordination of all activities—had a majority consensus at the .90 probability level. Another likelihood, the (voluntary) formation of risk-bearing consortia, was also well supported. Combining the responses to item (a) of Table 15.1 and items (e), and (l)-(q) of Table 15.4, the panel seemed to envision a strong trend toward formal interhospital arrangements, in which the autonomy of separate hospitals will be substantially altered but not totally submerged to complete merger.

A somewhat diffused pattern of forecasts is evident in respect to medical staff organization. Continuation of the existing basic form of hospital medical staff is seen, with relatively low likelihood that physicians will either be limited to one medical staff or be expected to practice in a generic staff that spans many institutions and is sponsored by a "third party." Yet, commonalities between two or a few hospital medical staffs is seen as quite likely. Instead of important new relationships among several medical staffs, the panel sees stronger relationships between each medical staff and its hospital, definitely including greater physician responsibility for hospital operations, with that relationship backed by new economic reimbursement schemes that treat a medical staff and a hospital as a single economic dyad.

With respect to organized ambulatory care, panelists' responses to the combination of item (z), Table 15.4, and items (e)-(g), Table 15.1, suggests a future of hospital-based neighborhood satellite clinics, staffed primarily by teams of generalists and family practitioners who are organized in part-time group(s) that hold specific relationships to hospitals.

CONCLUSION

The Delphi reported herein had substantial impact on the hospital for which it was performed. It buttressed the case for a change in hospital direction from exclusive orientation to inpatient operations to one that includes ambulatory care. The hospital shelved its plans for a traditional medical practice building as its next major physical expansion, and actively considered alternate forms of health care delivery, including sponsorship of an ambulatory clinic designed for service to its immediate neighborhood, and sponsorship of a health maintenance organization. The study added to the general understanding of and responsiveness to health care trends by the hospital in a way that more traditional approaches do not, probably because of the increased credence accorded the expert panelists and the thorough examination and extension of future trends that are inherent in the Delphi process [13].

As for other applications of Delphi, opportunities are widespread. Almost any one of the numerous forecasts reported here could be taken as the starting point of a more refined Delphi that would update and improve our perception of the future of a field characterized by extreme complexity and shortage of quantifiable measures. Yet, we are also concerned that Delphi not become misused, in the manner of a fad. It will quickly outlive its usefulness if it is used for purposes other than those for which it was designed, is conducted with inappropriate panelists, or is improperly processed. Clearly, the situation calls for careful, innovative, and continued experimentation with the technique, coupled with responsible interpretation and use of results.

NOTES

1. O. Helmer, Social Technology (New York: Basic Books, 1966).

2. N. Dalkey, The Delphi Method: An Experimental Study of Group Opinion (Santa Monica: Rand Corporation, RM-5888-PR, 1969).

3. It has been shown that consensus usually develops and stabilizes after this number of rounds. N. Dalkey, B. Brown, and S. Cochran, The Delphi Method, IV: Effect of Percentile Feedback of Relevant Facts (Santa Monica: Rand Corporation, RM-6118-PR, 1970).

4. A. Bender, A. Strack, G. Ebright, and G. VonHaunalter, "Delphic Study Examines Developments in Medicine," Futures (June 1969):289-303.

5. R. Judd, "Use of Delphi Methods in Higher Education," Technological Forecasting and Social Change 4 (1972):173-86.

6. M. Riesenfeld, R. Newcomer, W. Dempsey, and P. Berlant, "Perceptions of Public Service Needs: The Urban Aged and the Public Agency," The Gerontologist 12 (Summer 1972).

7. This comment about the need for bona fide experts is based in part on experience gained by one of the authors in a follow-up resurvey of round 3 of this study, as described in the text, coupled with a related application of the same Delphi to several groups of masters students in health administration. When round 3 was resubmitted one year after its original use to the expert panel, there was little variation of response—evidence of survey reliability. Also, the predictions of futures that evolved in the original three rounds did not vary as much by the four different backgrounds of panelists as they did by other (unexplained) dimensions. Yet, when round 3 was submitted to panels of students of graduate programs of different sponsorship (public health, business, public administration, medicine), the responses varied substantially by background and setting. One explanation of the difference in results is the relative expertness and experience of the professional versus student panels. The students appeared to be more gripped by the conventional wisdom of their different academic setting and less capable of separating their personal preferences for what the future should hold from their prediction of how it will likely be.

8. B. Brown, S. Cochran, and N. Dalkey, The Delphi Method, II: Structure of Experiments (Santa Monica: Rand Corporation, RM-5957-PR, 1969).

9. The authors are indebted to officials of St. Francis Memorial Hospital, San Francisco, for permission to extract some of the data reported herein from a larger study conducted by Gelwicks and Walls and Associates, Architects and Planning Consultants of Los Angeles, California.

10. A fifth realm relating to local circumstances has been eliminated from this paper.

11. This round was redistributed to panelists one year after its original distribution, as a reliability check. Variations in responses between years were minor, in only one case exceeding

a shift in the distribution of probability assessments by more than 5 percent. The second set of round 3 responses is reported here, making the Delphi forecast current to late 1973.

12. The response rate for round 1 was 100 percent. For round 2 it was 96 percent, and for round 3, 92 percent. All panel members contributed to at least two rounds.

13. As evidenced by the following comment by the hospital's long-range planning committee: "The Committee was impressed with the thoroughness and comprehensiveness of this study . . . and the assessment of probable trends in the forseeable future . . ., and hopes that this report can be given wider distribution in the San Francisco health care community."

16

GRAVITY MODEL

INTRODUCTION

This paper explores the patterns of patient flow to hospitals in rural areas. A patient-origin survey was conducted in the state of Idaho. "Hospital trade areas" were mapped out by searching through each hospital's admittance records for patients' place of residence. A gravity model was then applied to obtain another service area map of the same region. The gravity model is based on Newtonian theory which states that the potential attraction force between two bodies increases with the product of their masses and decreases with the distance between them. In this study, the mass is the number of beds, physicians, and facilities a hospital has with respect to other adjacent hospitals. The larger the hospital, the greater the drawing power it will have on the patient population. A comparison of the gravity model map and the patient origin map revealed a 96.5 percent match between the two. This showed that the gravity model is a powerful forecasting tool for health planners.

Introduction to Technique

The gravity model is a distribution model based on theories derived from Newton's law of gravitation, which states that there is a power of gravity pertaining to all bodies, proportional to the several quantities of matter which they contain and the force of gravity toward the several equal particles of any body is inversely related to the square of the distance from the particles.

The model has now been developed into a tool which aids planners in the process of site evaluation for a proposed facility.

David Huff's formulation (see Lambe reference) of the gravity model states that the attraction exerted on a consumer in area i by a retail center at location j is directly proportional to the size of the retail center and inversely proportional to the customer's distance from the center. The focus of this model is on the activity of the consumer, rather than on the activity of the firm. Increasing size of a center is a utility to the customer, as it generally means a larger product assortment. Increasing distance, however, is a disutility as it represents a cost. An individual wishing to be an efficient shopper will be attracted to a particular center in proportion to the ratio of utility to disutility.

REFERENCES

Catanese, A. J., Scientific Methods of Urban Analysis. Urbana, Ill.: University of Illinois Press, 1972. Pp. 223-28.

Dickey, J., et al., Metropolitan Transportation Planning. Washington, D.C.: Scripta, 1975. Pp. 199-209.

Kotler, P., Marketing Decision Making: A Model Building Approach. New York: Holt, Rinehart and Winston, 1971. Pp. 316-23.

Lambe, T., "The Opportunity, Gravity and Thurstone Models of Individual Choice," Socio-Economic Planning Sciences 3 (September 1969):411-19.

Nakanishi, M., and L. G. Cooper, "Parameter Estimation for a Multiplicative Interaction Model—Least Squares Approach," Journal of Marketing Research 11 (August 1974):303-11.

Render, B., and G. L. Shawhan, "A Spatial Interaction Model for the Allocation of Higher Education Enrollments," Socio-Economic Planning Sciences 2 (1977):43-48.

Stanley, T. J., and A. S. Sewell, "Image Inputs to a Probabilistic Model: Predicting Retail Potential," Journal of Marketing 40 (July 1976):48-53.

Stopher, P., and A. Meyburg, Urban Transportation Modeling and Planning. Lexington, Mass.: D. C. Heath, 1975. Pp. 140-58.

A MATHEMATICAL MODEL FOR DERIVING HOSPITAL SERVICE AREAS

James Meade

The basic premise explored in this paper is that patient flow in rural areas is based on the proximity to medical care. The hospital is defined as the center of care, and hospital catchment areas are defined by patient movements. A methodology is described to analyze patient flow among an assemblage of hospitals. Finally, a model which mathematically replicates patient movement is introduced to act as an aid in the hospital planning process.

In studying hospital spatial efficiency, the hospital planner must consider the resources of the existing hospital systems to provide patient care. Equally significant is the pattern of patient flow to each hospital. Therefore, it is important that the hospital planner know as much as possible about the spatial distribution of patients.

This paper has four objectives: (a) to discuss the concept of a patient-origin study as a means of hospital service area delimitation; (b) to acquaint the reader with the pattern of patient flow among an assemblage of hospitals; (c) to establish a foundation that the pattern of patient flow represents a construct of proximity to care; and (d) to establish the validity of the gravity model as a simple but efficient means of replicating the actual pattern of patient-hospital interaction in a group of dispersed rural hospitals.

METHODOLOGY

Study Area

The area selected for study in this paper is the state of Idaho. Idaho was selected because the needed data were available, this

Reprinted with permission from International Journal of Health Services Research 4, No. 2 (1974). Copyright 1974 by Baywood Publishing.

researcher was familiar with the area, and the population distribution in Idaho is amenable to study by a gravity-type equation.

Patient-Origin Survey

Among the various methods by which hospital service or trade areas may be established, the most accepted means is to search the hospital admittance records for patient place of residence. This type of search is known as a patient-origin survey. Once the record survey has been completed, the locations of patients are mapped with regard to the hospital. The hospital planner then has an accurate pattern of that specific hospital's trade area.

The data used in this paper were collected in Idaho hospitals during the months April through June, 1968. The sample included all patients discharged from each of the state's 46 general hospitals from September through November of 1967. It is felt that in most areas, the same time period is indicative of what one could expect under normal conditions during any time of the year. However, some localities may provide exceptions. For instance, the Snake River Valley during harvest time has an unknown number of migrant farm workers whose presence might not be reflected by these figures.

For the sake of simplicity only general hospitals or those not financed entirely by public funds have been included in this paper. The reason for excluding other hospitals is that these do not necessarily admit all types of patients, that is, mental hospitals usually treat mental patients exclusively.

The data were coded by patient zip code addresses. Therefore, it was necessary to select a scale to represent patient flow into different hospitals from one zip code area. For example, Homedale, Idaho (zip code 83628) has no hospital; therefore, it acts as a patient supply center to nearby cities that have hospitals. The data indicate that Homedale supplies patients to Caldwell (335 patients; distance from Homedale 13 miles), Nampa (43 patients; distance from Homedale 24 miles), and to Boise (40 patients; distance from Homedale 44 miles). Clearly, the majority of Homedale patients go to Caldwell, the nearest medical center for hospital care.

The scale selected to determine to which hospital service area a place without a hospital is assigned is as follows: A place that supplies 60 percent or more of its patients to one hospital is considered to be part of that hospital's service area. The figure of 60 percent was selected because, while patients in rural areas would normally go to the closest hospital, there may be other reasons such as referral, irrational choice, or an amenity which attracts them to another hospital further away. Sixty percent is larger than a simple majority

TABLE 16.1

Percentage of Patient Flow from Hospital to Nonhospital Areas[a]

Places with No Hospitals	Boise[b]	Nampa	Cald-well	Places with Hospitals					Mountain Home
				Weiser	Emmett	McCall	Council	Cascade	
Eagle	70.4	4.4	20.1		1.8	3.3			
Glenns Ferry[c]	53.3	5.0	2.1						39.6
Grandview	10.1	7.5	6.3						76.1
Homedale	9.5	10.2	79.1			1.2			
Horseshoe Bend[c]	39.3	2.2	5.5		48.1	2.7		2.2	
Kuna	15.6	60.0	22.0			2.4			
Marsing	6.2	20.2	73.6						
Melba	4.6	86.8	8.6						
Meridian	68.9	24.3	6.8						
Murphy[c]	34.8	43.5	21.7						
Parma	14.3	2.9	81.2	0.7		0.9			
Wilder	1.6	4.0	94.4						
Cambridge	6.3			29.2		2.0	62.5		
Idaho City	76.2				23.8				
New Meadows	17.8				2.8	46.1	28.3	2.2	
Riggins	21.6					75.0			
Midvale[c]	37.8			26.0			36.2		

[a]Source, Idaho Hospital Association and Washington–Alaska Regional Medical Program. Patient–Origin Study. Unpublished data, 1969.
[b]Major Regional Hospital Center.
[c]Places with less than 60 percent of the total patients not going to the closest hospital.

FIGURE 16.1

Location of Hospitals and Patient Supply Centers in Southwest Idaho, 1973

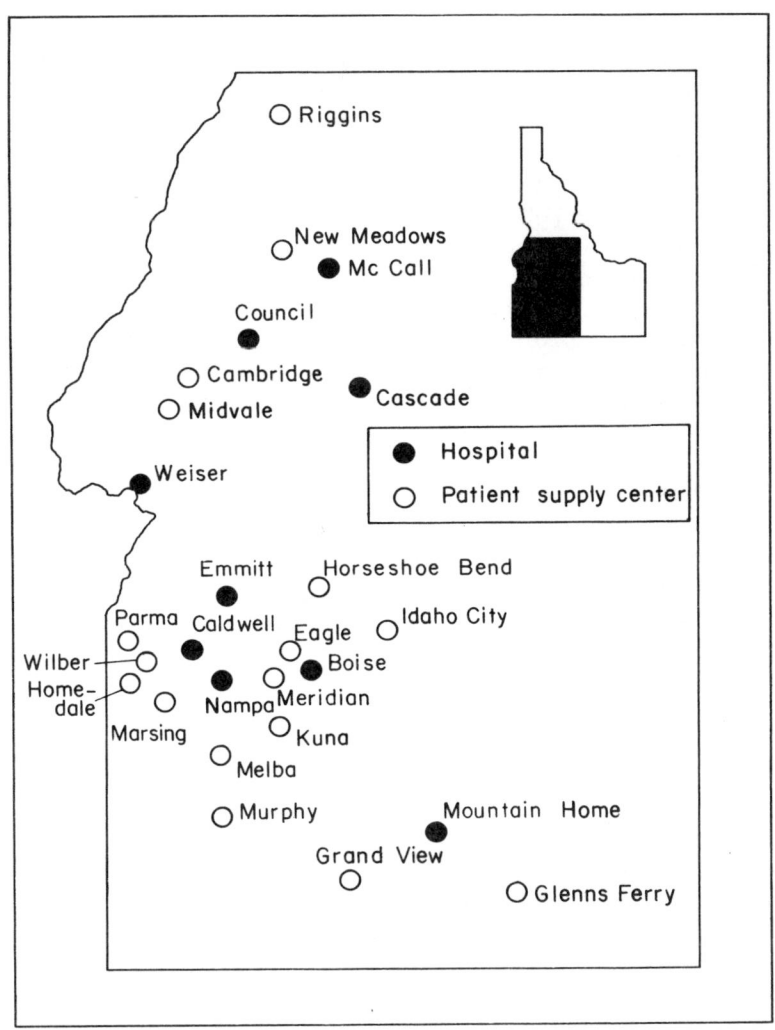

and seemed to be an acceptably large figure. Table 16.1, a data matrix showing the hospital centers on one axis, and places without hospitals on the other, supports the selection of the 60 percent patient figure. Figure 16.1 shows the location of hospitals and patient supply centers.

Table 16.1 indicates that in over 75 percent of the cases (13 of 17 places selected) patients do go to the closest hospital. With regard to the four places that do not fit this pattern (Glenns Ferry, Horseshoe Bend, Murphy, and Midvale), in two—Glenns Ferry and Murphy—simple majorities of their patients go to the closest hospital; in all four, however, there is a tendency for patients to go to Boise. This is not surprising when one realizes that Boise is the largest hospital center in the area and contains a great deal more in relation to hospital facilities or physician specialties than any other place in the region. Indeed, for patients to obtain equal or greater access to facilities or physician specialties, they would have to travel 428 miles to Portland, Oregon, or 349 miles to Salt Lake City, Utah. The chances that patients would travel this far are remote, although, no doubt, some do. More important, however, is the fact that the data in most instances support the original hypothesis that, in Idaho, a majority of patients do go to the closest center for hospital care.

Mapped Patterns: Patient-Origin

In mapping the patient-origin pattern, care was exercised in accounting for residents and establishing the service area boundaries in populated areas. However, due to the grouped manner in which the data were received, it was not always possible to account for each individual. Also, in the extreme rural areas where population was very sparse, the lines were either placed along rivers or some other natural boundary, or simply extended to maintain the symmetry of the line.

A patient-origin survey of all Idaho general hospitals has been utilized in this study.* The actual pattern of spatial interaction between the hospital facilities and the dispersed patient population has been mapped using the raw data from that survey (see Figure 16.2). The resulting pattern of hospital service areas indicates a variety of

---

*The patient-origin data were collected and compiled under the joint auspices of the Idaho Division of the Mountain States Regional Medical Program, the Idaho Hospital Association, and the State Comprehensive Health Planning Agency.

FIGURE 16.2

Hospital Service Areas in Idaho As Derived from Raw Data of an Idaho Hospital Association Patient-Origin Survey

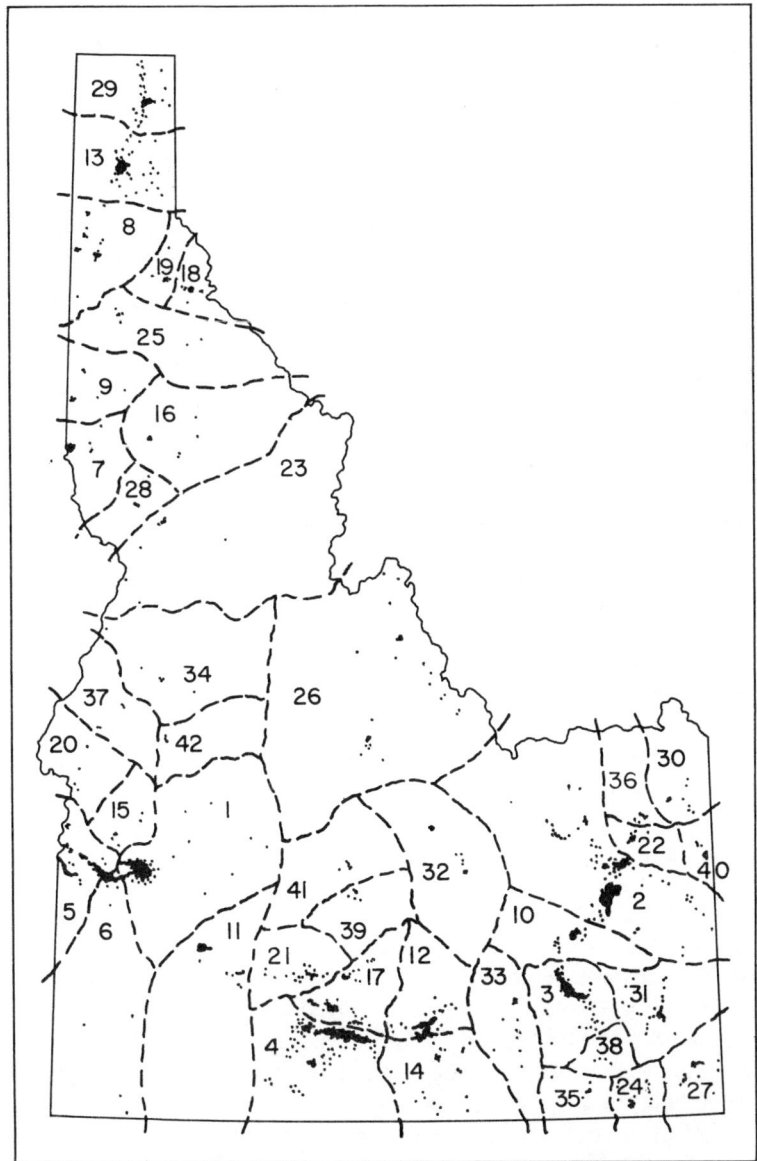

Note: Numbers are assigned to areas by population size. Service area 1 has the largest population, area 42, the smallest. One dot equals 100 people.

TABLE 16.2

Selected Hospital Service Areas and Population[a]

Hospital Service Area Number	Population	Area in Square Miles
7	27,966	925
8	27,756	1,425
16	11,547	2,925
17	11,519	1,275
18	11,501	800
21	9,261	1,150
22	9,117	575
33	4,111	1,625
34	4,141	3,475
39	2,500	1,150
40	2,539	400

[a]Source, Idaho Division, Mountain States Regional Medical Program. Idaho Health Profile, p. 4. Boise, Idaho, July 1969.

different sizes, shapes, and areas. Table 16.2 reviews some selected hospital service areas. These were selected to show differences in area population. Clearly, although two or more service areas may have the same population, they do not necessarily correspond in size. Nor are their populations always similar if they cover the same area, as a comparison of service areas 21 and 39 indicates.

The mapped pattern also reveals several spatial features. First, the larger hospital service areas are found either in sparsely populated areas or around the larger centers of population. The reason for large size in the case of areas deficient in population is due to the long distances between individual hospitals. An example of this is found by noting the distance between hospitals in areas 23 and 34 (see Figure 16.2). The reason for the big areas around the larger urban places such as Boise, Twin Falls, and Idaho Falls, may be attributed to the clustered nature of the state's population, especially around the major urban foci. Also, these centers are located in close proximity to the state's wilderness areas.

Since the actual patient-hospital pattern has been briefly examined and we wish to obviate further studies of that nature, it follows that a procedure to replicate that pattern is needed. Rather than selecting one method for analysis as a hospital service area replicator, this writer tried several mathematical methods including game theory, linear programming, regression, simulation modeling, and an adaptation of the gravity model. Because of the brevity of this paper, no explanation is offered to show why the first four methods were deleted. The reader is instead referred to the analyses of Earickson (1) and Meade (2).

GRAVITY MODEL

The method that was accepted to delimit the health service areas of Idaho is provided by an adaptation of Reilly's gravity model [3]. Reilly's model is based on the premise that a place will attract trade from an individual in its adjacent area in direct proportion to the size of the service center and in inverse proportion to the square of the distance away from the service center. The reason for selecting the gravity model adaptation stems from an analysis of the model's weak points as described by Converse [4] in the "New Laws of Retail Gravitation." He concluded that: (a) "the law does not seem to apply accurately in determining the trading areas of towns that differ greatly in size"; (b) "the accuracy was greatly reduced when the population of one town was twenty times the other"; and (c) "there is a problem of applying Reilly's law in suburban areas where the consumer travels through several separate communities." These are all admitted weak points of Reilly's law. However, they do not apply to Idaho because Idaho is a rural state in which the population of no one city is ten times greater than the ones it would be measured against. Converse's figure was twenty times as great, so the smaller figure satisfies the first point. Also, Idaho has a very limited number of suburban areas. Finally, Reilly's law was developed to measure the impact of rural trading centers. Therefore, there is no reason why it cannot measure primarily rural hospital service areas.

As stated, the delineation method to be used will be an adaptation of Reilly's law of retail gravitation. Accordingly, Reilly's formula will be changed from the original form where:

$$\frac{\text{miles between A and B}}{1 + \sqrt{\frac{\text{size of A}}{\text{size of B}}}} = \begin{array}{l}\text{distance of breaking point} \\ \text{from smaller trade area}\end{array}$$

to:

$$\frac{\text{miles between A and B}}{1 + \sqrt{\frac{(H+F+P)A}{(H+F+P)B}}} = \begin{array}{l}\text{distance of breaking point}\\ \text{from smaller hospital service area}\end{array}$$

where: H = number of hospital beds
F = sum of hospital facilities
P = sum of physician specialties
A = community
B = community
breaking point = maximum distance outward that, according to the gravity formula, a place exerts an attractive force

In the equation, A and B are separate and distinct communities, each containing a hospital. The total number of hospital beds contained in either place is indicated by H. Hospital beds were chosen because total beds are often used as an indicator of hospital size [5]. Furthermore, large size in hospitals as reflected by number of beds implies a wider range of functions performed by that hospital. Thus, HA = sum of hospital beds of community A.

The following list of hospital facilities was chosen because it reflects certain specialized equipment and personnel that major hospitals should contain. As such, the list reflects a high level of sophistication as to price, use, and availability.

Selected Hospital Facilities (F)	Number Contained
Cardiac catheter	0 to N
Intensive coronary care unit personnel	0 to N
Electroencephalograph	0 to N
Laboratory tests	0 to N
Diagnostic x-ray	0 to N
Therapeutic x-ray	0 to N
Radioactive isotopes	0 to N
Closed circuit television	0 to N
Bedside monitors	0 to N
Defibrillator	0 to N
Pacemaker	0 to N
Major operating room	0 to N

Physicians were placed in the expanded equation because they are the keystone to medical care. However, physicians were not broken down by specialty because of the lack of specialists in many of the state's hospitals. As such, the sum of physician specialties equals the total number of distinct specialties of each physician in the community, for example,

                12 general practitioners   12
                 3 surgeons   3
                 1 orthopedic surgeon   1
                                                 ──
                                                 16

Thus, PA = the sum of physician specialties of community A.

It is felt that by changing the sum of hospital beds and selected hospital facilities, plus by including the number of physician specialties, one will be able to obtain a more accurate hospital service area. The reason is that Reilly dealt essentially with an economic population. The expanded formula deals with a patronage function, that is, a service function as opposed to Reilly's economic function, although the two are closely interrelated.

The manner in which the gravity model map is derived is relatively simple. In fact the concept on which it is based dates back to Newtonian physics in that the potential attractive force between two bodies increases with the product of their masses and decreases with the distance between them. In the frame of this paper, size of the mass is related to the number of beds, facilities offered, or physicians that a specific hospital contains. In short, the more beds, facilities, and physicians a hospital has with respect to other adjacent hospitals, the more drawing power the larger facility exerts on the patient population.

Since the numerator of the equation is expressed as miles between two points (A and B), all one has to do is to fill in the appropriate numbers (beds, facilities, and physicians) and compute. The result will be the distance outward that the larger center exerts its attractive force. In essence, all that is accomplished is the derivation of a simple ratio where:

numerator: distance between two hospital centers
denominator: sum of hospital beds, facilities, and physicians of hospital A
1 plus the square root of
divided by
sum of hospital beds, facilities, and physicians of hospital B

= distance of breaking point from smaller hospital center

For example, assume two places as in Figure 16.2. Both places, A and B, contain hospitals. The dots represent patients who potentially would go to one or the other center for hospital care. Under the criteria of the formula, hospitals A and B have the following attributes:

hospital A: beds   250
             facilities   75
             physicians   81
                        = 406

hospital B: beds   50
             facilities   21
             physicians   7
                        = 78

Placing these attributes into the formula:

$$\frac{100}{1 + \sqrt{\frac{406}{78}}} = \frac{100}{1 + \sqrt{5.21}} = \frac{100}{1 + 2.28} = \frac{100}{3.28} = 31 \text{ miles}$$

Therefore, the smaller place (B) exerts its influence 31 miles toward place A. Other things being equal, the potential patients within the 31-mile radius will probably come to place B for hospital care; those outside the radius will probably go to hospital A for care.

In reality, however, there may be more than one path to go from point A to point B, as places are not always connected by just one road. In this instance, the formula should be calculated along all possible routes and the proper breaking points ascribed. Once all points have been calculated, they should be connected and thus the service areas of the hospitals are generated.

When connecting the breaking points that have been calculated, one should consider several factors, for example, alternate routes and topography or other surface features, such as lakes and rivers, as these might act to influence patient movement to hospitals. It would also be wise to consider the season because traveling conditions deteriorate in many places during the winter or rainy season. The point here is to be cognizant of the entire area before connecting points, as often a straight line is not correct. This is especially true the farther the points are from one another.

The method by which the gravity model maps were derived in this paper was by repetitive process. In fact, it was suspected, prior to their generation, that some form could be calculated by using any variety of criteria. After all, Reilly, in his original calculations, used floor space of retail centers to generate areas.

In this paper the first generation of the formula used bed size of hospital centers alone. The pattern or area generated was similar to the actual patient-origin areas but not closely enough. Successive repetitions added other criteria, such as hospital facilities and physicians, until the areas generated assumed the shape, or very nearly, of the actual patient-origin areas. In short, with each additional refinement of the model the areas generated more closely approximate reality.

MAP ANALYSIS

A map has been derived from the gravity equation. A comparison of the gravity model (Figure 16.3) and patient-origin map (Figure 16.4) indicates similarity. It was originally though that an acceptable match between the two maps should be about 75 percent. That is, the areas of both maps should be roughly equal in size and shape so that the map derived from the gravity equation should not over- or underpredict the area of the patient-origin map by more than 25 percent of the total land area. Actual mapping reveals that the match between the regions is 95.6 percent.

The method used to determine the match between the two maps is simple. A 5-square-mile grid system was imposed over the map, and the areas that did not align were demarked (Figure 16.5). The nonaligned area was totaled and compared to the total grid area. The comparison revealed that the area of nonalignment was 3,006 square miles. This figure is 3.5 percent of the total land area of 82,708 square miles.

The reasons for selecting the figure of 75 percent to be an acceptable replication between the two maps are as follows. First, by explaining 75 percent of the actual service area, one would have explained more, by mathematical means, than had ever been explained before. Second, it was a new use of an old predictive tool, but something that had never been attempted in Idaho or, for that matter, anywhere in the United States. Tyroller [6] has stated that "at the present time hospital planners cannot, with any degree of accuracy, predict more than one fourth of their actual hospital service area." Finally, it was decided that a larger figure than 25 percent would be desirable, a figure large enough to shock Idaho hospital planners so that they might review this method of analysis. Therefore, 75 percent was selected because it was three times the old amount.

An important feature the maps reveal is that the places of greatest variance occur in sparsely settled areas. Indeed, if measurements are derived from just the areas of map nonalignment (those areas where the methods do not align), the following information may be extrapolated. Idaho encompasses an area of 82,708 square land miles. The area in question covers 3,006 square miles or 3.5 percent of the state's total land area. Also, the population contained in the questionable area is 15,700, or 2.2 percent of the state's total

FIGURE 16.3

Hospital Service Areas in Idaho As Derived
from Results of a Gravity Model

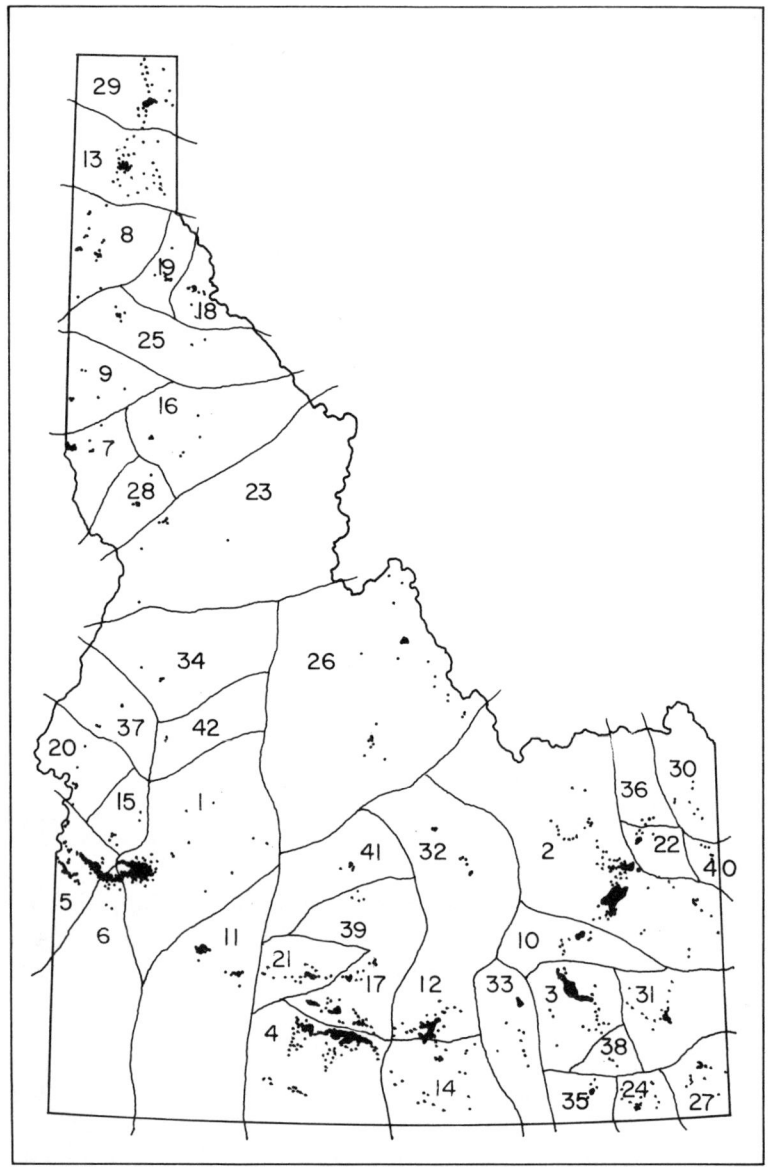

Note: Numbers are assigned to areas by population size. Service area 1 has the largest population, area 42, the smallest. One dot equals 100 people.

FIGURE 16.4

Comparison of Hospital Service Areas in Idaho

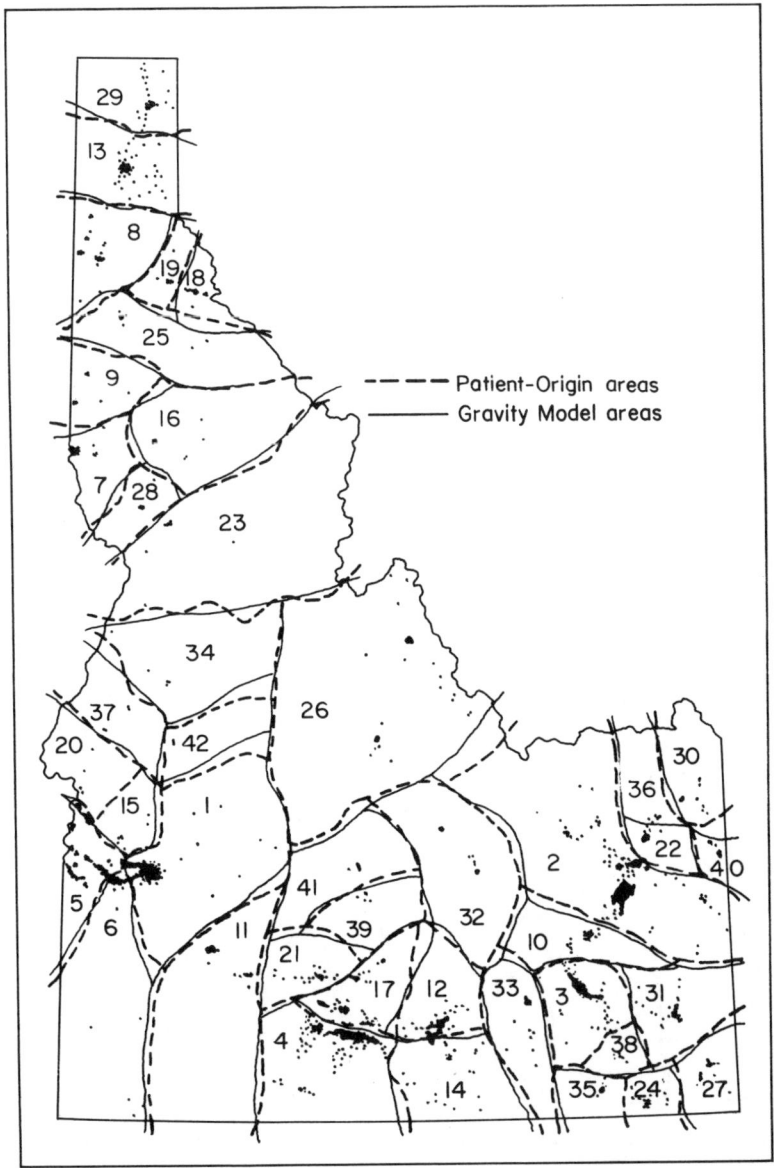

Note: Numbers are assigned to areas by population size. Service area 1 has the largest population, area 42, the smallest. One dot equals 100 people.

FIGURE 16.5

Service Area Nonalignment

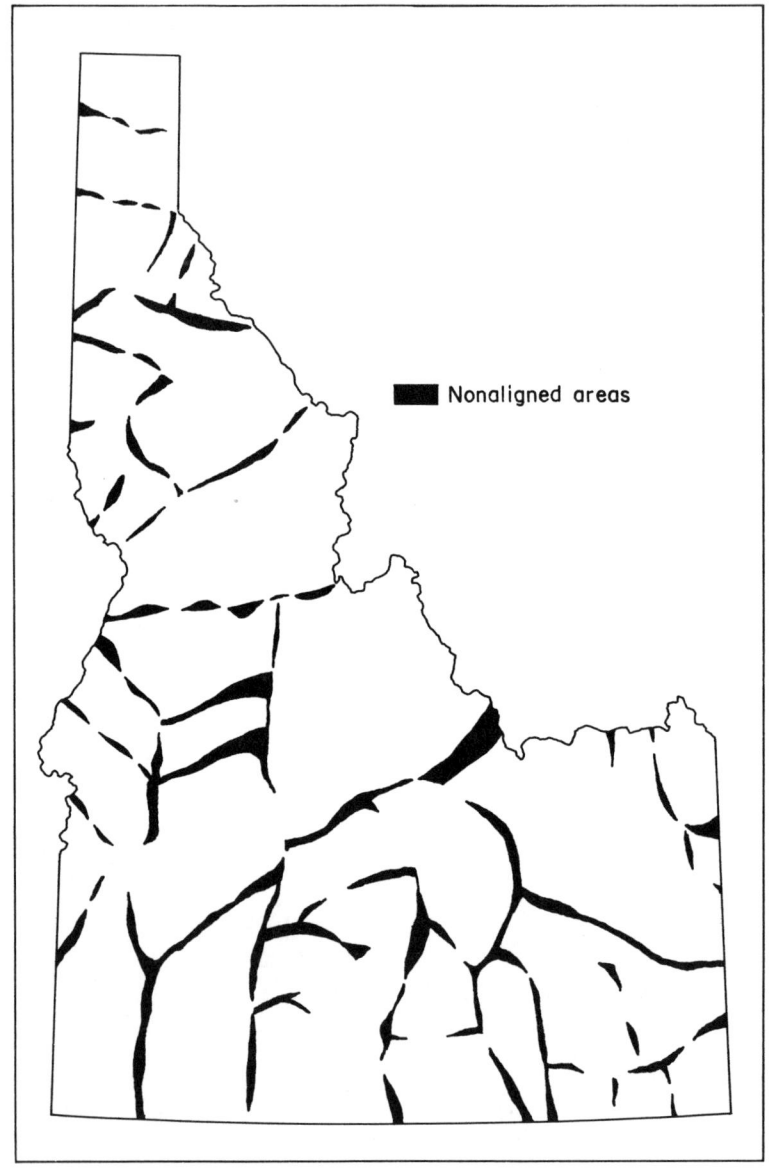

population of 704,600. Both figures are small and should not affect the model's validity since they do indicate close agreement between the two methods.

The success of the gravity model in predicting hospital service areas is clear. As such, several inferences may be drawn with appropriate cautions. One is that now any further hospital service area studies undertaken in Idaho have the potential to be accomplished faster and at much less expense than in the past. It is recognized that this model must be tested further to ascertain its reliability. However, such testing could be accomplished on a simple basis to hold costs to a minimum. Moreover, if future testing of the model proves its applicability, areas with a similar population pattern, such as most of the rural west, could find this method useful in planning new hospital facilities. Finally, the gravity model is simple to explain to lay people concerned with the planning process.

REFERENCES

1. R. J. Earickson, A Behavioral Approach to Spatial Interaction. Chicago: University of Chicago Press, 1970.

2. J. M. Meade, "Spatial Efficiency of Hospital Service Areas in Idaho: A Geographic Approach," unpublished doctoral dissertation, University of North Carolina, Chapel Hill, 1971.

3. W. Isard, Methods of Regional Analysis: An Introduction to Regional Science. Cambridge, Mass.: MIT Press, 1960. Pp. 499-566.

4. P. D. Converse, "New Laws of Retail Gravitation," Journal of Marketing 14 (1949):379-84.

5. J. Palmer, Measuring Bed Needs for General Hospitals: Historical Review of Opinions, with Annotated Bibliography. U.S. Public Health Service. Washington, D.C.: U.S. Government Printing Office, 1965.

6. H. M. Tyroller, personal communication, April 1969.

17

COST EFFECTIVENESS AND COST-BENEFIT ANALYSIS

INTRODUCTION

In the first article a decision model to evaluate the cost effectiveness of early diagnostic test programs is presented. The decision rule is based on the likelihood of the occurrence of the disease and the probability of test error. The cost of the test and treatment following early detection are matched against the economic benefits from a societal point of view. The backbone of the model consists of a simple decision tree. The model is illustrated by applying it to the Pap test for cervical cancer. The model can be adapted to a wide range of health problem areas.

In the second article, cost-benefit analysis is discussed. The authors applied a cost-benefit approach to a PKU (a hereditary condition) screening program in Mississippi. The costs and benefits associated with the PKU screening program were defined and quantified. Both retrospective and prospective approaches were used in the analysis. The retrospective approach measured the direct and indirect costs of the current PKU population and then compared this with the estimates of costs of screening, detection, and treatment. The prospective approach calculates the cost of screening, detection, and treatment of all the live births in a given year. The future savings of prevention were compared with the cost of screening and detection. The results from both approaches indicated that the program was beneficial not only to individuals but also to society in general.

Introduction to Technique

Cost-benefit and cost-effectiveness analyses are concrete ways of assessing the desirability of projects and programs. The questions to be addressed in cost-benefit analysis are:

1. Which costs and which benefits are to be included?
2. How are they to be valued?
3. At what interest rate are they to be discounted?
4. What are the relevant constraints?

In most cases, determining costs and their magnitudes is not a major problem since market prices are readily available. The main problem lies in determining what the benefits are and which values to assign to them.

Cost-effectiveness analysis is used in cases where costs can be measured in dollar terms, but benefits cannot. Alternative courses of action are compared in terms of their costs and their effectiveness in attaining some specific objective. Usually it consists of an attempt to minimize dollar cost subject to some mission requirements, or to maximize some physical measure of output subject to a budget constraint.

REFERENCES

Boggs, D. C., "Applying the Techniques of Cost-Effectiveness to the Delivery of Dental Services," Journal of Public Health Dentistry 35 (Fall 1973):222-37.

Dewhurst, R. F., Business Cost-Benefit Analysis. London: McGraw-Hill, 1972.

Goldman, T. A., Cost-Effectiveness Analysis. New York: Praeger, 1967.

Klarman, H. E., "Application of Cost-Benefit Analysis to Health Systems Technology," Journal of Occupational Medicine 16 (March 1974):172-86.

Singer, N., Public Microeconomics. Boston: Little, Brown, 1972.

COST EFFECTIVENESS OF EARLY DETECTION OF DISEASE

Stuart O. Schweitzer

A methodological framework for the cost-effectiveness evaluation of diagnostic tests for mass screening is presented. The decision rule is based on disease incidence, probabilities of test error, the cost of the test and of treatment for found cases, and the economic value (expected lifetime earnings or equivalent) of additional length or quality of life for those cured of the disease. The decision rule is applied to the Pap test for cervical cancer, with results showing that as a one-time screening device the test is cost-effective from society's standpoint. Extensions of the method would permit estimation of the disease incidence at which a given test or treatment would be cost-effective; would permit estimation of the break-even price of test and treatment with given disease incidence; and would allow determination of optimal testing frequency.

The purpose of this paper is to present a methodological framework that permits the evaluation of early diagnostic tests in terms of their cost effectiveness. The decision rule is based on aspects of the test in question (the prevalence of the disease and the cost of medical procedures used to treat a diagnosed condition) and the value of improved or prolonged life in the population to which the test is administered.

Reprinted with permission from Health Services Research 9, No. 1 (Spring 1974). Copyright 1974 by the Hospital Research and Educational Trust, 840 North Lakeshore Drive, Chicago, Ill. 60611.

Gratitude is expressed for many helpful suggestions from Hubert Alpert, M.D., Aaron Altschul, Ph.D., Robert Huntley, M.D., David Rabin, M.D., Ralph E. Smith, Ph.D., Robert Chambers, M.D., and Arthur Hoyte, M.D. Remaining errors are the sole responsibility of the author.

The value of one's own life is nearly infinite to the individual (although if the value of life were in fact infinite we would never take risks such as crossing a street or driving a car), and the value of pain and suffering is significant as well. But this analysis is restricted to societal decision making, and society, unfortunately, places a far more conservative value on our lives. Society places no monetary value on pain and suffering unless, perhaps, they cause a missed day of work, and external effects between individuals are not readily quantifiable. What this means is that many decisions that individuals justify would not be made by society.

Our private decisions concerning preventive health care are molded by media advertising from the large number of health foundations and associations whose sole purpose is the elimination of a particular disease, such as the American Cancer Society and the Society for the Prevention of Blindness. We are urged to have annual checkups, rectal examinations, eye examinations, chest x-rays, and so on. The narrow objectives of these special-purpose organizations mean that they have never had to justify their recommendations on economic grounds. It might be rational for individuals to purchase a large amount of diagnostic health services—annual health checkups, immunizations, and the like; neither the right of individuals to make such judgments nor the judgments themselves are questioned here. Today, however, a broader possibility presents itself. This is the possibility of offering government-financed third-party payment for most outpatient medical services. The same pooling-of-risk principle would occur on a smaller scale within the context of a health maintenance organization. Whenever others pay (directly or indirectly) for one's health services, they are entitled to ask if the return to them justifies their expenditure.

Only recently has informed thought begun to question the desirability of offering massive amounts of preventive health care. Kaiser Permanente, for instance, has abolished its annual multiphasic screening examination in favor of a less frequent testing program supplemented by special examinations when symptoms appear. Preventive health care comes at a high cost in terms of resources utilized, and planners must be well aware of the trade-offs and costs inherent in any new health program.

There is another view, perhaps more heretical, that preventive and episodic medical care have had little impact on society's health, as measured by longevity, morbidity, or man-days of work lost [1]. The implication of this line of reasoning is that resources presently directed toward medical services should be diverted into areas such as nutrition, pollution control, job safety, and housing. Though decision theory is equally applicable to these broader issues, such global questions are beyond the scope of this paper.

The term "preventive medicine" does not represent a single act of diagnosis and treatment; rather it represents a bundle of services that have to be analyzed both singly and jointly to account for differing diagnostic and treatment parameters. Even in the case of illnesses that are amenable to diagnosis, effective intervention, and cure, complications abound in the areas of disease patterns, diagnosis strategy, and treatment procedures. This paper will analyze the cost efficiency of a single medical strategy under uncertainty.

DEVELOPMENT OF THE DECISION RULE

A Simplified Test Situation

To make clear how a criterion is developed, prior analysis [2] is applied first to a simplified world in which an individual is in either of two states of health: he either has a disease, State D, with probability θ, or he does not—State D_0, with probability $1 - \theta$. He does not know his state, but he can choose between two acts: A, to take a diagnostic test, or A_0, not to do so. If he takes the test (assumed to be error-free, for this simple example) and is shown to have the disease, treatment will be administered that will effect a complete cure. If the patient has the disease and treatment is not administered, premature death will occur. This simple world may be represented by a table of consequences:

		Consequences	
		Act	
State		A	A_0
	D	Full life remains	Dies early
	D_0	Full life remains	Full life remains

This may be converted to an outcome table by specifying the consequences in more detail. Let ΔL denote the value of additional and/or improved life beyond the time of the decision concerning the test; T is the cost of the test; and p is the cost of the medical procedure effecting cure:

		Outcomes	
		Act	
State		A	A_0
	D	$\Delta L - T - p$	0
	D_0	$\Delta L - T$	ΔL

FIGURE 17.1

Simple Decision Tree

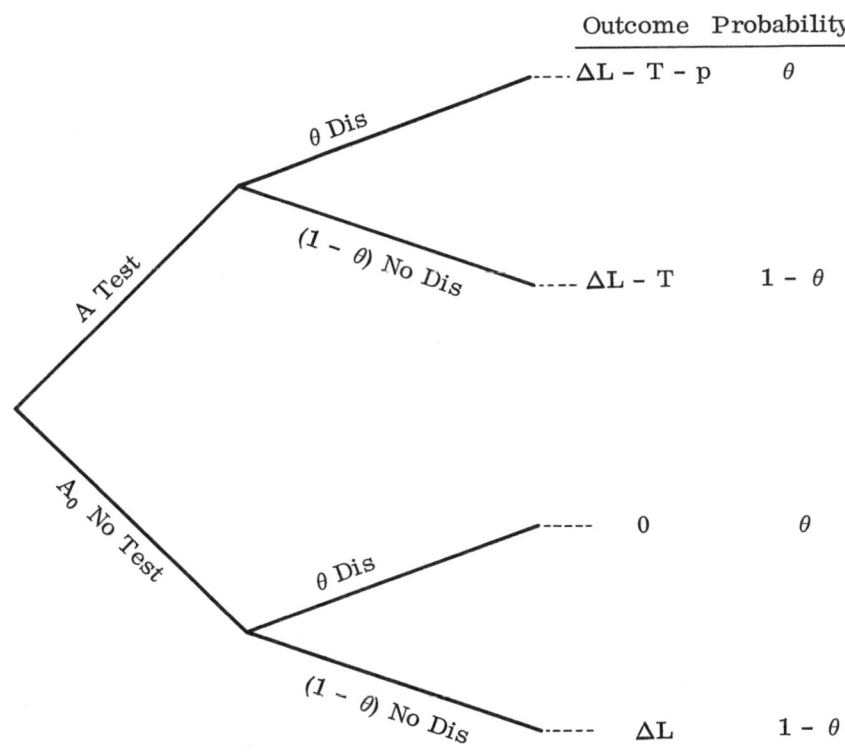

As mentioned, the probability of State D is θ (the disease incidence) and the probability of D_0 is $1 - \theta$. Then the expected value of act A, $E(A)$, is given by $E(A) = \theta(\Delta L - T - p) + (1 - \theta)(\Delta L - T)$ or, simplified,

$$E(A) = \Delta L - T - \theta p \tag{1}$$

Similarly, $E(A_0) = \theta \times 0 + (1 - \theta)\Delta L$, or

$$E(A_0) = \Delta L - \theta \Delta L \tag{2}$$

FIGURE 17.2

Decision Tree with Test Errors

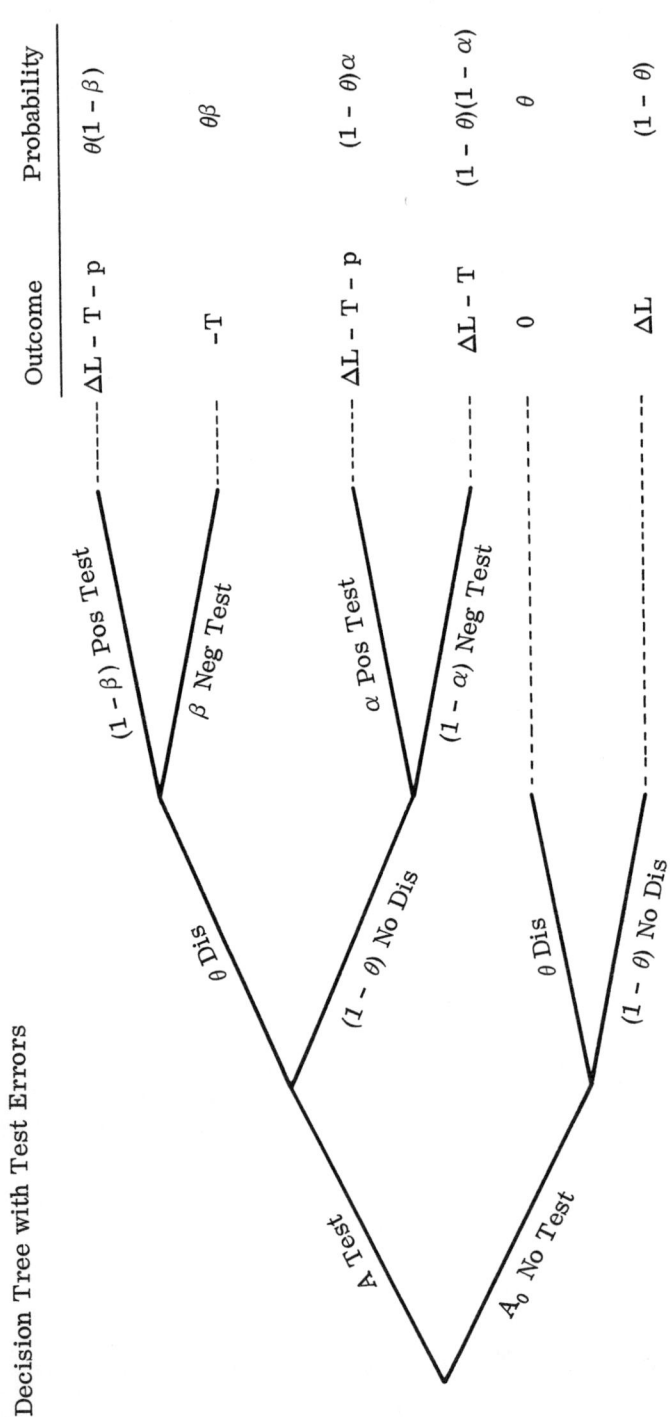

The "best" act depends on the comparison of Eqs. 1 and 2. Let λ denote the cost criterion to be established, where

$$\lambda = E(A) - E(A_0) \tag{3}$$

Obviously λ must be greater than zero, and this requirement generates a family of inequalities showing the conditions for the cost effectiveness of the test. One is that $T < \theta(\Delta L - p)$.

The lower the cost of the test, the higher the prevalence of the disease, the greater the value of prolonged or improved life, and the lower the cost of treatment, the more cost-effective the test will be.

This simple decision process showing outcomes may be diagrammed on a decision tree as shown in Fig. 17.1.

Tests Liable to Error

This simple illustration rests on the assumption that the test is infallible, so that it accurately reflects the probability θ that the disease was present. Real tests, however, make errors, which create other outcomes. Tests indicate false positives (Type I error, whose probability is denoted here by α) and false negatives (Type II error, whose probability is denoted here by β).

A more complete decision tree, including test errors, is shown in Fig. 17.2. The expected value of an act is the sum of outcomes each multiplied by their respective probabilities; thus $E(A)$, the expected value of taking the test, simplifies to

$$E(A) = \Delta L(1 - \beta\theta) + p[\theta(1 - \beta) - \alpha(1 - \theta)] - T \tag{4}$$

and the expected value of not taking the test is

$$E(A_0) = \Delta L(1 - \theta) \tag{5}$$

Again, for the test to be cost-effective it is necessary that $E(A) > E(A_0)$, or, from Eqs. 3, 4, and 5,

$$\lambda = \Delta L(1 - \beta\theta) + p[\theta(1 - \beta) - \alpha(1 - \theta)] - T - \Delta L(1 - \theta) > 0$$

Upon simplifying, the criterion is that

$$\lambda = [\theta(\Delta L + p)(1 - \beta) - (1 - \theta)\alpha p - T] > 0 \tag{6}$$

The magnitude of λ is directly related to the value of additional life ΔL and the disease prevalence θ and is inversely related to the cost of the test T, the probability of test errors α and β, and the cost of the procedure p (assuming that $\theta(1 - \beta) < (1 - \theta)\alpha$, that is, that the number of sick persons who are properly diagnosed and treated is less than the number of well persons who are properly diagnosed and thus not subjected to treatment).

Other Complicating Factors

The model depicted by Fig. 17.2 can be extended to fit a real world that is still more complicated. There are tests, for instance, that are inherently dangerous themselves (for example, sigmoidoscopy), so that an additional outcome is possible: harm (and cost) for those tested.

In some situations the early detection of a disease may not call for a treatment as such but only, perhaps, for a diet change, so that p may be nearly zero. Alternatively, some diseases will exhibit the same course and outcome regardless of whether or not they are detected. In this case, the loss in future lifetime earnings is suffered by all who have the disease, regardless of the test or detection, so that ΔL resulting from diagnosis and treatment = 0. The value of additional or improved life, ΔL, need not represent avoidance of premature death, of course. Perhaps only partial disability or inconvenience is caused by a disease (or a treatment), so that benefit may be represented by $\gamma \Delta L$, where γ is a disability index, $0 < \gamma < 1$. It is possible that γ may in fact be a function of the stage of the disease when detected; that is, $\gamma \Delta L$ may be dependent on the frequency of the test.

Time Dependency

From these points, it seems naive to talk about the efficacy or cost effectiveness of a diagnostic test outside of a time framework. A test that is cost-effective if done once (for example, in childhood, as is the PKU test on the newborn) may be superfluous if repeated. Analogously, tests done annually for some rapidly spreading diseases may be too infrequent to be cost-effective but might be cost-effective if done more frequently.

Time dependency may be incorporated into the analysis by replacing θ, the probability of disease, with the conditional probability $P(\theta_t)$, which is defined to be the probability that an individual has a disease, given that he was free of the disease t periods before. Thus $P(\theta_t) = \theta | P(\theta_{-t}) = 0$.

The critical probability of morbidity, θ_c, that will render a diagnostic test cost-effective can be determined by setting the expression of λ in Eq. 6 equal to zero. One can replace θ with θ_c and solve explicitly for θ_c. Gathering terms in Eq. 6,

$$\theta_c(\Delta L - \Delta L \beta + p\alpha + p - p\beta) - p\alpha - T = 0$$

Then

$$\theta_c = \frac{T + p\alpha}{\Delta L(1 - \beta) + p(1 + \alpha - \beta)} \quad (7)$$

In order to determine the optimal frequency of a test, one needs to determine θ_c on the basis of all parameters. Note that the dependency of θ_c on ΔL makes θ_c, and hence the optimal frequency, dependent on the age of the individual. Once θ_c is determined, the initial test is signaled when the individual enters the age group for which the age-dependent probability of disease, θ(age), is equal to θ_c. Then one may consider not θ(age) but $P(\theta_t)$, the conditional probability of θ given that the disease was not present previously.

For a disease that progresses slowly, $P(\theta_t)$ will remain small and below θ_c for an extended period of time, indicating a long spacing between tests. For diseases that begin suddenly and progress rapidly, such as lung cancer, $P(\theta_t)$ will rise to θ_c more quickly, so that more frequent testing will be indicated.

AN EMPIRICAL EXAMPLE

The application of this decision rule can be illustrated with an actual disease detection test widely accepted as a successful preventive health action: the Papanicolaou (Pap) smear test for cancer of the cervix. The economic value of the Pap test as a mass screening tool has been questioned, especially in Britain, on the grounds that widespread use of the test has not been conclusively shown to be associated with reduced mortality and that it detects not only the life-threatening invasive cancer of the cervix but also its presumed precursor, carcinoma in situ [3, 4]. The latter, which is not itself a clear menace, is reported to be far more common than invasive cervical cancer [3], but cases are followed up as if they would in fact develop into invasive cancers. The statistical data, unfortunately, are inadequate for judging the probability of this transformation [4], so the problem remains a medical rather than an economic one, outside the scope of this work. The model could be easily accommodated to any new data that proved relevant. The Pap test meanwhile serves

FIGURE 17.3

Decision Tree for Cervical Cancer Diagnosis Strategy

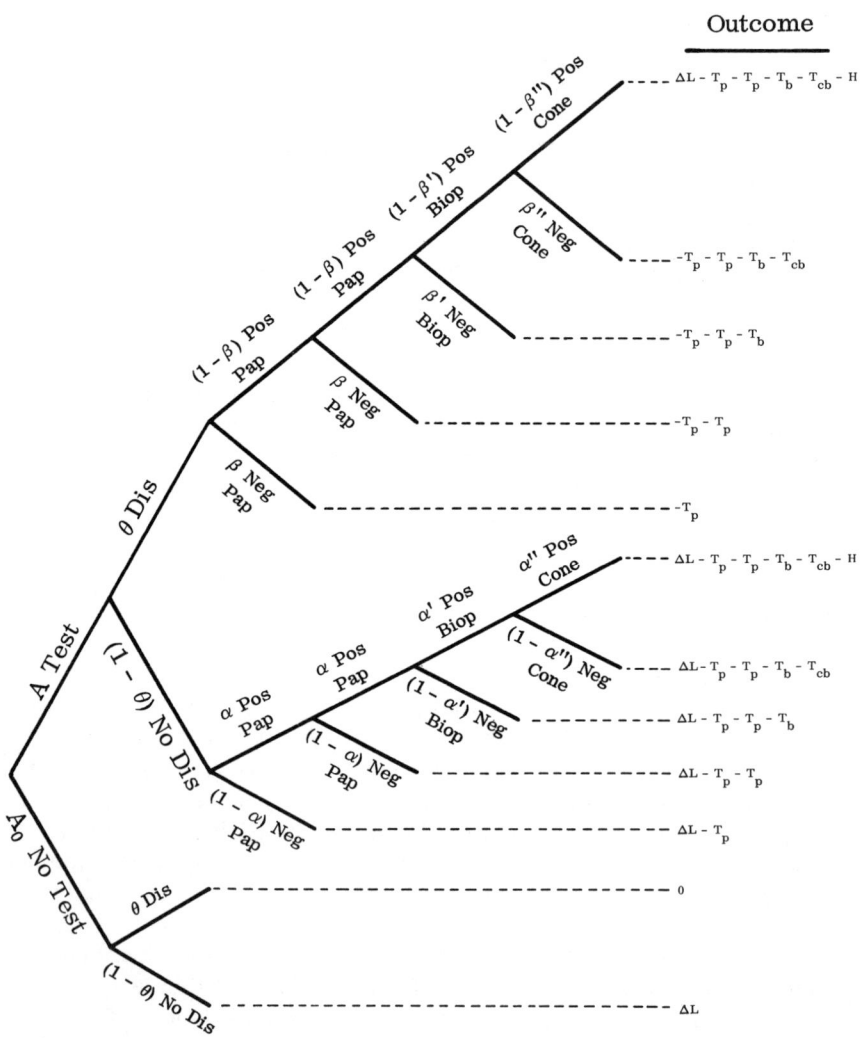

very well as an example for the empirical application of this model. To simplify matters, the Pap test will be considered in use as a one-time screening test.

Cancer of the cervix in the United States is variously reported to occur in women at the rate of 31.5 [5] or 30-40 per 100,000 women [6]. Although the incidence of cervical cancer rose 9 percent between 1950 and 1960, the mortality rate fell dramatically (41 percent) during this period [5]. The morbidity rate rises sharply after age 20 and peaks at about 100/100,000 at age 50. Thereafter the rate levels off and remains essentially constant [6]. For the present purpose, 35/100,000 is taken as the estimate of θ.

Briefly, and with some simplification, the strategy for testing and treating the disease is as follows. The presence of cancer cells can usually be detected by the relatively simple and inexpensive Pap test, which is usually administered in a physician's office annually. If the test is positive, a second test is performed. If this retest confirms the results of the first, a punch biopsy is performed to confirm the cytological (Pap) diagnosis. If the biopsy yields negative results, no further action is taken other than more frequent diagnostic testing. If the biopsy is positive, but not indicative of the more serious, invasive cancer, a cone biopsy (removal of a portion of the cervix) is performed in a hospital. If the cone biopsy shows that the disease has become invasive, either radiation therapy or various surgical procedures proposed in the literature are usually thought indicated. The more conservative surgical approach is partial removal of the cervix and uterus; the more radical is total removal of the cervix and uterus (radical hysterectomy). The choice is essentially based on one's view regarding probabilities of recurrence. Radical hysterectomy is assumed in this example, following the recommendation of Graham [6]. The question of radiation therapy versus surgery is still controversial among physicians; the decision model could, of course, take into account any alternative diagnosis/treatment strategies.

With the diagnosis/treatment strategy for cervical cancer described here, the decision rule is more complex than that shown in Fig. 17.2 and Eq. 6. The more realistically elaborate decision tree needed is shown in Fig. 17.3. The notation used in this extended decision tree is as follows:

T_p = cost of Pap test

T_b = cost of punch biopsy

T_{cb} = cost of cone biopsy

H = cost of hysterectomy

The parameters α and β are the probabilities of Type I (false positive) and Type II (false negative) errors, respectively, of the Pap test; α' and β' denote the similar probabilities for the punch biopsy, and α'' and β'' denote those for the cone biopsy.

The decision rule—that is, the equation that defines λ for this more complex situation—will not be given here. It is derived from the outcomes shown in Fig. 17.3 and their relevant probabilities, just as Eq. 6 is derived from Fig. 17.2, and is analogous to Eq. 6 in every respect except for the greater number of terms.

Cost and Probability Data

The incidence of cervical cancer has already been mentioned, with the value of 35/100,000 chosen for θ. There is some disagreement as to the error parameters of the Pap test. Graham [6] reports that 86 percent of women who have early-stage cancer will be so diagnosed; Dickinson [7] reports that the Mayo Clinic finds 96.7 percent of the true cases. Thus the probability of Type II error, β, ranges from 14 percent to 3.3 percent. For simplicity the midvalue, 8.7 percent, is taken. This is possibly a very conservative estimate, as estimates of β have been as high as 33 percent [8].

On the other hand, the Pap test will also produce some false positives. The probability of this Type I error, α, is 5 percent according to Graham and 0.2 percent according to Dickinson. Here also the midpoint, 2.6 percent, will be used. It is assumed that where a retest is indicated, the first and second applications of the Pap test are independent of each other in a statistical sense.

The next parameters are the error probabilities of the punch biopsy. Evidence indicates that the probability of a Type I error of the punch biopsy is on the order of 3.3 percent, while probability of Type II error is approximately 10 percent [6], so that α' and β' are 3.3 percent and 10 percent, respectively. Direct measures of the error probabilities for the cone biopsy are not available, so reasonable assumptions are made: $\alpha'' = 2$ percent and $\beta'' = 4$ percent.

The cost of the Pap test varies, of course. The California Medicaid (Medi-Cal) program reimburses the physician $12 for the procedure and lab test [9], whereas Mayo Clinic reported the cost to be $3.53 in 1968 [7]. The Medi-Cal allowable fee is undoubtedly in the low range of usual and customary fees; the Mayo Clinic cost appears to reflect only laboratory costs, not total costs of the test. The patient's time cost must be included too. It is estimated that the Pap test requires $1\frac{1}{2}$ hours total patient time (including waiting time, travel time, and procedure time) and that the diagnostic biopsy takes 2 hours. Both estimates assume that the tests are performed by themselves and not in conjunction with other services. A wage figure of $3 is used as the average hourly earning of women employed full time, with the assumption that women not in the labor force will still have to hire temporary help. Thus using the Medi-Cal figure for the Pap test and adding time costs gives a total cost of $16.50.

The direct cost of the punch biopsy is $36 according to the California Relative Value Scale, which, with patients' time cost, gives a total cost of $42. The cone biopsy costs $138, according to the CRVS, plus 1 day of hospitalization and 2 days of incapacitation. A rate of $78 per hospital day is assumed, based on Feldstein's data adjusted to 1970 prices [10]; $24 per day is allowed as time cost for the patients' recovery, for a total cost of $264.

The final surgical procedure that completes the model, radical hysterectomy, is expensive. In 1961 the procedure cost $870 at Mayo Clinic [7], including hospitalization. Inflating this figure by the rate of increase of the medical care component of the Consumer Price Index between 1961 and 1970 raises it to $1502 [11]. The CRVS cost is $384. Adding 5 days of hospitalization and 10 days of disability leads to a total cost of $1014, which is used here.

With these parameter estimates and a decision rule adapted from Eq. 6 according to the situation depicted in Fig. 17.3, one can find the value of λ that renders the Pap test diagnosis and treatment strategy just described cost-effective. Calculated thus, $\Delta L = \$36,667$, and the criterion for cost effectiveness of the Pap test as a one-time mass screening procedure is satisfied.

Another way of analyzing the diagnosis and treatment strategy is to determine the expenditure per case diagnosed and treated. This analysis, using the same parameters, yields an average of $44,241 per case treated. The difference between the average cost per treatment and the $36,667 expected outcome of the diagnosis and treatment strategy results from the different way in which extended life is treated as outcome for those who do not have the disease but are given the test.

Interpretation: The Cost-Effectiveness Decision

Whether or not the stated decision criteria are or would be met in practice depends on a number of factors, all pertaining to the way economic value is assigned to the lives and well-being of the population. Since the resurgence of human capital research in the 1960s [12], many studies have measured output of human investment programs by estimating foregone earnings of injured parties. This approach has been recognized in courts for a number of years in cases involving wrongful injury.

The expected lifetime earnings approach was taken by Dickinson [7] in assessing the total benefit to be derived from a screening program for cervical cancer; however, this approach leaves much to be desired. The most obvious gap, and that most easily corrected, is the imputed value of household services performed by the out-of-labor-force component of the female population. Also, an estimate of purely personal consumption may be deducted from earnings. Weisbrod [13] performed computations similar to this; his figures have been updated here to arrive at an estimate of economic loss due to early death from cervical cancer. Two alternative rates of discount, 4 percent and 10 percent, are used for the calculations. The value of ΔL by this methodology is approximately \$72,000 at 4 percent and \$50,000 at 10 percent. Thus the strictly economic assessment of ΔL yields the conclusion that as a one-time mass screening procedure the Pap test is cost-effective. These figures are based on the entire female population. Risk of contracting cervical cancer is not uniform across all age groups, of course. Whereas θ would be appreciably greater for older women, ΔL declines in middle age, leaving the choice of the most cost-effective group a far from trivial question.

DISCUSSION

One could consider this strict lost-earnings evaluation of ΔL as a lower bound on a more complete measure that would account for such unmeasurable concepts as the value of pain and suffering, externalities, fear of diagnosis, and so forth. An attempt to include these intangibles in a measure of program effectiveness is being made by Torrance et al. [14, 15]. Using standard gamble techniques, direct utility measurements are made, and these utility levels are applied to estimates of duration of various states of health as produced by medical programs. Measurement of lost earnings is a subset of this utility approach, with various states of health dichotomized into only two categories—able to work or unable to work. The simplicity of this methodology, its general applicability to all health programs, and its appropriateness for much governmental decision making warrant its continued application. One can make a case, however, for the narrow economic measure of ΔL as the appropriate tool for public policy involving direct expenditure of public funds. If the psychic and intangible benefits of a program are positive, rational people will engage in an activity beyond the level of government support. With a cost-effective test, the most efficient allocation of public and private funds might result from public subsidy of the procedure through a national health insurance scheme, with the consumer left to pay the remainder of the cost of the test and the full cost of more frequent tests, if desired. A system of subsidies rather than full payment might well be incorporated into a health delivery and financing system. This analysis provides an indication of the appropriate payments involved.

The decision rule formulation developed here can be adapted to a wide range of medical situations—different diagnosis/treatment strategies, different outcome possibilities for the treated and untreated, and various test parameters. The rule can determine the economic basis for several aspects of testing strategies; optimal spacing, selection of target population groups, and the payment or subsidy policy that might be warranted.

It cannot be emphasized strongly enough, however, that the gaps in the methodology used are serious. This is meant as an economic analysis only; as such, it omits important nonquantifiable aspects of the problem, such as a more complete value of human life and pain and suffering. Policy planners considering these other criteria might well make social decisions contrary to that indicated by the single economic dimension. Additionally, as indicated earlier, these factors almost certainly would lead to individual decisions different from those of society. There is, however, real and current need for this sort of analysis as one input into the social decision-making process.

The highly advanced state of technology in the health industry today leads to a wide range of services that may be purchased. Society will never be able to afford all the care that researchers can make feasible, so choices are extremely difficult. Economic analysis cannot provide a total answer to society's allocation decision, but it can provide information to assist in making this decision.

REFERENCES

1. A. L. Cochrane, Effectiveness and Efficiency: Random Reflections on Health Services. London: The Nuffield Provincial Hospitals Trust, 1972.

2. M. Hamburg, Statistical Analysis for Decision Making. New York: Harcourt, Brace and World, 1970. Chap. 13.

3. H. S. Ahluwalia and R. Doll, "Mortality from Cancer of the Cervix Uteri in British Columbia and Other Parts of Canada," Brit. J. Prev. & Soc. Med. 22 (1968):161.

4. L. J. Kinlen and R. Doll, "Trends in Mortality from Cancer of the Uterus in Canada and in England and Wales," Brit. J. Prev. & Soc. Med. 27 (August 1973):146.

5. W. E. O'Donnell, E. Daye, and L. Venet, <u>Early Detection and Diagnosis of Cancer</u>. St. Louis: Mosby, 1962. P. 152.

6. J. B. Graham, L. S. J. Sotto, and F. P. Paloucek, <u>Carcinoma of the Cervix</u>. Philadelphia: Saunders, 1962.

7. L. Dickinson, "Evaluation of the Effectiveness of Cytologic Screening for Cervical Cancer," <u>Mayo Clinic Proc</u>. 47 (August 1972):550.

8. J. B. Graham, L. S. J. Sotto, and F. P. Paloucek, "The Value of Cervical Cytology," <u>Lancet</u> 287 (December 9, 1972):1236.

9. Committee on Fees of the Commission on Medical Services, <u>1964 Relative Value Studies</u>. San Francisco: California Medical Association, 1964.

10. M. S. Feldstein, <u>The Rising Cost of Hospital Care</u>. Washington, D.C.: Information Resources Press, 1971. P. 17.

11. U.S. President's Council of Economic Advisers, <u>Annual Report</u>. Washington, D.C.: Government Printing Office, 1972. P. 249.

12. "Investment in Human Beings," <u>J. Polit. Econ</u>., Supplement, Vol. 70, October 1962.

13. B. A. Weisbrod, "Costs and Benefits of Medical Research: A Case Study of Poliomyelitis," <u>J. Polit. Econ</u>. 79 (May-June 1971):527.

14. G. W. Torrance, D. L. Sackett, and W. H. Thomas, "Utility Maximization Model for Program Evaluation: A Demonstration Application," in R. L. Berg (ed.), <u>Health Status Indexes</u>. Chicago: Hospital Research and Educational Trust, 1973.

15. G. W. Torrance, W. H. Thomas, and D. L. Sackett, "A Utility Maximization Model for Evaluation of Health Care Programs," <u>Health Serv. Res</u>. 7 (Summer 1972):118.

APPLICATION OF COST-BENEFIT ANALYSIS TO A PKU SCREENING PROGRAM

Kenneth C. Steiner
and
Harry A. Smith

Although the cost-benefit model had its primary origin and application in this country in the Department of Defense, its theoretical base, which combines welfare economics, public finance, and resource economics, has been used indirectly for centuries [1, 2]. It was one means of evaluating a proposed project; therefore, the approaches used were alternately called "investment planning" or "project appraisal." The cost-effectiveness model is a variation of the original cost-benefit model.

Both cost-benefit and cost-effectiveness models are pragmatic approaches to very real problems and have little abstract theory underlying their development and application. Certain assumptions are necessarily somewhat theoretical in nature, but this need not detract from the use of the models. The decisions based on the data resulting from these analyses are far better than the intuitive decisions that otherwise would be made. The purpose, then, of cost-benefit and cost-effectiveness analyses is to improve the decision-making process in very real situations.

Cost-benefit analysis is based on the assumption that the problem can be identified; the cost of its consequence can be measured within a permissible range of accuracy; the problem can be eradicated or controlled at some predetermined level by a new program; and the

---

Kenneth C. Steiner, M.S. is a graduate student in the Department of Health Care Administration, University of Mississippi School of Pharmacy (University, Mississippi 38677).

Harry A. Smith, Ph.D. is Professor of Pharmacy Administration, University of Kentucky College of Pharmacy.

The research reported in this paper was supported by the Research Institute of Pharmaceutical Sciences, University of Mississippi. Reprinted, with permission of the Blue Cross Association, from Inquiry 10, No. 4, pp. 34-40. Copyright 1973 by the Blue Cross Association. All rights reserved.

cost of the new program also can be measured. Thus, the costs associated with the old problem become the benefits against which the costs of the new program are compared. Conceptually, this is sound when the assumptions made are reasonably true, the calculations are accurate, and the methodology is reasonably acceptable. Cost-benefit analysis requires more definitive assumptions than cost-effectiveness, but it is an easier model to use where its application is valid.

Cost-effectiveness, on the other hand, is based on a more fluid conceptual framework. In fact, Quade [3] defines cost-effectiveness analysis as "any analytical study designed to assist a decision-maker identify a preferred choice from among possible alternatives." Even Quade, however, states that this definition is too broad. A more precise definition would be that cost-effectiveness analysis is a methodical approach of identifying alternative solutions to a problem (or courses of action) in terms of costs and their effectiveness in attaining some specific objective. While the costs of the alternatives are always measured in terms of dollars, the effectiveness may be measured in any of a number of terms as long as the term selected is applicable to the alternative under study. One can readily see the wider scope of factors and measurements opened to the investigator in a cost-effectiveness study; for example, comparable rates of incidence of diseases, mortality rates, fewer physician visits, etc., just to mention a few in the health field. One may compare the relative rates of effectiveness against a standard or budgeted cost, or even against variable costs as long as the ratios remain comparable and the results aid in the decision to be made.

Solutions to certain public health problems are more amenable to one model, while solutions to other problems require the other approach. Equally sound decisions may be reached by either method, while some problems will not yield to either. The choice of the best model or analysis is not always clear-cut; however, one of the models usually is best suited for a particular problem.

Usually the cost-benefit model is the best approach for screening programs for diseases. Use of this model in screening programs assumes first of all a valid test; that is, a relatively high rate of success in detection of the disease and a reliable statistical estimate of the success of the test. Second, the model assumes there is a cure for the disease or that it can be controlled to the extent that the patient may live a productive life, or at least a measurable percent of cases can be cured or controlled. Third, it assumes that estimates of the cost of the various parameters can be measured.

COST-BENEFIT ANALYSIS OF A PKU SCREENING PROGRAM

The cost-benefit approach was used successfully to measure the cost-benefit parameters of a phenylketonuria (PKU) screening program for Mississippi and relating the costs to the benefits.

Phenylketonuria is a hereditary condition in which the patient possesses a simple Mendelian autosomal, recessive gene. It is caused by a rare, inborn error of metabolism and usually results in mental retardation. This disease is somewhat unique in the area of mental deficiency as it is readily detected, and when diagnosed early in life, the deficiency can be modified or prevented with dietary treatment. PKU develops because of the patient's inability to metabolize phenylalanine properly. The result is a deficiency in the amount of phenylalanine that is converted to tyrosine, and large amounts of phenylalanine are found in the blood and spinal fluid. There are no physical standards for comparison in the diagnosis of children with suspected PKU at birth. The child will be apparently normal, but at three or four months of age signs of retardation will appear. The first noticeable change will be the infant's loss of interest in his surroundings, followed by a decrease in mental development, which finally ceases at the age of 10 to 14.

Costs of PKU

The costs associated with PKU were categorized into two areas: direct costs and indirect costs. Direct costs were defined as the actual expenditures for medical and other services attributable to the disease, reflecting the use of resources. These include both personal and nonpersonal costs. Personal service expenditures included the cost of hospital care, professional medical care, and pharmaceutical services, to list the major items. Nonpersonal service expenditures included medical supplies, drugs, medical research cost, government grants, charges for depreciation of facilities, and any other nonpersonal cost associated with the disease [4, 5].

Indirect costs were defined as a loss of economic productivity attributable to the disease, resulting from either death or disability. These indirect costs were calculated on the basis of the annual loss of production as measured by the loss of wages for the work years or months attributable to disease. It was presumed that the patients would have been gainfully employed in a full employment period [6]. The median incomes of the population segmented by age and sex were used in this study. Future earnings were discounted at the rate of 4 percent to ascertain their current value [7].

The total cost per case, direct and indirect, served as the measure of benefits derived from preventing that case. Three types of benefits are identifiable: 1) reduction in the use of health resources; 2) gains in economic output; and 3) satisfaction from better health. Much too little attention has been given to the latter benefit, according to some economists [8, 9]. But this benefit, the satisfaction or feeling of well-being of the patient, is very difficult to measure, especially in economic terms. Thus this factor is normally treated as a bonus or windfall to society after all the other calculations are made.

There are two basic approaches in the application of the cost-benefit analysis—the retrospective and the prospective approaches. Both approaches were used in this study. The retrospective approach measures the direct and indirect costs of the current population with a disease entity, PKU in this instance. After these calculations are made, an estimate of the costs of screening, detecting, and treating these patients from among the entire population encompassing the life spans of the patient population is calculated.

The other technique, utilizing the prospective approach, calculates the cost of screening, detecting, and treating all of the live births in a given year. The future savings (cost to society) of preventing the direct medical cost of the people who are successfully detected and treated plus the indirect costs of future economic productivity of these patients are compared to the cost of screening and detection.

RESULTS OF THE RETROSPECTIVE METHOD

Information from the three mental institutions in Mississippi provided the data for computing the direct and indirect costs associated with PKU patients. Demographic characteristics of the patients provided the base line data as shown in Table 17.1. The direct costs for all mentally retarded patients in the three institutions are summarized in Table 17.2.

Since PKU patients were not identified among the retarded patients in the three Mississippi institutions, the direct cost of maintaining PKU patients had to be estimated by the most reliable means available. First, the personal service costs for all patients in the institutions were calculated on a per patient per year basis. These figures were multiplied by the known number of mentally retarded patients in all the three institutions. This gave an overall annual cost of $3,762,398 for personal services for all mentally retarded patients in the three institutions. The total non-personal service cost per year for the three institutions was $367,748. In addition, $73,346 in research grants was awarded to other institutions to study mental retardation during the baseline

TABLE 17.1

Age and Sex Distribution of Mentally Retarded Patients
in Mississippi Mental Institutions in 1967

Age	Male	Female	Total
Under 5	3	0	3
5-9	32	36	68
10-14	83	49	132
15-19	158	74	232
20-24	176	74	250
25-34	260	148	408
35-44	234	175	409
45-54	201	210	411
55-64	148	234	382
65+	84	109	193
Total	1,379	1,109	2,488

year. The total annual direct cost was $4,203,492. Based on the reported statistic that 1 percent of all mentally retarded patients are PKU patients [10], the best estimate of the direct cost per year per PKU patient was 1 percent of $4,203,492 or $42,035. PKU patients have been reported to be institutionalized 30 years on the average [11]; therefore, the estimated total direct cost for PKU patients was $1,261,050.

Indirect costs are measured by the loss of income. It was assumed that once a mentally retarded patient was institutionalized, he remained incapacitated for life and was a complete loss to the work force. The indirect costs for all the institutionalized mental retardates were computed and reported in Tables 17.3 and 17.4.

The total estimated indirect cost for the mentally retarded population was $105,354,512. One percent of this amount, $1,053,545, was allocated to the PKU patient population. The sum of the direct and indirect costs was summarized in Table 17.5.

The total cost (the sum of direct and indirect costs) to society to care for the 25 PKU patients (1 percent of the 2,488 institutionalized mentally retarded patients) was $2,314,595.

TABLE 17.2

Summary of Direct Costs for Institutionalized Mentally Retarded Patients

	Whitfield	Ellisville	Meridian	Total
Personal services				
Cost/patient/year	$ 1,847	$ 1,241	$ 1,322	$ 1,512[a]
Number of patients[b]	1,094	1,248	146	2,488
Total	$2,020,618	$1,548,768	$193,012	$3,762,398
Nonpersonal services				
Depreciation	$ 83,510	$ 78,215	$ 13,041	$ 174,766
Imputed interest	113,991	66,951	12,040	192,982
Research grants	—	—	—	73,346
Total	$ 197,501	$ 145,166	$ 25,081	$ 441,094
Total direct cost	$2,218,119	$1,693,934	$218,093	$4,203,492

[a]Rounded average for the three institutions.
[b]The numbers represent the mentally retarded patient population; there were other patients with various mental disorders in these institutions.

TABLE 17.3

Adjusted Present Value of Lifetime Earnings for Males: Amount Discounted at 4 Percent, Adjusted to 1967 Dollars and for Mississippi, by Age

(1) Age	(2) Earnings[a]	(3) Inflator Factor[b]	(4) Inflated Lifetime Earnings[c]	(5) Lifetime Earnings Deflated[d]	(6) Number of Mentally Retarded[e]	(7) Adjusted Lifetime Earnings for Mentally Retarded[f]
0-4	$ 62,026	1.090	$ 67,608	$34,480	3	$ 103,440
5-9	79,333	1.090	86,473	44,101	32	1,411,232
10-14	97,736	1.090	105,442	53,775	83	4,463,325
15-19	114,613	1.090	124,928	63,713	158	10,066,654
20-24	126,688	1.192	151,012	77,016	176	13,554,816
25-34	125,801	1.141	143,539	73,205	260	19,033,300
35-44	104,629	1.158	121,160	61,792	234	14,459,328
45-54	71,676	1.178	84,434	43,061	201	8,655,261
55-64	37,168	1.143	42,483	21,666	148	3,206,568
65+	6,560	1.155	7,577	3,864	84	324,576
Total						$75,278,500

[a]From: Rice, D. P. Estimating the Cost of Illness, Health Economics Series, No. 6, Publication #947-6 (Washington, D.C.: GPO, May 1966) Table 24, p. 93.
[b]Ratio of 1966 median income to 1963 median income.
[c]Column 2 times column 3.
[d]Column 4 times ratio of 1967 median income for Mississippi to 1967 median income for U.S.
[e]Obtained from Table 1.
[f] Column 5 times column 6.

Source: Column 3 derived from: U.S. Bureau of the Census. Current Population Reports, Series P-60, No. 43, "Income of Families and Persons in the United States: 1963" (Washington, D.C.: GPO, September 29, 1964) Table 20, p. 36; and ibid., No. 53, "Income in 1966 of Families and Persons in the United States" (Washington, D.C.: GPO, December 28, 1967) Table 20, p. 38.

TABLE 17.4

Adjusted Present Value of Lifetime Earnings for Females: Amount Discounted at 4 Percent, Adjusted to 1967 Dollars and for Mississippi, by Age

(1) Age	(2) Earnings[a]	(3) Inflator Factor[b]	(4) Inflated Lifetime Earnings[c]	(5) Lifetime Earnings Deflated[d]	(6) Number of Mentally Retarded[e]	(7) Adjusted Lifetime Earnings for Mentally Retarded[f]
0-4	$36,280	0.964	$34,974	$17,837	0	$ 000,000
5-9	46,289	0.964	44,623	22,758	36	819,288
10-14	56,422	0.964	54,391	27,739	49	1,359,211
15-19	64,936	0.964	62,598	31,925	74	2,362,450
20-24	67,960	1.150	78,154	39,859	74	2,949,566
25-34	65,608	1.110	72,825	37,141	148	5,496,868
35-44	58,801	1.119	65,798	33,557	175	5,872,475
45-54	47,634	1.130	53,826	27,451	210	5,764,710
55-64	33,816	1.116	37,739	19,247	234	4,503,798
65+	12,525	1.361	17,047	8,694	109	947,646
Total						$30,076,012

[a] From: Rice, D. P., Estimating the Cost of Illness, op. cit., Table 24, p. 93.
[b] Ratio of 1966 median income to 1963 median income.
[c] Column 2 times column 3.
[d] Column 4 times ratio of 1967 median income for Mississippi to 1967 median income for U.S.
[e] Obtained from Table 1.
[f] Column 5 times column 6.
Source for Column 3: Same as in Table 3.

TABLE 17.5

Total Costs for Institutionalized PKU Patients in 1967*

Direct costs	
30-year extended direct costs	$1,261,050
Indirect costs	
Present value of lifetime earnings lost	1,053,545
Total direct and indirect costs	$2,314,595

*Determined by taking 1 percent of the respective costs for mentally retarded patients.

TABLE 17.6

Retrospective Analysis of Program Costs

Number of screening tests required	660,000[a]
Cost of initial screening	$ 561,000[b]
Cost of retesting within six weeks	$ 561,000[b]
Number of confirmation tests required	3,300[c]
Cost of confirmation tests	$ 12,375[d]
Cost of retesting while on special diet	$ 3,937[e]
Cost of special diet for seven years	$ 127,750[f]
Administrative cost (10% of other costs)	$ 126,606
Total program cost	$1,392,668

[a] Figure rounded to the nearest 1,000.
[b] Based on mean cost of $.85 per test from a survey of 42 health departments.
[c] Based on national statistic of 0.5 percent cases requiring confirmation test.
[d] Based on mean cost of $3.75 from survey of the health departments.
[e] Based on average cost of $3.75 per test once every two months for 7 years.
[f] Based on national statistics of an average cost of $2.00 per day per patient.

Estimated Detection Cost

This cost was compared to the estimated program cost to have detected this number of PKU patients and maintained them at a self-supporting status in society. This estimated cost was computed retrospectively as follows. The incidence rate of PKU among a white population is 1:15,000 [12], while the incidence rate among the nonwhite population is 1:100,000 [13]. The 1967 ratios of live births among white and nonwhite populations in Mississippi were 49 percent and 51 percent, respectively. Based on 46,714 live births in 1967, 1.76 PKU cases would have been detected if all 46,714 newborns had been tested, or 1 case of PKU could be found in 26,542 newborns. Therefore, testing approximately 660,000 newborns over a period of 14 years would have been required to have detected the 25 institutionalized PKU patients. The cost of screening the newborns and treating this number of patients has been outlined in Table 17.6.

This total, $1,392,668, is the estimated cost to detect and treat the 25 suspected PKU patients in the Mississippi mental institutions. This figure can then be compared to the total cost of institutionalization and earnings lost of $2,314,595. The resulting cost-benefit ratio was calculated to be 1 to 1.66. Stated positively, each dollar spent in the detection and control of the disease would have yielded a net gain of $0.66 above the cost of the detection and control program.

RESULTS OF THE PROSPECTIVE METHOD

The prospective method based on 1967 live births in Mississippi was thought to yield more valid results than the retrospective method. As previously noted, testing the 46,714 live births in 1967 would have detected an average of 1.76 PKU cases. The total costs to conduct such a screening program were tabulated in Table 17.7.

It was assumed that the total number of live births would be tested initially and again within six weeks. Also, it was assumed that an average number of confirmation tests would be made, and a test monitoring the PKU urine level would be performed every two months. A diet cost of $2.00 per patient per day was used in the computations, which is the highest cost reported in the literature [14]. The statistics used in Table 17.7 maximized the cost of the detection and treatment program.

Based on the data used in the retrospective method, the direct cost of institutionalized care was estimated at $1,690 per case per year. If the 1.76 cases had been detected in 1967, it would have cost $89,232 for institutional care for 30 years, the minimum expected length of time of institutionalization, or $210,588 for the 70.8 years

TABLE 17.7

Program Costs for Live Birth Data

Number of live births in Mississippi in 1967	46,714
Average cost per screening test	$ 0.85
Number of confirmation cases	233.6
Number of cases of whites	1.52
Number of cases of nonwhites	.24
(A) Cost of initial screen test	$39,707
(B) Cost of retest at six weeks	$39,707
(C) Cost of confirmation at $3.75 per test	$ 876
(D) Diet cost of 1.76 cases for seven years	$ 8,994
(E) Cost of retest while on diet	$ 278
(F) Administration cost	$ 8,956
Total cost of program	$98,518

of normal life expectancy of a one-year-old child born in 1967. The indirect cost for loss of future earnings, discounted at 4 percent per annum [7], totaled $45,830. The total direct and indirect costs were $135,062 for 30 years of institutional care and $256,418 for 70.8 years of institutional care. These data yielded cost-benefit ratios of 1 to 1.37 and 1 to 2.60, respectively.

Again, the gain to society using live-birth data and the prospective method was substantial, even if we use the minimum of 30 years of institutionalization. In all of the calculations, costs of the detection and control programs were maximized, while direct and indirect costs (benefits) were minimized.

CONCLUSION

The conclusion to be drawn from this study is that a PKU screening program is beneficial not only to the person who has the disease but also to society. The retrospective approach yielded a cost-benefit ratio of 1:1.66. Using the more valid prospective approach, the cost-benefit ratio was 1:1.37 when the direct costs were minimized to correspond to the 30 year average time a patient is institutionalized. A ratio of 1:2.60 resulted when the full life expectancy was used.

Neither the time and money spent for a PKU preventive program nor the economic benefits derived from such a program reveal the additional financial burden and amount of personal care required by the families of the undiagnosed patients. In addition, the emotional stress which is inflicted upon the families cannot be measured in economic terms.

Cost-benefit analysis proved to be a satisfactory technique in evaluating a PKU screening program as it has in several other diseases. It provides the model to determine the social validity of such programs as family planning, day care centers, preventive dental care, fluoridation of water supply, and vaccination against communicable diseases. Cost-benefit estimates have been made of cancer and other major diseases. Both models have been applied to various aspects of maternal and child health. This enumeration is not exhaustive, but does represent some of the more obvious applications of the models.

The cost-effectiveness model could also be used to determine the desirability of using nonphysicians in limited areas of primary health care; this category could include the pediatric nurse, physician's assistant, the clinical pharmacist, and the emergency paramedic. Cost-effectiveness analysis might also be applied to cardiac emergency ambulance service.

One area in which cost-effectiveness analysis can and should be applied is to new health care delivery systems such as the health maintenance organization concept. One of the weaknesses in these emerging government-sponsored experimental health care models is the internal evaluation included in the grant. The evaluation, using the cost-effectiveness model, should be performed by an outside agency.

Special education for the various categories of mentally deficient children is another field in which cost-benefit analysis would provide proof of the social value of these programs. It is the opinion of the authors that the programs in special education could have one of the highest benefit-to-cost ratios of all the various social programs.

The application of cost-benefit and cost-effectiveness models is far-reaching. It seems axiomatic that more money should be funded for this type of research before appropriating huge sums of money for the many supposedly worthwhile social projects.

REFERENCES

1. A. R. Prest and R. Turvey, "Cost-Benefit Analysis: A Survey," The Economic Journal 75 (1965):683-735.

2. A. W. Marshall, "Cost-Benefit Analysis in Health," paper presented in Monterey, California, November 10, 1965, and reproduced by the Rand Corporation.

3. E. S. Quade, "Cost Effectiveness: An Introduction and Overview," paper presented at a Symposium on Cost Effectiveness Analysis, June 14-16, 1965, sponsored by the Washington Operations Research Council and reproduced by the Rand Corporation.

4. D. P. Rice, "Estimating the Cost of Illness," American Journal of Public Health 57 (1967):424-40.

5. D. P. Rice, Estimating the Cost of Illness, Health Economics Series No. 6, PHS Publication #947-6. Washington, D.C.: U.S. Government Printing Office, May 1966. P. 3.

6. R. Fein, Economics of Mental Health. New York: Basic Books, 1958.

7. Rice, Estimating the Cost of Illness, Parts II and III, Appendix B.

8. Marshall, "Cost-Benefit Analysis in Health," p. 3.

9. H. E. Klarman, The Economics of Health. New York: Columbia University Press, 1965.

10. D. Y. Y. Hsia, "Recent Developments in Inborn Errors of Metabolism," American Journal of Public Health 50 (1960): 1653-61.

11. G. C. Cunningham, "Two Years of PKU Testing in California," California Medicine 111 (1969):11-16.

12. R. P. Hormuth, specialist in services for mentally retarded children, Children's Bureau, Department of Health, Education, and Welfare, personal communication.

13. H. P. Katz and J. H. Menkes, "Phenylketonuria Occurring in an American Negro," Journal of Pediatrics 65 (1964):71-74.

14. W. R. Centerwall, S. A. Centerwall, P. B. Acosta, and R. F. Chinnock, "Phenylketonuria. I. Dietary Management of Infants and Young Children," Journal of Pediatrics 59 (1961): 93-101.

18

COMPUTER APPLICATIONS

INTRODUCTION

The strength of this paper lies in the wealth of current information about (1) the status of computer applications in the health care industry, (2) guidelines for managers to follow in choosing a computer system which meets institutional needs, and (3) types of hospital information systems presently offered by suppliers of computer systems. The authors stress that an effective hospital information system is essential if a hospital is to survive in its complex environment. The authors also emphasize that a computerized information system must integrate both administrative and clinical functions, and that the hospital must keep up to date on the "state of the art" of computer systems.

REFERENCES

Ball, M., "Medical Data Processing in the United States," Hospital Financial Management 28 (January 1974):10-30.

Ball, M., and G. L. Hammon, "The Who, What, When, Where of Health-Care Consulting," Hospital Topics 54 (November/December 1976):50-52.

Ball, M., How to Select a Computerized Hospital Information System. New York: S. Karger, 1973.

Collen, M. E., Hospital Computer System. New York: Wiley, 1974.

Ferderber, C. J., "A Standardized Solution for Hospital Systems," Datamation (September 1975), pp. 52-53.

Fields, C., About Computers. Cambridge, Mass.: Winthrop, 1973.

Frankfurter, G. M., A. E. Jelmert, C. C. Pegels, J. P. Seagle, and E. L. Wallace, "A Computer-Based Blood Inventory Information System for a Regional Blood Distribution Center," Transfusion 10 (July-August 1970):203-14.

Graham, J., Making Computers Pay. New York: Halsted Press, 1976.

Hammon, G. L., "Information Systems," Hospitals 48 (April 1974): 83-86.

Schmitz, H., "A Protocol for Evaluating Hospital Information Systems," Hospital and Health Services Administration 22 (Winter 1977):45-56.

OVERVIEW OF COMPUTER APPLICATIONS IN A VARIETY OF HEALTH CARE AREAS

Marion J. Ball
and
Gary L. Hammon

Referee: Glenn Anderson

PREFACE

It is the intent of the authors to present to the reading audience a broad overview of the fast emerging field of computer applications to the entire health care delivery system in the United States. Certain subspecialties have been well-represented in the literature and, for that reason, will be summarized in this paper and referenced for the reader for further inquiry. This paper pertains to the clinical and communication application of computers in medicine, with a detailed

Reprinted from CRC Critical Reviews in Bioengineering 2, No. 2, January 1975. Copyright CRC Press, Inc., 1975. Used by permission of CRC Press, Inc.

state-of-the-art description on radiology systems as well as the entire area of financial and management alternatives available to the health care industry.

The authors have made every effort to present accurate and timely information. Due to the normal delays between the preparation and the publication of the paper, some new information may have occurred in the interim.

We would like to thank the various suppliers of computer systems in medicine who have helped in verifying the data and assisting us in presenting, as of the summer of 1974, the current status of hospital information systems.

Key Words

Computers, Health Care, Cost Justification, Selection, Financial, Clinical, Applications, Installation, Management, and Automation.

PRESENT STATUS OF MEDICAL DATA PROCESSING IN THE UNITED STATES, 1974

Hospital Information Systems appear to be a hospital's only way of survival in today's complex and dynamic world. The areas of patient care, medical audit, and financial management benefit from this approach. United States hospitals spend between 7 and 10 billion dollars annually to acquire and communicate information, which represents 25 to 33 percent of the total hospital budget. Estimates indicate that over 50 percent of this hospital communication burden can be effectively automated.

In a recent report (issued by Battelle Columbus Laboratories and KMB Health Systems, Inc., of Palo Alto, California, a subcontractor to Battelle) entitled "Evaluation of the Implementation of a Medical Information System in a General Community Hospital," some basic issues were discussed. The report was funded by the National Center for Health Sciences Research and Development, and an interim report was issued September 30, 1973. The system discussed is the Technicon Medical Information System (MIS) at El Camino Hospital in Mountainview, California. The following five hypotheses are addressed. A computer based Hospital Information System

1. induces significant changes in procedures or organizations;
2. increases the effectiveness or efficiency of the hospital service functions;

3. is acceptable to the staff;
4. reduces the cost of hospital services to the patient;
5. is cost-effective for the hospital.

The following trends are becoming evident as regards the above hypotheses:

1. Significant procedural changes were evident in going to such a system.
2. As for the effectiveness or efficiency, a positive response was found among nurses, one very mixed reaction from the physicians, and some improvement in turnaround from certain ancillary areas.
3. Acceptance varied by type of hospital.
4. On cost reduction to the patient, at the moment no change is apparent due to lack of time to determine such a statistic.
5. On MIS cost effectiveness—"The <u>predicted</u> average potential savings (FY 72-76) range from $83,000 to $88,000 per month, which exceeds the system's contract cost to the hospital of $82,750 per month."*

With the above trends in data available, it behooves us to very carefully begin planning to incorporate whatever efficient and cost-effective computerization is available into our overtaxed health delivery system. To start with, we must recognize that communication is the cornerstone of effective health care delivery. If the request for service issued by the physician is "lost in the shuffle," then all of the expensive ancillary expertise has no way of being responsive to the patient's needs. It is for this reason that this paper will place special emphasis on computer assisted information systems to integrate the medical and administrative information needed in hospitals.

CLINICAL APPLICATIONS

At this point, brief discussions will follow on computer involvement in: (a) clinical laboratory, (b) pharmacy, (c) medical records, (d) admission, (e) radiology diagnosis and therapy, (f) outpatient clinic, (g) dietary, (h) patient history, and (i) the administrative areas.

---

*Report issued by Battelle Columbus Laboratories and KMB Health System, Inc., Palo Alto, California, entitled "Evaluation of the Implementation of a Medical Information System in a General Community Hospital."

Clinical Laboratory

The computerization of the clinical laboratory has been one of the recognized successes of computers in clinical medicine. It has been said that "it [the computer in the laboratory] has survived a rocky infancy and is now a healthy, rapidly growing youth."

In the laboratory marketplace we see a "shake-out" underway. The underfinanced and/or less successful vendors of computerized laboratory systems are moving on to other fields of computerization or have gone out of business.

Laboratory medicine today comprises all subfunctions relating to the discipline of pathology, including clinical pathology, gross and microscopic specimen analysis (also cytology), and forensic pathology. Not only are the commonly automated areas of hematology and serum chemistry included, but also urinalysis, histopathology, and microbiology. It also encompasses quality control, trend analysis, laboratory instrument monitoring, and all aspects of specimen control, including intradepartmental file management techniques when applicable. One area still lacking is positive specimen identification. The use of computers in laboratory medicine is usually quite successful, particularly with the small dedicated computer systems now available. At the onset of computerization, there is no reduction in cost, but rather a smaller increase of cost. As the rate of test procedure grows, the cost remains essentially constant in the computerized laboratory. Many labs performing over 300,000 tests a year are beginning to consider a dedicated turnkey lab system or some form of computerization.

Pharmacy

Pharmacy departments are one of the ancillaries that cut across categorical organizational boundaries. Computerization can protect patients from adverse drug reaction, drug to drug interaction, drug to food interaction, drug to lab test interaction, and allergies.

Pharmacy must be considered in conjunction with other systems such as accounting, admissions, and laboratory. Some of the pharmacy systems currently available perform pricing, charging, inventory control, formulary listing, purchase order preparation, and other administrative procedures. Subfunctions relate to therapeutic agents and their usage. These include drug inventory control, prescription formulation, maintenance of a formulary, and appropriate aspects of clinical pharmacology, such as usual dosage, order checks and reminders (inpatient), contraindications, and hypersensitivity reactions. In addition, appropriate aspects of clinical toxicology and acid base (fluid) therapy are included as subfunctions.

Some of the vendors in this area are B-D Spear Medical Systems, Searle Medidata, International Business Machines, Burroughs, Technicon, Honeywell, and Health Data Corporation.

Medical Records

The medical record is becoming more and more important as national legislation on acceptability is being developed. The medical records department must be considered an integral part of a hospital information system of any size or description. In the future, more requirements will be imposed on and more requests for information will be asked of the medical records administrator. Professional Standards Review Organizations (PSRO) and other controls are already causing a strain on the medical records department.

Medical record administration is a huge problem to be faced and conquered before we are really successful in achieving a "hospital information system." The area is ill-defined and usually has a low status. The hospital administrator will be forced to spend more time in managing this activity because of the vital nature of this department.

Indexing is a big problem for medical record administrators. Also, the choice of the patient identifier, as to whether it should be the social security number, hospital unit number, or sequential systems, is constantly under discussion. The conversion of the record to some form of machine-readable media is very costly and requires a great deal of planning and supervision. One of the true pioneers in this field as it pertains to reconstructing the medical record is Dr. Lawrence Weed.

There are no easy solutions to the automation of the medical records department today. It appears that we need to devote more attention to the design and implementation of a good system, that is, first manual, then computerization.

Admission

The automation of the admitting function has come into the spotlight. One of the "stumbling blocks" to the effective automation of this area is the need for accurate, current, and available medical record information. Here, one sees again the interrelationships between and among systems.

There are several vendors interested in developing and implementing systems for this area. Some are: Sperry Univac Company; B-D Spear Medical Systems; Shared Medical Systems; Systems Development Corporation; Four Phase Systems, Inc.; Genetron, Inc.;

McDonnell Douglas Automation Co.; Health Data Corporation; and Technicon Medical Information System.

Radiologic Diagnosis and Therapy

Work is being done in administrative applications, radiological information systems, and radiographic diagnostic systems. This includes all subfunctions relating to diagnostic radiology, including the conversion of requests to facility and technician schedules, patient preparation notices and reminder systems for reporting on individual roentgenograms, and maintenance of a film file locater. In addition, all subfunctions relating to therapeutic radiology are included, such as the calculation of isodose curves, patient treatment schedules, and tabulation and maintenance of the results of treatment (tumor registries).

However, it appears that more work is required before this area will be ready for a "turnkey" implementation. William R. Glou states in the December 1973 issue of Medical Electronics and Equipment News:

> The automated report system* may well become the most important improvement in overall radiology department services since the introduction of automated film processing. It reduces administrative time and speeds x-ray reports to the referring physician. With our system we can describe 85% of all pathological findings without a dictating machine. Our bed capacity is expected to grow from 350 to 1,000 beds with a projected work load of 180,000 radiological exams by 1974. More than ever, we must be efficient.
>
> The Department of Radiology at the University of Missouri-Columbia Medical Center has been using the Missouri Automated Radiology System (MARS) for reporting and retrieval of a patient's clinical history, previous studies and reports, radiologic diagnoses in the department and the display of these reports to terminals located on the patient's ward. Computer terminals in the Department allow radiologists access to a central computer. Department-developed programs aid in diagnosing bone tumors, heart diseases, gastric

---

*General Electric Raport Radiological Reporting System.

ulcers, and lung lesions. Use of MARS at the Medical Center has saved from 2.3 to 3.3 hours from the time a patient arrived in the Department for examination and the time a written report is available to the referring physician.

Other systems can be found at: Johns Hopkins Hospital Radiology Reporting Systems, University of Nebraska Medical Center Radiology Reporting System, University of Arkansas (DRIS), and Beth Israel CLIP Radiology System.*

Outpatient Clinic

There is renewed interest in computerizing the outpatient clinic functions. The federal government appears to be the prime reason for the new emphasis. Health Maintenance Organizations (HMOs) are another reason for the concern for finding new methods and procedures. Also, third-party payers are moving toward the reimbursement of outpatient services to reduce the use of inpatient services for some items.
Scheduling and billing are two applications in the clinic today. Honeywell has a system at Boston Children's Hospital. Univac appears to be interested in the automation of the area also. Automated health testing seems to be finding a place in the overall area of preventive medicine. Searle, Mediquip, IBM, and Medlab are among the companies involved in this area.

Dietary

Computerized dietary systems were quite popular a number of years ago, but appear to have lost some of the initial impetus. There are two reasons for the apparent slowdown in dietary computerization. One reason is the cost-justification factor, and the second reason is the trend to contract food services.

---

*A detailed article on Diagnostic Radiology Reporting/Information Systems will be discussed in this regard by Gerald S. Lang in an upcoming issue of CRC Critical Reviews in Bioengineering.

Transtech, Inc. (now a part of American Hospital Supply) is one vendor that appears to be doing well today. The CAMP* software is being used by a number of hospitals also.

Patient History

A patient history system has been under investigation and experimentation for some time. The University of Wisconsin-Madison Hospitals have been working on this for eight years. They now have a LINC (Laboratory Instrument Computer) that "talks" to psychiatric patients via three terminals.

IBM has announced a field developed program (FDP) for patient history taking under their Health-Care Support package. This should provide the impetus for more installations.

Dr. Stephen Yarnell and Dr. Warner Slack are very actively working on further developments in this field. Searle is the leader in this marketing effort with Meratec, Control Data Corporation, Mediquip, and IBM among others also in the business.

Administrative Area—Automation Alternatives

One would think that by 1974, research and study would have made available clear-cut answers to such questions as

Should we use a computer at all?
Should we install an "in-house" machine?
Is sharing or shared service the better choice?
Is a facilities management (FM) agreement the most viable alternative?

One is continually amazed that these questions still have no sure answer. At a recent meeting, a hospital financial officer asked for advice as to the best course of action for his hospital in the perilous area of computers and data processing. The institution's bookkeeping machines were in need of replacement due to extensive use over a number of years. The hospital was in the 200-bed range and anticipated expansion within three to five years. He wanted to know if the bookkeeping machines should be replaced with new units; or should

---

*The diet planning aspect was originally developed by Tulane University and has been emulated by several vendors.

he consider the use of "someone's" shared system; or could the installation of an "in-house" computer be justified? One does not suggest the concern and/or questions are inappropriate or out of order; rather, one points out that a similar question was posed to me in 1963 at a meeting of the American Hospital Association. It appears that in the years between the two discussions, we should have developed some guidelines, checklists, or something for the "new venturer" in this bewildering area.

It must be pointed out that such a decision is no easier today, with or without the checklists, etc.; the proliferation of vendors, products, and third-party payers has increased the number of alternatives. Our "new venturer," trying to make an informed decision, is caused fear and trembling just from viewing the variety of vendors which market hardware and/or software. One reason is suggested for the lack of a checklist or form to follow in this activity: It is impossible to stay up to date on the alternatives, let alone to maintain an updated, widely circulated document on their relative virtues. It appears that the informed use of knowledgeable consultants is the best approach for the health care institution without internal expertise. Hopefully, these consultants possess current knowledge on the "state of the art" and can evaluate the institution's needs, real and imaginary, and make intelligent recommendations to top management.

This paper will cover the points to consider if one is interested in automating the functions of a health care institution. The three approaches to be discussed are an "in-house" computer system, a shared system, and facilities management. One does not indicate a best choice, but will provide items for consideration in your search for a solution to your computerization problems.

The "in-house" computer system to be discussed herein is not of the mini-computer type. The vendors in this market are, for the most part, well-known and have been with us for a number of years. Some reasons for and against the acquisition of an "in-house" computer are listed here; a comparison to a shared approach is found in another section.

"In-House" Computer System (Central Facility)

Reasons For

1. Have needs (real) that cannot be met by a shared center or FM.

2. An FM firm and/or shared center does not appear to be responsive to users in your area.

3. Concern for confidentiality of patient information and desire to keep patient files within your physical control.

4. Institution has competitive salary rates and can attract and retain competent personnel.
5. Just want your own computer.

Reasons Against

1. High start-up costs, even with vendor-supplied software that works.
2. Requires large dollar commitment for a definite period of time.
3. Uncertainty of results from the effort.
4. Computer personnel salary level causes problems with other hospital employees.
5. Training costs for computer are high and are increased by the turnover rates.
6. Recruitment of skilled data processing personnel, especially those with hospital experience, can be difficult.

Shared Systems

The concept of shared computer centers has been with us for a number of years. The types of organizations one may find serving as a shared center are

1. A single hospital with a computer may provide service to other hospitals.
2. A nonprofit corporation may be formed by a group of hospitals.
3. A religious order may establish a data processing center for its hospitals.
4. A state Blue Cross agency may operate a center.
5. A state or metropolitan area hospital association may operate a center.
6. A general service bureau that processes data for all types of business enterprises may provide the center.
7. A shared hospital computer company or "hospital computer utility" may be the operator.

The first five types listed above are usually nonprofit organizations, while the other two types are usually operated for a profit. With the nonprofit types, hospitals usually participate in establishing priorities, in determining new applications for development, and in similar decisions. The hospital also may participate to some degree in the activities of the last type—the hospital computer utility. However, very little hospital participation is possible in the sixth type— the general service bureau. Such an organization may have acquired its applications packages from a software house. It may not have the technical capability to modify programs as required by events.

As one would expect, there are certain advantages and disadvantages to the shared computer center when compared to an "in-house" computer operation. They include the following:

Advantages

1. Developmental and operational costs per hospital are reduced.
2. Larger and more efficient computers can be utilized.
3. A more qualified and diversified data processing staff can be employed. However, fewer personnel are required on a per hospital basis. Because fewer personnel are required, there is less strain on the local labor market.
4. Salaries for data processing staff do not upset salary and wage scales in the hospitals.
5. In some cases, multiple central computers provide a better back-up capability in the event of computer failure.
6. Management information can be shared.
7. Costly surveys to procure comparative management information can be eliminated.
8. Space can be saved in the hospitals.
9. Building modifications necessary to establish a computer room in the hospital are eliminated.
10. In shared systems in which the hospitals actively participate in systems design, the ideas and experiences of a number of hospitals may lead to better systems.

Disadvantages

1. Less freedom—or no freedom—for the individual hospital to influence systems design and priorities.
2. Achieving consensus concerning system design, priorities, and goals may be a slow process.
3. Either hospitals lose some individuality in terms of report formats, documents, codes, and so on, or the computer programs must be more complex in order to meet the demands of individual hospitals.
4. The time period required to introduce new applications is longer, since applications usually are not introduced to all participating hospitals at once.
5. Confidentiality of patient information can be compromised due to loss of direct physical control.
6. Center may decide to discontinue the addition of new applications, forcing the hospital to abandon its plans or causing the hospital to change vendors.

A more comprehensive discussion of shared computer systems can be found in the Hammon and Jacobs article [1].

Facilities Management

Professional management of an organization's data processing activities by an outside firm is known as facilities management (FM) [2]. The idea or approach dates back to 1962, and FM firms appear to specialize in particular industries. The reason for this specialization is the obviously desirable enhancement of the transferability of people and software.

In order to understand more fully the discussion that follows, another definition for FM should be considered. FM is "an information processing service in which an outside supplier assumes some level of line responsibility for the operation of the (client's) computer facility" [3]. This implies that top management must still be involved—determining what systems are needed, setting priorities, and establishing constraints—and is still essential for the success of the partnership.

The types of FM arrangements can be categorized as follows:

Location of Computer

The computer may be

1. in the hospital;
2. at the FM firm site;
3. small computer(s) in the hospital with the main computer at the FM site;
4. in another hospital which is a client of the FM firm.

Supplier of the Computer and Related Hardware

The computer and related hardware may be

1. entirely supplied by the hospital;
2. supplied by the FM firm, whether the equipment is located in the hospital or not;
3. supplied by the FM firm and the hospital, each providing equipment at its site.

Supplier or Developer of New Applications

New applications may be

1. developed by the hospital;
2. developed by the FM firm;
3. turnkey programs supplied by the FM firm, which would make necessary modifications for the hospital;

4. developed by systems analysts and programmers on the hospital staff under the supervision of key personnel provided by the FM firm.

Supplier of Systems Analysts and Programmers

Personnel may be

1. provided by the hospital, except for supervisory or key personnel. (The American Hospital Association engaged in this type of arrangement in 1970 in order to tide it over a difficult situation created by turnover of key personnel.) The FM firm may be given authority to terminate the employment of unsatisfactory personnel;

2. provided by the FM firm. (The FM firm may hire personnel previously on the payroll of the hospital.)

Computer Room Operations

The equipment may be operated by

1. the hospital;
2. the FM firm;
3. the hospital under supervision of the FM firm.

A logical question is often asked about the reason for facilities management. Numerous surveys and studies have indicated that a significant number of hospitals are disappointed with the performance of their computer department and experience higher than anticipated costs. It appears that there are basically three reasons why hospitals choose FM arrangements—to solve management, cost, and/or people problems.

It must be pointed out that if management problems are the result of incompetence at the top levels of hospital management, an FM arrangement is doomed to failure. An institution must face up squarely to this type of problem before making a decision on a future course of action. In some instances, a hospital would never have had a data processing problem if the chief financial officer and/or hospital administrator had possessed the leadership and management qualities required of him in this day and time.

In hospitals with their own data processing departments, there may be dissatisfaction with the disparity between promised benefits and achieved results and with missed deadlines, poor documentation, mounting costs, personnel turnover, etc. Management might also recognize its inability to keep pace with a rapidly advancing technology.

If personnel problems are the reason for exploring FM, are you ready to discipline, fire, or reassign employees and/or department heads who are not performing the tasks necessary to insure success of the automation effort? If the answer is no, FM will be faced with the same obstacles and difficulties as the previous operation. It is important to face these challenges (problems) squarely, resolving them in favor of the hospital as a patient-care institution.

In hospitals with no previous EDP experience, management recognizes FM as a solution to lack of expert guidance for the hospitals' data processing programs. An FM firm's expertise can provide more running applications in a shorter period of time. This means the hospital has the opportunity to benefit from automation at an earlier date.

FM offers a solution to the management problem and provides better advice and guidance than an internal EDP staff or hardware and software salesmen can offer.

The cost problem is solved, at least in comprehensive FM arrangements, because management knows exact costs for the duration of the contract.

If the correct vendor is chosen, the results to be expected can be matched against the expected costs for a realistic evaluation.

The people problem amounts to this: It is difficult for the hospital to attract EDP people, to select the best qualified, to pay the demanded salaries without upsetting hospital pay scales, and to retain good personnel. There is frequently a very high turnover rate among better EDP personnel. Parnell points out that one reason for this is that they tend to identify with the profession rather than with the employer. They are ready to change jobs for better salary, challenge, promotional opportunity, or more satisfying relationships with their peers [4].

FM firms have exhibited the ability to attract EDP personnel: They have the know-how to select the best qualified; they can pay high salaries; they can demonstrate a career path within the company; they can provide challenging assignments; and they do a pretty good job of retaining the best. This is important, for there are tremendous qualitative differences in the abilities of EDP personnel. It is the high quality of personnel that enables the FM firm to develop better systems at less cost than could the average in-house staff.

Some other advantages of FM include

1. Ability of the FM firm to reconfigure hardware, software, and personnel to conform to actual needs. Because of its knowledge of hardware and software, the firm is in a much better position than the hospital to deal with vendors and procure the right hardware/software for the job—no more, no less.

2. More stringent documentation, security, and operating standards.

3. Management access to proficient data processing advice, as from a consultant.

4. Availability of back-up people and back-up equipment (the latter in cases where equipment is duplicated at FM firm site).

A number of disadvantages to FM are cited in the literature. Actually, these are potential dangers resulting from the relationship itself. These are listed for hospitals which engage in FM to recognize and avoid:

1. Management may abdicate its responsibility to set data processing goals and to insure that they are being achieved.
2. The profit motive may cause the FM firm to cut corners and fail to develop optimal systems.
3. The FM firm may fail financially.
4. There may be breaches in security and confidentiality by involving outsiders.

The advantages and disadvantages of using facilities management have been covered. In further exploration of this approach, one suggests consideration of the following:

1. What is the source of the hospital's data processing problems? If problems attributed to data processing actually originate in other departments, a change to facilities management will not solve them, as stated earlier.
2. What is the primary concern? Is it a large developmental effort for the future, or is it to improve current operations? Might the need be to start up a new system or to make major repairs to existing systems?
3. Can the needs be defined in detail and for the duration of the contract? Are the needs specific enough? Are they likely to remain fairly stable, or are they susceptible to significant change? [3]
4. What arrangements are desirable? Full or partial service? On-site or centralized remote operations? With or without takeover of existing data processing equipment, or software, or staff?
5. Investigation of FM firms. Once preliminary matters have been determined, the hospital can begin to evaluate the suitability of various FM firms. It is stressed that the evaluation must be thorough. A poor choice can result in monetary loss, litigation, or lack of satisfactory progress. Following are some of the factors to be investigated.
6. Nature of the firm. Is this firm primarily in the FM business, or is FM a subordinate activity? Does it specialize in the hospital industry?
7. Financial stability. Is the organization adequately funded and has it reached or exceeded the break-even point? In many areas, the competition is quite keen. It is probable that some of the financially insecure firms will fail.

8. Management competence. Do the principals of the firm have adequate management experience in the data processing business? Are they experienced with hospitals? It is pertinent to review the past experience of the principals and, where possible, to solicit opinions from former employees.

9. Technical competence. Are the employees experienced with hospitals? Do they possess the requisite breadth and depth of experience?

10. Stability of work force. Has the firm experienced heavy turnover of professional personnel? Such would indicate management problems and would weaken reliability of the determination of technical competence.

11. Satisfaction of other clients. Are other clients, especially hospitals, satisfied with the services they are receiving? Do they plan to continue the relationship?

12. Can you work with the firm? Will the firm be comfortable to work with? Is the proposed relationship a good fit? Are the employees to be assigned to the hospital fully qualified?

13. Visit to firm's site or sites of operation. This may not seem to be a very important point. However, facility security, neatness and orderliness, visible schedules, and proper documentation are conspicuous indicators of adherence to "basics." Of course, the FM firm's manner of performance should be discussed with client management, auditors, and user personnel.

The next area of concern for a hospital considering the use of facilities management is the contract for service. Legal counsel is strongly advised. A definitive contract can be of great assistance in lessening the incidence and severity of conflicts [2]. Parnell states, "a fair and flexible contract—protecting both parties—is difficult to execute [5]." It is said that the contract is a "communication vehicle" and provides a mechanism to prevent disagreement over minor points. It should be as long as necessary to completely describe the proposed relationship. Again, the use of legal counsel is encouraged.

Since the contents of a contract for FM will vary with the level of service, assumed responsibility, goals and objectives of the hospital in entering the arrangement, and many other factors, a checklist of items to consider is appropriate (no order of importance is conveyed by the sequence):

1. Terms of the contract
2. Basis of charges
3. Basis for negotiation of fees for a new contract
4. Basis for negotiation of new systems development and major systems changes
5. Termination procedures

6. Basis for early termination of a contract
7. The right to audit the operations of the FM firm
8. Protection against patent or copyright infringement suits against the FM firm
9. FM firm liability for losses resulting from faulty programs and operating errors
10. Transfer of equipment, if applicable
11. Arrangements and charges for physical space
12. Supervisory arrangement, in the event the FM firm supervises client staff
13. Security arrangements (both physical and data)
14. The nature and extent of the system to be developed and/or operated
15. Performance milestones
16. Nonperformance clauses with penalties defined
17. Setting priorities
18. Provision for audit of systems by an independent agency
19. Necessity for approval by third-party payers or auditors for certain applications developed
20. Responsibility to include back-up and restart procedures for all systems designed
21. Minimum response time to terminal inquiries
22. Frequency of file updates
23. Input and output requirements
24. Scope of the documentation, including user manuals
25. Training for user's staff by the FM firm
26. Ownership of software developed under the contract
27. Careful definition of all terms used in the contract
28. Grievance procedures with time schedule

Under an FM arrangement, the hospital administrator must still manage his data processing activities. With FM, the administrator may be able to fulfill his responsibilities more easily. However, he cannot sit back and say, "Good, now I can stop thinking about EDP." He still is responsible to the board for the overall operations of the hospital—including data processing. He still must establish the hospital's EDP goals and follow up on the progress by and performance of the FM firm to insure that the goals are being achieved and benefits realized.

HOSPITAL INFORMATION SYSTEMS

Hospital information systems (HIS) will be discussed in the following section and divided into three distinct areas: (a) systems handling primarily data collection and message switching, with nine major companies involved in this effort; (b) systems that do the above and incorporate certain medical record functions, and eight companies marketing this approach; and (c) the introduction of the mini-computer functional processing concept into HIS development, which is at present in the conceptual stage.

Systems Handling Primarily Data Collection
and Message Switching

This section will discuss the lower level Hospital Information Systems, which primarily offer a data collection and message switching capability. The following is a definition of these types of systems: They can transmit orders; they can capture the charges for one day; they can prepare a census; they may be used for results reporting or employee time recording; and they can be interrogated regarding charges for the current day. However, they do not maintain an electronic patient medical record file.

The following companies will be discussed in this section: Automated Systems Corporation; B-D Spear Medical Systems; Diversified Numeric Applications; International Business Machines (IBM); Medelco, Inc.; Medilogic Corporation; National Cash Register Company; Searle Medidata, Inc.; and Standard Register Company. All of these suppliers have made a contribution to the approach defined above.

Automated Systems Corporation (ASC)

This Data Acquisition and Communication System is based on two computers, one suited to the on-line, real-time exigencies dictated by data acquisition and communications, and one oriented to the basic administrative, fiscal, medical records, and data management function. The two computers may be linked so that they can transmit data back and forth at high speeds. One of these is the Data Communications Controller (DCC) supplied by ASC, and the other is any central processor available to the hospital.

ASC uses a Varian 620/L mini-computer with a Pertec D3000 disk drive and a National Cash Register Century 200 computer at St. John's Hospital in Tulsa, Oklahoma. The former is linked to input/output terminals throughout the hospital. Here, input/output terminals are linked to a mini-computer for daily operations. The system supports cathode ray tube (CRT) terminals, typewriter terminals, and card input. Patient information is recorded on the disk, transmitted to various departments within the hospital, and sent to the central computer for processing and accounting functions.

The on-line system will perform the following hospital functions:

1. Message switching
2. Employee time-keeping
3. Admissions, transfers, dismissals, preadmission, inpatient
4. Outpatient, transfers, dismissals, room bed updates
5. Service transactions, central supply, pharmacy, laboratory, radiology, inhalation therapy, dietary, orthopedic charges, physical therapy, intensive care and recovery room, emergency room, outpatient, special charges.

B-D Spear Medical Systems

B-D SPEAR CYBERMEDAC allows for automatic input to the computer. This system is built according to the following distinct processing activities: (1) servicing of remote on-line video terminals sending requisitions/messages to the system in a real-time mode; (2) communication with central work station in a real-time mode and processing of basic system functions such as new admissions, bed status, and current charges; and (3) execution of batch mode programs such as census, daily charge activities, and departmental activity lists.

It is designed in a manner that will allow expansion of the system functions without making changes necessary to the basic functions. The following are independent subsystems; therefore, any combination of the functions may be included in the desired configuration: (1) bed control; (2) admitting and census; (3) printed requisitions delivered electronically; (4) automatic, uniform pricing; (5) computer input; (6) inventory control information; (7) time-keeping by work center; and (8) pharmacy package. This is the foundation of a modular approach.

Other features of the system are automatic security check on all entries; validation of all entries; automatic message routing to all "need-to-know" locations; catalogues and prints lab requisitions by unit, type, and sex; automatic generation of secondary messages such as "hold tray"; procedure and service summaries available by department; all transactions recorded on magnetic tape; allows use of plastic card or keyboard for input at terminals; and all messages reflect date, time, and employee identification. This system is currently operational at Central Kansas Medical Center at Great Bend, Kansas, and Pinehurt Hospital in North Carolina.

Diversified Numeric Applications HOSPITROL

HOSPITROL is a computer based hospital communications system which coordinates and channels communications and information from one department to another. With terminals located on all nursing stations and in most clinical areas, as well as in many ancillary departments, orders, charge collecting and reporting, information for admission, discharge or transfer, and retrieval of patient data can be accomplished.

At North Memorial Hospital in Minneapolis, Minnesota, the prototype is automating preadmission and admission activities, including inpatients, outpatients, emergency room, and repeat patient, and it provides a current census. Requests for patient services are automatically communicated from terminals at nursing stations to the ancillary departments concerned.

The HOSPITROL equipment consists of two DNA Med/16 computers, core memory, disk and drum storage units, magnetic tape units, card reader, line printer, operator's console, and numerous hospital oriented communication terminals. A mass storage unit contains 25 million characters of information on patient orders, etc. Thirty-five terminals are designed specifically for the hospital area in which they are to operate. All patient accounting information in the HOSPITROL system will be generated on magnetic tape for subsequent processing by the NCR/200 computer in the North Memorial Data Processing Department.

International Business Machines (IBM)

Several avenues have been followed by IBM as they have approached the computerization of hospital information systems. One major attempt at data collection was the IBM 1800/2790 installed and operating at South Fulton Hospital in Atlanta, Georgia. This is a system very similar to the Medelco approach, and it concentrates on requisitioning and routing functions. It seems, however, that the modular packages to be discussed in the next section under the heading of IBM are the most current approach for the company.

Medelco

The Medelco Total Hospital Information System (T*H*I*S) handles patient, room, and bed information on a real-time basis, in addition to message switching and storing of financial transactions. Terminals consisting of a file of edge-punched cards, an optical card reader for input of data into the system, and a teleprinter for hard copy output are located at each nursing station and ancillary department.

Prepunched cards for each order, service, or product available in the hospital are in the card files, as are cards for patients. The central processor, designed for message switching and data storage, has limited computing capability.

This system can be seen at Deaconess Hospital in St. Louis, Missouri. This is one of 28 installed operational systems.

Medilogic Corporation

The system developed by Medilogic addresses the handling of hospital business and operations data to provide control, on-line ordering and message switching, billing, charge collection, management reporting, and financial operating information. The record-keeping functions and cost analysis requirements imposed by price control agencies, Medicare, Blue Cross, insurance companies, hospital associations, and others are serviced by the system as well. It is aimed at the hospitals that are big enough to need help, but too small to do it efficiently alone.

The Local System consists of a mini-computer with large-scale disk storage and a network of terminals throughout the hospital for continuous data collection, communications, and processing of time-critical data. The Remote System serves several hospitals, with each participating hospital having its own Local System.

The equipment for the Local System consists of purchased components as well as items manufactured by Medilogic. The major equipment elements are:

1—Data General Nova mini-computer with 48,000 character, high speed memory.

2—56.6 million character Century Data Model 244 mass storage disk drives.

1—Multiplexer in 32-channel modules for up to 128 channels (manufactured by Medilogic).

2—Disk controllers (manufactured by Medilogic).

1—Data Printer Corporation Model V-306 line printer—300 to 600 lines/min as required.

TEC Model 420 cathode ray tube (CRT) terminals—as many as required.

Centronics Model 306 character printer terminals—as many as required.

1—Paradyne MARQ 48 modem for transmitting to and receiving from the Remote System.

The Remote System equipment consists of a Medilogic communications terminal and an IBM 370 with appropriate disk drives and tape units.

The Local System mini-computer programs consist of an Executive System, designed and developed by Medilogic, that manages all the applications programs and interaction with the terminals.

The National Cash Register Company

The National Cash Register Company is in the midst of writing a hospital interactive data collection and message switching system. The system will utilize a combination of terminals for input and communication.

The input from the nursing station will be with the use of a fibre optic pen strobing color bar codes. By selecting a specific type transaction, "lead thru lights" will be displayed to guide the operation with separate descriptors for each type, for example: service orders, census, transfers, discharge, check in/out.

Class 260 thermal printers would be used in ancillary departments to receive or send messages. Either 260s or a teletype-compatible CRT would be used in the admitting area.

The NCR Company has a pilot on-line admissions, preadmissions, admits, room selection, and sign in/out of doctor messages at Kettering Memorial Hospital in Dayton, Ohio. This has been installed as of November 1974.

The NCR Company is orienting its activities to an intelligent on-line data terminal system geared toward hospital nursing station use. Model 275-200 terminal has a 4K core and is a programmable unit for data entry and communication with any hospital wide computer system. In operation, a data wand is passed over encoded symbols signifying each instruction given by a doctor. An accompanying keyboard allows for manual data entry. The equipment routes these instructions to the involved departments, and creates records for subsequent accounting. At present, the company is most active in the fiscal area of hospital data processing, but is becoming actively involved in other areas.

Searle Medidata Inc.

The Searle Medidata Network 320 Hospital Information System is a modularly expandable communications and applications computer system. It is designed to control census, route orders, collect charges and other financial information, and return results directly to a nursing station.

The heart of the system is a unique "touch-terminal." The terminal presents 320 patient order choices at one time to the operator on a single terminal panel. The nurse can place 90 to 95 percent of her orders from that common order panel and the rest from other overlay sheets. An order is entered by touching the phrase (or phrases) describing the order on the "touch-terminal." The computer prints the order immediately at every "need-to-know" terminal, including a confirming printout at the originating station. The printer operates at 30 characters per second.

In addition to the "touch-terminal," other terminals are attached to the system. Cathode ray tubes are used to input textual and extensive numeric data in the admitting office and financial areas. A receive-only version of the "touch-terminal" is available for installation in areas where it is not necessary to enter orders; maintenance, housekeeping, and dietary are typical sites. A complete financial package is available with the system to process the data base that has been collected by the network.

This system is being installed at Baptist Memorial Hospital in Jacksonville, Florida, and Children's Hospital in Buffalo, New York.

The Standard Register

At present, Standard Register has made its mark with its Source Record Punch. This is an off-line system for data collection using a standard Hollerith card. This system is installed in approximately 200 U.S. hospitals. Standard Register plans to have a central processing unit (CPU) that can interface with all terminals currently available in hospitals, and a special Standard Register terminal. The CPU they plan to use is a Texas Instruments 960A, with a variety of other vendors supplying the tape and disk drives, controllers, and printers. The overall system, however, will be marketed under the name of Standard Register. They consider themselves a mini-computer system vendor, and are aiming at providing the service of dissemination of information from the nursing station for approximately $1 per patient day. As the reader can see, the newer efforts are leaning heavily on the mini distributed approach, which will be discussed in more detail later in the paper.

Systems that Handle Data Collection and Message Switching and Incorporate Certain Medical Record Functions

This section will discuss those systems incorporating certain medical record functions in conjunction with all of the functions discussed above. The costs for the former systems are of the order of 1 to 2 dollars per patient day. For the higher level systems discussed below, 2.50 to 4 dollars and up per patient day are realistic.

In this section, the following vendors will be discussed: Burroughs Corporation; Control Data Corporation; Datacare; Honeywell Information Systems; International Business Machines; McDonnell Douglas Automation; Spectra Medical Systems Inc.; and Technicon Medical Information Systems.

Burroughs Corporation

The Burroughs/Medi-Data Hospital Information System (BHIS) was developed jointly with Medi-Data, Inc. The system provides information processing with an On-Line-Real-Time Data Base, available to the user on inquiry, including complete automatic communications capabilities in the area of patient care, from reservations through discharge. Pertinent information is provided as a by-product "off-line" for administrative accounting, research, and statistics.

On-line terminals, consisting of a CRT unit with keyboard and teleprinter, are connected to the center computers by means of leased telephone lines. The following hospitals are served or will be served on a service basis from Charlotte: Charlotte Memorial Hospital, which has been operating fully on the inpatient system for three years; Duke University Medical Center in Durham, North Carolina, which completed its inpatient system and has future plans for an outpatient system; and Memorial Hospital of Jacksonville, Florida, which began installing the full system for both inpatients and outpatients simultaneously in the spring of 1974.

The Burroughs/Medi-Data System now automates and offers on demand, via display or print basis, many hospital routines, including: 1) complete census, preadmissions, reservations, admissions; 2) transmitting doctor's orders and communications to appropriate ancillary departments and service departments; 3) nurses' notes; 4) hourly departmental scheduling for surgery and physical therapy, with further capabilities as required; 5) transmitting test results and diagnosis to the proper location; 6) recording and updating data on the patient's medical record; 7) floor stock resupply and on-line drug profiles; 8) diet and nourishment census; and 9) all fiscally oriented procedures.

Action is initiated via the physician's handwritten orders. The ward secretary, located at the terminal, then enters through the keyboard all patient-related information in the doctor's words. These data are displayed on the CRT screen along with the stored dictionary counterparts, and a hard copy is also produced for verification. Upon confirmation, patient files are updated, and requisitions are generated in the appropriate action points throughout the hospital as required on a specific time basis, with multiple orders of a single procedure generated from one entry. The system prepares all care and medication schedules for each nursing station, pharmacy, laboratory, and other ancillary departments.

Test results from ancillary departments are entered directly into the computer, and they are printed out at corresponding nursing stations to be posted on the patient's chart. All entries are validated by the patient number and room and bed number by the system to confirm the contents. Laboratory results are summarized daily and printed in descending date order by patient by procedure for the chart.

Outpatients can be entered into the system through an outpatient registration system similar to that for inpatients. Medical orders can be entered in the same manner as inpatient data, and requisitions are sent to applicable departments, and charges are posted. Results may be sent to the requesting clinic or department. Outpatients may stay on the system for a predetermined period of time or as scheduled for repeat visits. This system can be seen at Charlotte Memorial Hospital in Charlotte, North Carolina.

In addition, Burroughs is also entering the hospital information field with a somewhat different approach, using a new display, small and compact for use at the nursing station. This system is called the Burroughs Hospital Information Processing Systems (BHIPS), and can be seen at Wesley Hospital in Wichita, Kansas.

Control Data Corporation

Control Data Corporation's concept of an integrated medical information system is to coordinate all health related activities—patient care, administrative, education, and research—via a hospital communications system based on TOTES, a Transaction Oriented Terminal Executive Operating System utilizing a Distributed Data Base Management System. In this concept, various small computers with either shared or dedicated applications are tied together through TOTES and a hospital communications controller. Each computer retains all patient data necessary for efficient operation for its application, and passes on all data necessary to a large central Data Base Management Computer.

This system—MEDICOM—is a hospital communications and patient file management system. TOTES is a new operating system designed to manipulate data via a touch-sensitive CRT terminal—DIGISCRIBE. All medical application programs are to operate independently for TOTES, enabling the user to create his own applications.

Currently, the dedicated systems for medical computer applications offered by CDC include: (1) Medlab, an intensive care patient monitoring system which includes heart catheterization, intensive care unit, coronary care unit, surgery monitoring, preadmission screening and history, and a laboratory reporting system; (2) computer assisted electrocardiography, a scaler ECG system developed by CDC and CEIS, Denver, Colorado; (3) Pathlab, a clinical laboratory management and automation system; and (4) MEDISHARP, an administrative data processing system.

Various parts of the previously mentioned applications can be seen at Latter Day Saints Hospital, Salt Lake City, Utah; St. Lukes Hospital, Phoenix, Arizona; Mercy Hospital, Pittsburgh, Pennsylvania; Bethesda Naval Hospital in Maryland; and CEIS/ St. Lukes in Denver.

Although all of the above systems have the capability of standing alone, they are being planned so they can be combined with TOTES to form an integrated system. No complete system is in operation at this time, but one under development is St. Louis University Hospital in Missouri; another is at Flinders Hospital in Australia.

Datacare

Datacare has adopted the principle that all communication is through one central processing unit into which all terminals are linked. Presently, the terminals are IBM's 2760, which uses the 2740 as a control unit, with plans to upgrade to a Datacare developed CRT and printer attached to the PDP-8 computer which handles the Laboratory System at Roanoke Memorial Hospital. Medication, diets, treatment, laboratory requests, and radiology are entered via these terminals.

Upon admission, the patient's identification, vital statistics, and personal and financial information are recorded in the system file. Once these files have been established, daily activity relating to the patient's treatment and progress can be applied to them and used by the system to facilitate patient care. For example, when an X-ray is ordered in the Datacare System, medications are automatically ordered, diets are changed, and treatments prescribed. After a reading is reported in radiology, diets are restored, etc.

This system is presently operational at Roanoke Memorial Hospital, Roanoke, Virginia.

Honeywell

National Data Communications (NDC) concluded agreements in September 1973 with Honeywell, giving them worldwide rights to market the VITAL (REACH) System. NDC will continue to operate as a company developing software and applications for the VITAL System, plus maintenance and facilities management. (B. Wilson Whiteside, V.P. Marketing)

The VITAL System, marketed by Honeywell Information Systems, Inc., is a clinically oriented medical information system. The CRT display terminals and associated printers are located at the nursing stations, in ancillary departments, and in the business areas.

This affords hospital personnel the capability of inputting and displaying both fiscal and medical information on a patient.

At the same time that the nurse or doctor enters a service request for laboratory work or X-ray, a charge is immediately and automatically made on the fiscal record of the patient's bill and is recorded on the patient's medical record. In addition, as a by-product of ordering through the system, inventories are updated, and volume and statistical reports are automatically maintained for each hospital department. Laboratory tests can be ordered from the nursing stations, and schedules for laboratory sections are generated on a regular basis. This is said to provide optimum use of staff and facilities. Upon discharge of the patient, the medical record is stored on magnetic tape or hard copy, and a complete bill is created for the patient.

The VITAL (REACH) System utilizes the Honeywell 1695/1697 series central processing units located in the hospital. The system offers the hospital service and back-up by using one processor on-line and one off-line in a batch processing mode.

The on-line system consists of four functions: (1) patient registration and bed census management, (2) patient order entry, (3) results reporting from ancillary departments, and (4) nursing service charting.

Honeywell Information Systems uses the BOL Language for the off-line application programs. In summary, VITAL has three components: (1) an operating system, (2) application modules, and (3) a compiler in which applications are written.

The VITAL (REACH) System is installed at Deaconess Hospital in Evansville, Indiana; Lakeland General in Lakeland, Florida; and Baptist Hospital of S.E. Texas (including Women's and Children's Hospital in Beaumont, Texas). VITAL (REACH) is being installed at Huntington Memorial Hospital in Pasadena, California.

Presently, all transactions are spooled from a disk each night to the patient accounting system, and the plan is to handle the work on-line. Systems of similar design will be implemented at Morton Plant Hospital, Clearwater, Florida, and University Hospital, Tampa.

In addition, a similar system has been developed at Mansfield General in Mansfield, Ohio, with an almost identical computer and terminal configuration. This one has a mini-computer message concentrator and switching front-end.

However, rather than using a catalog of service codes to enter preformatted messages, Honeywell has developed "menu" formats for admission, laboratory, and radiology. Here the CRT operators call up the screens of orders: lab, for example, which shows CBS, hematocrit, sed rate, SMA-12, Kahn, etc., each with a one-digit code. The operator enters the one-digit code for the test desired from the screen. This initiates the order to lab and the audit trail at the ordering nursing station.

This system is between a Level I and Level II system, but leaning more in this section's direction.

International Business Machines Corporation (IBM)

IBM Corporation's concept of an integrated medical information system utilizes the System/370 processor to form the foundation for:

1. A communication system that centrally controls the flow of source data to ancillary locations through the hospital.
2. A central information system that electronically receives, transmits, and stores data for immediate access.
3. A real-time system that processes and provides data in a desirable format.

IBM's medical systems are designed to assist many different service areas in the hospital. These include nursing stations, admissions, pharmacy, clinical laboratories, X-ray, dietary, electrodiagnostics, operating room, central supply, medical records, business, etc.

IBM Health Care Support (HCS) Family of programs for System/370 include:

1. HCS/Accounting System: Provides a financial management system for a hospital or group of hospitals. The program provides patient billing, accounts receivable, and general ledger applications.
2. HCS/Laboratory Information System: Is intended to assist laboratories in hospitals, clinics, and medical schools to reduce paperwork and devote more time to planning and testing. The program attempts to minimize clerical tasks of manually counting, sorting, transcribing, and preparing laboratory test reports.
3. HCS/Data Communications Program: Permits users of the accounting system and laboratory information system to link remote terminals to a central computer.
4. HCS/Admission System: Provides for patient preadmissions, admissions, transfers, and discharge. Maintains a hospital census and alphabetic patient name index.
5. HCS/Order Communications System: Is planned to provide for the entry and communication of doctors' orders, requisitions, and general messages. Utilizes hospital defined information.
6. HCS/Pharmacy Order Entry and Scheduling System: Is intended to provide for entering medication orders, scheduling medical administration (either unit dose or individual prescription), confirming PRNs given and noting exceptions to regularly scheduled drugs, maintaining the patient drug file, automatically charging for medications, updating inventory, and displaying drug information.

7. HCS/Pharmacy Inventory Control System: Has the object to provide for inventory controls, including multiple locations and individual drug security.

8. HCS/Patient History System: Also hopes to provide for automated patient history-taking, utilizing flexible formats for the creation of a patient medical history data base.

9. HCS/Electrocardiogram (ECG) Analysis Program: Provides significant assistance to the cardiologist in the measurement, interpretation, and reporting of the electrocardiogram.

10. HCS/Coordination of Benefits: This relates to the accounting system, where insurance coverage is also allocated correctly.

11. HCS/Revenue Management System: This also relates to the accounting system.

12. HCS/Patient Data Base System—HCS/DL/1: Includes the following: (1) patient registration system, (2) a new admission system, and (3) updates order communication system.

The HCS programs use the Customer Information Control System (CICS) and the IBM 3270 Information Display System. CICS provides the Communication Control and Support for the system. The IBM 3270 system includes CRTs, which have lightpen and badge reader capability and printers.

The patient can be located by displaying the current nurse station census on the CRT. After identifying the patient, the required order can be entered by using a "menu" selection process. When the order has been completed, it can be verified on the display before transmission to the required departments. Alternately, an order may be entered directly via a keyboard. A single copy of the selection screen is maintained within the system.

The IBM 2790 Hospital Communications and Control program for the System/7 computer is designed to integrate all major nursing and service areas into an interactive network of IBM 2791 terminals, which are used to route messages and service orders to a specified destination. The system controls this network and automatically captures charge data for posting to the proper patient account. At this time, it is difficult to place this system into the first category. It seems to be developing into a Level II system.

McDonnell Douglas Automation Company

The McDonnell Douglas Hospital Patient Care (HPC) System is an on-line, real-time system designed to service the ordering, results reporting, and basic scheduling needs of the hospital. Originally installed in October 1969, the HPC System currently services four hospitals located remotely to the data center, utilizing the shared computer concept. Original application areas installed were admissions, clinical laboratory, radiology, and nursing (ordering and patient information retrieval). Since the original installations, pharmacy and laboratory instrumentation modules and central services have been installed and are currently in operation at St. Francis Hospital in Peoria, Illinois.

The system is designed for ordering to be done from the nursing station, with the clerical people on the station having the primary responsibility for order entry. Utilizing cathode ray tubes as the ancillary entry devices, results reporting from laboratory and radiology are operational. Laboratory tests being done on SMA 12/60 and 6/60 are automatically retrieved through an on-line IBM System/7, which is interfaced like a terminal into the CPU.

Currently, all ancillary departments and admitting use CRTs for entry devices, with an IBM 1092 keyboard at each nursing station. Development is presently underway to incorporate advanced four-phase terminals at the nursing stations. This system can be seen at St. Francis Hospital in Peoria, Illinois.

Spectra Medical Systems, Inc.

The Spectra 2000 is a real-time, on-line computerized medical information system. A dedicated "stand-alone" computer is located in the hospital. Modular in both hardware and software, the Spectra 2000 provides an information processing capability for entry, storage, and retrieval of medical data pertaining to the patient from admission through discharge.

This system was designed for use by medical people—doctors, nurses, medical technologists, and pharmacists. It is also used by most other people in the hospital who serve the patient in some way. These people, wherever they are, can use any nearby data station to reach and utilize patient information appropriate to their job responsibilities.

A data station generally consists of a video display device, lightpen, keyboard, and a printer. They are located at key hospital areas, normally including admitting, nursing stations, laboratory, pharmacy, dietary, and radiology. Doctor's lounges and adjacent medical office buildings are other convenient locations.

The system performs the following functions: admit/discharge/transfer; medical order entry; medication scheduling; medication charting; permanent chart document preparation; nurse scheduling; current census; patient drug profile; staff requirement report; utilization review report; and charge capture. Additionally, the system contains an extensive drug interaction library.

Nurses enter medication charting information, admitting clerks assign patients to empty beds, and other hospital people receive and transmit nearly all medical information that can be committed to automation via the color CRTs. Orders written into this system automatically generate an immediate printed confirmation at the station where entered, as well as requisitions in all appropriate ancillary services. This information is immediately entered into schedules reports (medication schedules, bed availability, nurse staffing, utilization, patient profile, etc.), since all data are updated in real-time. These reports print out automatically or at the request of authorized users.

Technicon Medical Information Systems Corporation

Technicon provides a modular medical information system consisting of several modules that can be installed separately, in various combinations, or as a total integrated system. The modules are: financial management; admission/transfer/discharge; pharmacy and medications scheduling; clinical laboratories; radiology and other medical ancillaries; and nursing-care planning and reporting.

The systems are available on two bases: (1) full service contract—Technicon provides terminals, software, and all computer facilities; and (2) support contract—Technicon provides terminals and leases the software for use in the hospital's own computer center.

When the total Medical Information System (MIS) is in use, all of the modules function as previously described, and the integration between the modules is complete and automatic.

At present, this system is fully operational at El Camino Hospital in Mountain View, California. Shortly, St. Barnabus Hospital in Livingston, New Jersey, will install the Technicon MIS, which will be replacing the current Hospital Information System managed by EDS.

The Introduction of the Mini-computer Functional Processing Concept into HIS Development

One of the distinct differences to be pointed out here is that the actual computer power is brought to the source of action. A descriptive term that will be used to emphasize this difference is herein called Functional Processing. What is functional processing and its advantages?

One of the underlying reasons for functional processing is the ability and necessity of the hospital administrator and his staff to be able to have various options in planning. The large, centralized systems demand that a major planning effort be undertaken long before the actual implementation of the proposed system. Since the use of an integrated data base is now considered an integral part of such systems, and multiple functions will be utilizing the data communications, processing, and storage capabilities, failure to conduct the required scope and depth of planning can lead to serious difficulties in later implementation. The result is often long lead times, cost overruns, and the ultimate shrinkage of systems objectives and performance.

Functional systems have unique merit in the hospital setting. Individualized systems can be built around mini-computers to more adequately serve the actual needs of discrete functions, the most likely areas being admissions, pharmacy, radiology, medical records, and certain phases of laboratory. In functional approaches, these systems can be implemented independently of each other as one area becomes ready to be computerized. By creating a collection of functional modules which have been custom-designed to focus sharply on specific needs within the user department, the success of the system is much more likely. Management gains, too, in the level of financial risk involved, since any one functional system represents a model cost when compared to larger, centralized systems. Also, the size of the financial considerations can be ascertained in advance. An underlying factor in this type of approach is that each hospital department has unique data requirements. This means that one can be oriented to an overall centralized planning concept, but have the flexibility of a functional implementation program. This is the strength of building a hospital information system with "mini" function processors. In order to have a unified system in the total management of the hospital, careful thought must be given to the integration of the various functional systems.

Summary

It seems appropriate to close this section with a quote by Alvin Toffler from his book, Future Shock:

> Rational Behaviour depends upon a ceaseless flow of data from the environment. It depends on the power of the individual to predict with at least fair success, the outcome of his own actions . . . The more rapidly changing and novel the environment, the more information the individual needs to process in order to make effective, rational decisions.

It is the opinion of the authors that computerized hospital information systems will be necessary to meet the need for "effective rational decision."

This paper has presented various computer applications in the health care field. The authors have also attempted to present the reader with some tools to intelligently select and implement the various systems discussed.

REFERENCES

1. G. L. Hammon and S. E. Jacobs, "Shared Computer Systems," Part 1, Hospitals 44 (1970):50; Part 2, Hospitals 44 (1970):72.

2. G. Anderson, G. L. Hammon, and S. E. Jacobs, "Facilities Management: Wave of the Future?" Hosp. Financ. Manage. 4 (1974):40.

3. B. Romberg, "Is Facilities Management for You?" Infosystems 19 (1972):32.

4. D. M. Parnell, Jr., "A New Concept: EDP Facilities Management," Admin. Manage. 31 (1970):20.

5. D. M. Parnell, Jr., "EDP Facilities Management: Abdication or Salvation?" From an address from the American Management Association's National Briefing, as reported by Data Process. Dig., September 1970.

19

INVENTORY CONTROL

INTRODUCTION

This paper describes a short-term blood inventory level forecast system for better blood inventory planning and control. The Inventory Level Projection Model presented projects daily inventory level fourteen days into the future so that appropriate management action can be taken if necessary. The system consists of four submodels: (1) blood expirations forecast model, (2) blood collections forecast model, (3) blood transfusion forecast model, and (4) blood inventory projection model. The model proved to be quite accurate in forecasting when it was applied at a Regional Blood Center. A cost-benefit analysis of the forecasting system is presented at the end of the paper.

Introduction to Technique

The classical approach to inventory control is to develop a prescriptive model which upon application will generate the required ordering decisions and provide satisfactory control.

An altogether different problem arises in inventory control of blood. Reordering or replenishment of supplies takes place through planned collections and these blood collections frequently must be planned with considerable lead time. Because of this situation, a different approach is required.

The blood inventory control approach uses a blood inventory forecasting model which consists of four submodels. Each submodel uses a different technique for forecasting. For instance, blood collections are forecast on the basis of prior experience while blood utilization is forecast by exponential smoothing. The forecast is made for several periods into the future. Management reviews the forecasts and on the basis of the forecasts, decides to increase, decrease, or maintain planned collection by short-term collection adjustments. These adjustments consist of extending or reducing blood collection hours and increasing or decreasing blood collection publicity prior to planned collections at certain blood collection sites.

Manipulation by management of the blood collections (the inflow) thus results in more desirable inventory levels, which in turn result in less wastage of blood and fewer incidences of blood shortages.

REFERENCES

Bierman, H., C. Bonini, and W. Hausman, Quantitative Analysis for Business Decisions. Homewood, Ill.: R. D. Irwin, 1969.

Frankfurter, G. M., A. E. Jelmert, C. C. Pegels, J. P. Seagle, and E. L. Wallace, "A Computer-Based Blood Inventory Information System for a Regional Blood Distribution Center," Transfusion 10 (July-August 1970):203-14.

Pegels, C. C., "Exponential Forecasting: Some New Variations," Management Science 15 (January 1969):311-15.

Rockwell, T. H., R. H. Barnum, and W. C. Giffen, "Inventory Analysis as Applied to Hospital Whole Blood Supply and Demand," Journal of Industrial Engineering 13 (March-April 1962):109-14.

Vollman, T., Operations Management: A System Modelbuilding Approach. Reading, Mass.: Addison-Wesley, 1972.

MANAGEMENT CONTROL OF BLOOD THROUGH A SHORT-TERM SUPPLY-DEMAND FORECAST SYSTEM*

George M. Frankfurter
Kenneth E. Kendall
C. Carl Pegels

Design, development, implementation, and operation of a short-term blood inventory level forecast system is described. The primary purpose of the forecast system is to alert blood center management to the short-term inventory level of blood supplies so that they can take corrective action to either reduce or increase blood collections. A test is performed on the system, and it is demonstrated that management took action to reduce collections in response to higher than necessary inventory levels and increased collections during a period when insufficient inventory levels were forecast.

This paper describes how a short-term computerized blood inventory level forecast system provides the management of a regional blood collection and distribution center with adaptive inventory planning information. The information consists of advance warning of potentially low or high blood inventory levels. Management utilizes this advance information and exercises its authority to increase blood

---

The research contained in this paper was performed pursuant to Contract No. PH-43-68-1281 with the National Institutes of Health, Department of Health, Education, and Welfare. Findings and conclusions do not necessarily represent views of the Public Health Service. Reprinted with permission from <u>Management Science</u> 21, No. 4 (December 1974). Copyright 1974 by the Institute of Management Sciences.

*Processed by Professor W. W. Cooper, Departmental Editor for Public Administration and by Professor M. G. Simpson, Associate Editor; received June 1971, revised August 1973. This paper has been with the authors seven months for revision.

collection efforts during the lead time if low inventory levels are projected and decreases blood collection efforts if high inventory levels are projected. As a result, the short-term blood inventory level forecast model enables management to control blood inventory levels and thus eliminate blood shortages and excessive expirations which result from excessively high blood inventory levels.

The regional blood collection and distribution center for which the model was developed and which currently uses it supplies blood to 54 hospitals in western New York and northwestern Pennsylvania, serving over two million people. Total blood collections amount to approximately 65,000 units annually, and about a two-week supply of blood is in inventory (available) in the region at any one time. The inventory is distributed over the regional blood center (about a four-day supply) and the 54 participating hospital blood banks (about a ten-day supply). All blood is collected by the regional blood collection and distribution center and thus passes through it at least once.

REVIEW OF BLOOD MANAGEMENT PROBLEMS

Human blood consists of a variety of therapeutic components not available in synthetic form. In addition, it serves as a replacement of blood loss incurred during surgery or because of internal and external injuries. Unfortunately, it is a perishable product and deteriorates over time. Some blood components must be used right after donation or at least within 24 hours of donation; other components should be used within seven days, and the legal life limit on whole blood and packed red cells is 21 days. Although the plasma of blood has some value after 21 days, for all practical purposes, the red cells lose most of their value after 21 days and as a result, the 21-day life of blood has become the common benchmark for marking the maximum lifespan of blood.

The only source of blood is the healthy human being who donates one unit (approximately one pint) of blood a maximum of five times per year at a time and place convenient to him or her. Certain times of the year, especially summer and midwinter, are time periods when donors prefer not to donate and because of the short lifespan, blood shortages occur. These blood shortages seldom cause fatalities of patients in need of blood, but they do severely disrupt the operation of usually scarce health care facilities. Surgery is frequently postponed and patients suffer from being forced to do with less blood than would otherwise be available for replacement (as in surgery) or for therapeutic purposes (as in hemophilia).

Because of the above problems, a variety of blood management research projects have been reported in the literature. Most of these projects report on inventory related studies. Elston, Pickerel and

Jennings [1, 2, 3, 5], individually and jointly, have used computer simulation to study the effect on shortages of a variety of inventory management policies. Pegels and Jelmert [7, 8] in two separate papers have evaluated by analytic means blood bank assignment (crossmatch) policies and the effect of assigning the same unit of blood to more than one patient. Individually, Pegels [6] has proposed an analytic blood bank collection scheduling and inventory control system. Rockwell et al. [11] have reported on a study using analytic methods to analyze blood inventory policies. Various parts of a large-scale regional blood bank management project have been reported by Frankfurter et al. [4] and by Pegels and Wallace [9, 10]. This paper is an outgrowth of the latter project.

Based on the above references to the literature the reader will have become aware that most of the concern has been on the inventory practices of blood banks. Most of the authors with few exceptions have started from the premise that traditional inventory management as practiced in industry can relieve the problems. To a considerable extent this is true. However, what has frequently been overlooked or ignored is the fact that both blood supply and blood demand on any given day are random variables with variances of considerable magnitude. Fortunately, with adequate lead time, the mean supply rate can be adjusted upward or downward. In addition, historical demand rates and inventory levels contain information that can be useful to forecast demand. Demand in this case consists of both the needs of patients and inventory wastage resulting from expirations (blood units aging beyond 21 days).

THE INVENTORY LEVEL PROJECTION MODEL

The inventory projection model discussed below is one that has evolved over time. An important consideration in the development of this model has been the requirement that it be responsive to current conditions for the Regional Blood Collection and Distribution Center which it serves. Another important consideration is ease of transfer to other regional areas. The model is operated daily through a time sharing computer system and is written in the BASIC computer language, and, therefore, ease of operation and ease of modification are important features of the implemented model.

The model projects daily inventory levels fourteen days into the future. On the basis of these projected inventory levels, appropriate management action is taken when necessary.

THE VARIOUS SUBMODELS

There are various submodels which together make up the total program or master model. These are (1) blood transfusions forecast model, (2) blood expirations forecast model, (3) blood collections forecast model, and (4) blood inventory projection model which also serves as the executive model which controls the other three submodels.

The inventory projection for each day into the future can be summarized by the following accounting identity:

Beginning inventory - transfusion forecasts - predicted expirations + forecasted collections = ending inventory

Note that in the above equation beginning inventory and ending inventory are inputs or products of the executive model. The other components are respectively determined by the submodels. A detailed discussion of the submodels follow below.

BLOOD EXPIRATIONS FORECAST MODEL

The forecast of blood expirations is made for a whole week, say on Friday, and is based on actual weekly collections during the past three weeks. A positive exponential function has been found to fit the relationship between expirations and past collections. Using this exponential function with empirically derived parameters, the weekly forecast of expirations, E, is $E = \exp(\alpha + \beta C)$ where C is the sum of the actual collections during the previous three weeks and α and β are parameters. Estimates of α and β, $\hat{\alpha}$ and $\hat{\beta}$ respectively were obtained by regressing the logarithm of actual expirations (E) on the three week sum of collections (C).

Suppose that actual collections during each of the past three weeks are 940, 1260, and 1300 units respectively. Total collections then sum to C = 3500. Also suppose that the expirations forecast, E, equals 56 units for the week. Since blood is collected on Mondays through Fridays, there will be no expirations on Fridays and Saturdays, but only on Sundays through Thursdays. As the model only operates on Mondays through Fridays, the weekly expirations file appears as shown in Table 19.1. The reader may observe that the same forecast is used for two subsequent weeks. Although this simplification may appear and may in fact introduce error in forecasts for specific days, the objective of the model to show trends is not affected. Even high accuracy of trends is not that important, since the primary objective of the model is to serve as a trigger for managerial action.

TABLE 19.1

Collections Forecast

Line Number	Collections and Expirations
100	02/23/73,
110	Collections,
120	245,
130	385,
140	230,
150	295,
160	415,
170	285,
180	390,
190	290,
200	350,
210	295,
220	245,
230	Expirations,
240	58,
250	29,
260	29,
270	29,
280	0,
290	58,
300	29,
310	29,
320	29,
330	0,

BLOOD COLLECTIONS FORECAST MODEL

Daily blood collections forecasts are made by committee and are entered into the computer to be available for the inventory projection model. Either daily or weekly forecasts of collections can be handled. If only weekly forecasts are available, a simple division by five produces daily forecasts. The collection forecasts are stored in a data file in Table 19.1.

BLOOD TRANSFUSION FORECAST MODEL

An exponential smoothing model with a weekly cyclical component is used to forecast daily transfusions in the large hospitals. The model forecasts a basic permanent component $\bar{S}_t$ which is based on current and historical transfusions. The formula used is $\bar{S}_t = \omega_e S_t / F_{t-L} + (1 - \omega_e)\bar{S}_{t-1}$ where S_t are the transfusions during the past 24 hours, ω_e is an estimated weight, $0 \leq \omega_e \leq 1$, $\bar{S}_{t-1}$ is the previous permanent component and F_{t-L} is a cyclical weight determined L days ago.*

The length of the cycle, L = 10 days, and the current cyclical weight F_t is found by the formula $F_t = \omega_F S_t / \bar{S}_t + (1 - \omega_F) F_{t-L}$ where ω_F is a weight, $0 \leq \omega_F \leq 1$.

The forecast for the next L days is $S_{t,i} = F_{t+i-L} \bar{S}_t$ where $S_{t,i}$ is the forecast for day $t + i$, $i = 1, 2, \ldots, L$. Hence the forecast for the current day, that is Monday if the forecast is made on Monday, is $S_{t,1}$ which then equals $S_{t,1} = F_{t-9} \bar{S}_t$. Since F_t is different for each day of the 10-day cycle, each of the ten F_t's must remain in the computer memory.

The transfusions forecasts for the next L days are then stored in an on-line file. The permanent component and the cyclical components as well as the estimated weights for the permanent component and the cyclical components of the forecast are stored in a separate file and called upon when needed by the program.

EXECUTIVE PROGRAM

Beginning controllable inventory in hospitals and in the blood center is entered into the computer at the end of previous day, day t. Hence, the ending inventory forecast for day t + 1 will be for the end of the day on which the forecast is being made. Then for day t + 1 or day 1,

Ending forecast (1) = Beginning inventory (1) - Transfusions (1)

- Expirations (1) + Collections (1),

---

*There are considered to be five days in a week and not seven. Transfusions on weekends are included in the Monday figure, Monday being the day on which they are reported. The length of the cycle L is 10 days and not 5 days to allow a forecast horizon of 10 days.

TABLE 19.2

Partial Output of the Forecast Model

	Short-term Inventory Forecast for Fri 07/21/72				
	Aggregate Total of All Types				
Day	Begin Inv	Trans-fusions	Expir-ations	Collec-tions	Ending Forecast
Mon	1882	273	52	280	1837
Tue	1837	195	26	130	1746
Wed	1746	193	26	275	1802
Thu	1802	227	26	225	1774
Fri	1774	195	0	270	1849
Mon	1849	239	52	220	1778
Tue	1778	202	26	255	1805
Wed	1805	174	26	330	1935
Thu	1935	199	26	340	2050
Fri	2050	153	0	245	2142
		B—			
Mon	39	6	1	6	38
Tue	38	4	1	3	36
Wed	36	4	1	6	37
Thu	37	5	1	5	36
Fri	36	4	0	6	33
Mon	38	5	1	5	37
Tue	37	4	1	6	38
Wed	38	4	1	7	40
Thu	40	4	1	8	43
Fri	43	3	0	5	45
		AB—			
Mon	28	4	1	2	25
Tue	25	3	0	1	23
Wed	23	3	0	2	22
Thu	22	3	0	2	21
Fri	21	3	0	2	20
Mon	20	4	1	2	17
Tue	17	3	0	2	16
Wed	16	3	0	3	16
Thu	16	3	0	3	16
Fri	16	2	0	2	16

and for day i = 2, ..., k it is

Ending forecast (i) = Ending forecast (i - 1) - Transfusions (i)
- Expirations (i) + Collections (i)

A forecast as generated is shown in Table 19.2.

The forecast made the next day, t = 2, will be for Tuesday and L days into the future. The only input required is the inventory in hospitals and in the blood center, and the previous day's (Monday's) transfusions. The weight file is updated and the collections and expirations file is updated by the formula: Expirations (i) = Expirations (i + 1) from the previous day's file, i = 1, 2, ..., L - 1, and Expirations (L) = Expirations (L - 5). The same updating procedure is followed for the collections portion of this file.

With all files updated the executive program is called and a new forecast for the next L days is made. The above procedure is repeated for Wednesday, Thursday, and Friday; the following Monday the total procedure is repeated.

HOW THE OUTPUT IS USED

As briefly mentioned before, the model described above is for short-term planning purposes only. It is not intended to provide high-accuracy daily forecasts but rather daily projections of inventory levels over the next L days (two weeks) into the future. In other words, each day an updated inventory level projection is generated. On the basis of the daily projections, management of the blood center is able to respond with appropriate management action.

Management action can take several forms, each dependent on the inventory level projection. If a high inventory level is projected, management can take no action and enjoy a plentiful supply of blood with a concomitant high percentage of expirations; or alternatively it can reduce the level of bloodmobile activity by possibly postponing a bloodmobile or combining two bloodmobile locations. Savings in operating costs are then, of course, realized. In case of average inventory level projection, no action is needed. However, in case of low inventory level, management can take appropriate steps to increase donations by notifying blood donor recruiters, by sending out additional flyers, and possibly by increasing the number of radio of T.V. spot announcements.

IMPLEMENTATION EXPERIENCE

When the forecasting model was initially introduced at the Regional Blood Center, there was a substantial amount of enthusiasm shown. Several meetings were held to explain the concept of the model and its potential. The Blood Center staff members not only understood the basics involved, but also even offered several suggestions which were immediately incorporated in the model. One of these was the breakdown of the daily forecasts by blood type, since the initial program merely yielded aggregate totals. Since the model needed a donation forecast for two weeks into the future, the committee responsible for that task agreed to modify their forecasting on a two-week basis in addition to their traditional one-week forecast.* Within a week of these introductory meetings, a daily forecast of the blood center's inventory by blood type for the next two weeks was available to the Blood Center. Three copies were generated each day. One to the assistant medical director, one to the regional blood program administrator, and the third to his assistant.

The most useful feature of the forecasting model is that it shows the various blood managers the trends, by blood type, for the next two weeks. Initially, several members of the Blood Center, due to their limited exposure with such concepts, looked not at the projected two-week levels, but at the next day's forecast in an effort to determine the model's accuracy. Fortunately, the model was quite accurate in forecasting the next day's inventory. However, it took time to point out that the former is not the primary function of the model when viewed as a management tool. Greater utilization of the model currently takes place since the Blood Center staff members have become more accustomed to its main function of supplying information for management control. In the next section a brief review is presented of the effect of the inventory level projections on management behavior.

MANAGEMENT CONTROL THROUGH FORECASTS

The effect the forecasts had on management's behavior in controlling inventory levels through modification of collection efforts was considerable. As observers of the management process, the researchers had advocated modification of collection efforts but had not expected the positive results that occurred.

---

*The committee's donation forecast seemed to be more efficient and accurate than any conceivable mathematical and/or statistical forecasting model.

In Table 19.3 is listed the inventory level forecast two weeks into the future, and this forecast is compared with the actual inventory level that resulted. The periods shown are consecutive periods, and the timespan was arbitrarily chosen. Note that during the first ten periods, when daily inventory level forecasts were below 1500 units, the resulting actual inventory levels were all higher and on the average about fifteen percent higher. Subsequent to period 10, the inventory level forecasts were all in excess of 1500 units and the resulting actual inventory levels were all lower and on the average over sixteen percent lower. Considering that the timespan was arbitrarily selected, the behavior of management and their success are quite remarkable All attempts at increasing collection while forecasted inventory levels were above 1500 units were successful.

Prior to development of the forecast system inventory levels would grow to wasteful levels in periods of high volume blood collections and drop to dangerously low levels in the traditional shortage period of midsummer and end of year holiday season. Although these shortage periods have not been eliminated yet, the forecast model provides management with an advance warning and triggers extra recruiting efforts to help increase the low blood inventory levels during shortage periods.

Management now consciously makes efforts to modify collections on the basis of the forecasted collections and considers an inventory level of 1500 to 1700 units a desirable range. Forecasts below this range trigger efforts at increasing collections; forecasts above this range cause collection efforts to be reduced.

COST BENEFIT ANALYSIS OF FORECAST SYSTEM

A forecasting model that provides estimates of future blood inventory conditions has the potential of producing a high benefit-cost ratio. The benefit of knowing future blood inventory levels consists of the ability to modify the inventory levels which produce the attendant savings in reductions of expirations and eliminations of deferred surgical operations. Deferred surgical operations are quite common in regions affected by blood shortages.

The costs of development and operating cost are listed below together with incremental benefits. The benefits are maximum potential benefits and are not being attained in their entirety.

Wider adoption of the system by other blood regions has been hindered by the lack of sound inventory information systems to serve as a foundation for a more general inventory management system. In addition the authors have been concerned with demonstrating feasi-

TABLE 19.3

Comparison of Forecasted and Resultant Inventory Levels

Period	Forecasted Inventory Level Two Weeks Prior	Projected Over-supply (+) or Under-supply (−)	Actual Inventory Level	Difference Between Actual and Forecast Due to Management Action
1	1483	−	1540	+57
2	1437	−	1530	+93
3	1247	−	1360	+113
4	1355	−	1426	+71
5	1281	−	1526	+245
6	1238	−	1844	+606
7	1252	−	1737	+485
8	1375	−	1548	+173
9	1362	−	1414	+52
10	1457	−	1534	+77

(continued)

11	2179		1842	-337
12	2100	+	1615	-485
13	1889	+	1809	-80
14	2071	+	1646	-425
15	2225	+	1695	-530
16	2669	+	2003	-666
17	2227	+	1729	-498
18	1984	+	1776	-208
19	1918	+	1693	-225
20	2223	+	1833	-390
21	2476	+	1935	-541
22	2196	+	1911	-285
23	2255	+	1818	-437
24	2237	+	1771	-466
25	2304	+	1983	-321
26	2512	+	1960	-552
27	2202	+	1923	-279

Incremental Costs

Developmental Costs	Personnel—5 man months	$ 7,000
	Computer time, storage, etc.	750
	Total developmental costs	$ 7,750
Annual Operational Costs	Computer time, storage, etc.	$ 400
	Total added operational costs	$ 400

Incremental Benefits

Maximum Potential Annual Benefits	Reduce outdating 2000 units at $26	$52,000
	Avoid 2 deferred surgical operations at $400	800
	Total maximum potential benefits	$52,800
	Percentage attainment: 50-60 percent	

bility of the system and not with the marketing efforts required to have the forecasting system become more widely adopted.

From the above discussion, it may be observed how a relatively simple group of management science models were combined to make a straightforward inventory level forecast or projection system. The inventory forecasts provided information to management which allowed them to smooth and control the critical blood inventory levels.

REFERENCES

1. R. C. Elston, "Inventory Levels for a Hospital Blood Bank Under the Assumption of 28 Day Shelf Life," Transfusion 8 (1968):19.

2. ——— and J. C. Pickerel, "Guides to Inventory Levels for a Hospital Blood Bank Determined by Electronic Computer Simulation," Transfusion 5 (1965):465.

3. ———, "A Statistical Approach to Ordering and Usage Policies for a Hospital Blood Bank," Transfusion 3 (1963):41.

4. G. M. Frankfurter, A. E. Jelmert, C. C. Pegels, J. P. Seagle, and E. L. Wallace, "A Regional Computer Based Inventory Information System," Transfusion 10 (July-August 1970):203.

5. J. B. Jennings, "An Analysis for Hospital Blood Bank Whole Blood Inventory Control Policies," Transfusion 8 (1968):335.

6. C. C. Pegels, "A Blood Bank Collection Scheduling and Inventory Control System," AIIE 1 (1969):51-55.

7. ———— and A. E. Jelmert, "An Evaluation of Blood Inventory Policies: A Markov Chain Application," Operations Research 18 (November-December 1970): 1087-98.

8. ————, "A Study of Two Blood Bank Crossmatch Policies," AIIE 3 (March 1971):69-75.

9. ———— and E. L. Wallace, "Analysis and Design of a Model Regional Blood Management System," in B. Avi-Itzhek, ed., Developments in Operations Research. New York: Gordon and Breach, 1971.

10. ————, "A Computerized Management Information System for Human Blood Utilization," Information Processing 71. Amsterdam: North Holland, 1972.

11. T. H. Rockwell, R. A. Barnum, and W. C. Giffin, "Inventory Analysis as Applied to Hospital Whole Blood Supply and Demand," Journal of Industrial Engineering 13 (March-April 1962):109-14.

20

INPUT-OUTPUT ANALYSIS

INTRODUCTION

The need to forecast cash flow and working capital needs accurately in a hospital, and hence to develop a sound hospital budgeting system, has increased tremendously over the past few years. The purpose of this article is to demonstrate the superiority of a hospital budget based on an input-output model over a conventional budget for management decisions on pricing, output determination, planning, and cost control. The input-output model is described in terms of the departments (final or intermediate) in the production system, the unit of output, and the relationship between outputs and inputs at departmental level. Regression analysis is used to estimate the coefficients for fixed and variable labor and other resources requirements. The results of the study indicated that the input-output budget could cause substantial changes in posted hospital rates for individual departments.

Introduction to Technique

Input-output analysis is a technique developed by the economist Wassily W. Leontief. It is used to study the flows over some particular time period of the value of goods and services used and produced by different industry sectors. Specifically, it is a breakdown of the total output of different industries into the portion which is sold to other industries for use as inputs in their production and the portion which is sold to final users of the product.

Input-output techniques can be used for accounting as well as forecasting. To illustrate input-output accounting, R. B. Platt (see references) uses a simplified three industry model: agriculture, manufacturing, and services. Some part of the output over some period of time of each of these industries may be sold to another industry or industries as raw materials or semifinished goods to be used as inputs in their production. The balance of output not sold as intermediates is sold to final users of the product. To produce its output, each industry requires some intermediate goods purchased from other industries (and perhaps uses some of its own products as well) and pays out to the "primary" factors of production their contribution to the industry's total output. In dollar value, each industry's total output equals its total inputs, that is, its total output is equal to the sum of the cost of production plus profits.

REFERENCES

Cich, B., "Regional Hospitals Need Projection: An Input-Output Approach," Socio-Economic Planning Sciences 10 (1976):37-42.

Dorfman, R., P. Samuelson, and R. Solow, Linear Programming and Economic Analysis. New York: McGraw-Hill, 1958.

Livingstone, J. L., "Input-Output Analysis for Cost Accounting Planning and Control," Accounting Review 44 (January 1969):48-64.

Platt, R. B., Major Approaches to Business Forecasting. Englewood Cliffs, N.J.: Prentice-Hall, 1974.

INPUT-OUTPUT ANALYSIS AND THE HOSPITAL BUDGETING PROCESS

William O. Cleverley

Two hospital budget systems, a conventional budget and an input-output budget, are compared to determine how they affect management decisions in pricing, output, planning, and cost control. Analysis of data from a

Reprinted with permission from Health Services Research 10, No. 1 (Spring 1975). Copyright 1975 by the Hospital Research and Educational Trust, 840 North Lakeshore Drive, Chicago, Ill. 60611.

210-bed not-for-profit hospital indicates that adoption of
the input-output budget could cause substantial changes
in posted hospital rates in individual departments but
probably would have no impact on hospital output determination. The input-output approach promises to be a
more accurate system for cost control and planning
because, unlike the conventional approach, it generates
objective signals for investigating variances of expenses
from budgeted levels.

The development of a sound hospital budgeting system is fast
becoming a matter of paramount importance in hospital administration.
Increasingly pressed by the exigencies arising from third-party
financing, hospital administrators find they must pay increasing attention to cash forecasting and management of working capital. Public
pressure over rising hospital costs has spurred the development of
hospital budget systems. Hospitals participating in the Medicare program now must prepare yearly operating budgets. Medicare legislation
also provides for further experimentation in prospective reimbursement, and the latest Mills-Kennedy national health insurance proposal
would require prospective reimbursement for all hospitals.

Although one of the major requirements for any successful prospective reimbursement system is a soundly developed and accurate
budget, most hospitals do not have very sophisticated budget systems.
The standard for acceptability has been the budget system recommended in the American Hospital Association (AHA) manual, Budgeting
Procedures for Hospitals [1].

The objective of this article is to assess the effect of two alternative budget systems on management decisions in an actual hospital
setting. Specific decision areas are pricing, output determination,
planning, and cost control. The two budget systems tested are the
conventional AHA system, in use at the study hospital, and a budget
system patterned after an input-output (I-O) model in which estimates
of technological coefficients are developed from past operating results
and used to project future costs. The use of I-O models in cost
accounting and budgeting has been the subject of much discussion in
the accounting literature during the past decade [2-5]; as applied to
hospital cost accounting, I-O analysis has been discussed briefly
under the general rubric of the simultaneous equation method [6].

The initial steps in using the I-O approach are the same as those
used in implementation of the AHA budget model.

The first step is to break down the production system into a set
of activity centers—industries in macro models, departments and
divisions in micro models. These departments are classified as either

final or intermediate centers. Final centers produce services that are consumed directly by the patient, and intermediate centers produce services that are consumed by other centers. In a hospital budget, the activity centers are revenue and nonrevenue departments.

The second step is to define the unit of output or service produced in each department. This step is essential to associate cost with level of service and to permit interdepartmental transfers to be quantified.

The third step is to define the relationships between outputs and inputs at the departmental level. There are two classes of inputs for which relationships must be specified: external and internal. External input relationships include the expected quantities of labor, supplies, and other direct costs required at alternative output levels. Internal input relationships include the expected quantities of intermediate departmental outputs or indirect costs required at alternative output levels.

The synthesis of all these steps in both budget models is a system of defined mathematical relationships that determine total and departmental costs for specified levels of service. The nature of specification and the formality of the mathematical systems are the major differentiating characteristics between the two budget models.

INPUT-OUTPUT MODEL APPLIED

The study hospital is a not-for-profit short-term general hospital with 210 beds and 40 bassinets located in northern California. The departmental and associated output structure used in the model is summarized in Table 20.1.

Ten of the departments are classified as intermediate product centers since they furnish no direct medical services to the patient; the remaining 17 departments are classified as direct or final product centers. With minor exceptions, this structure is in conformity with the structure employed in the hospital's budget. The hospital's pharmacy and inhalation therapy departments are not included because revenue data were not available at the time the analysis was conducted.

Hospital resources were divided into four major categories: labor, supplies, capital, and other. These categories represented 62, 14, 15, and 9 percent of total incurred cost, respectively. Labor was the only component of total cost for which records of physical usage had been maintained. To include this information in the model, individual labor resource categories were developed for each department. The other three components of total cost were measured in dollars only. Capital cost was simply unadjusted historical cost

TABLE 20.1

Output Measures for Hospital Departments

Department	Output Measure
Intermediate product centers	
Administration	Total employee hours*
Plant operation	Kilowatt hours
Plant maintenance	Requisitioned hours
General stores	Purchases
Housekeeping	Hours of service
Laundry	Pounds of laundry
Nursing office	Nursing hours
Admitting	Admissions
Medical records	Discharges
Dietary	Total meals
Final product centers	
Medical/surgical	Patient days†
Obstetrics	Patient days†
Intensive care	Patient days†
Nursery	Baby days
Elderly	Patient days†
Surgery	Surgery hours
Delivery	Deliveries
Radiology	Films
Radiation therapy	Treatments
Laboratory	Work units
EKG	Tests
Isotope	Tests
Physical therapy	Treatments
EEG, EMG	Exams
Pulmonary function	Treatments
Outpatient	Cases
Health screening	Patients screened

*Total hours worked by all employees including Administration.
†Patient days for the respective inpatient care center.

depreciation. Revisions for replacement cost values were included in the model to more properly state cost in current terms.

Simple regression analysis was used to estimate the fixed and variable labor requirements for the 27 departments. Hours worked during a given two-week period (H_t) were estimated as follows on the basis of units of output:

$$H_t = F + b \cdot X_t$$

where F = estimated fixed labor coefficient
b = estimated variable labor coefficient
X_t = units of output for a given two-week period

In all but four departments, the fixed term was significant at the 0.05 level of confidence; the variable term was significant at the 0.05 level in all but two departments. The estimates were derived from a sample study of 26 biweekly labor reports for May 1969 through April 1970.

Regression analysis was used in a similar fashion to determine the coefficients for the other resource categories (supplies, other). In many cases, the fixed term was not significant and a completely variable relationship was adopted. The sampled set was the twelve monthly cost reports from June 1969 through May 1970. Since the data could not be adequately adjusted for changes in prices, no attempt was made to extend the sample set. No physical unit data were employed.

Two sets of capital coefficients were estimated. The first set resulted from dividing departmental depreciation in 1969 by the budgeted department output. In the second set, price level-adjusted depreciation, stated in 1969 dollars, was substituted. The Consumer Price Index was used in making this adjustment. The primary purpose of adjusting depreciation charges according to price levels is to ensure that hospital capital is recovered from current revenue. (The AHA has formally recommended the use of price level-adjusted depreciation for fixed and movable equipment in its Statement on the Financial Requirements of Health Care Institutions and Services [7].)

Simple regression analysis was also used to estimate internal input coefficients where suitable records of interdepartmental service utilization were available. The dependent variable was the amount of output supplied by a service department to the user department, and the independent variable was the output of the user department. In departments in which no records of transferred output were available, the number of service department transfers was estimated on the basis of samples.

The required levels of production in the final product centers were taken directly from the hospital's budget. Specification of these output levels then generated the required output from the ten intermediate product centers. Forecast output levels for both intermediate and final product centers were then multiplied by the estimated input relationships to determine budgeted costs.

THE HOSPITAL'S BUDGET

The hospital's budget was developed from departmental cost forecasts. The costs of intermediate product departments are allocated to final product or revenue departments by using the step-down method of cost apportionment. This method is commonly used in the hospital industry because of its simplicity and acceptability to third-party payers.

DIFFERENCES BETWEEN THE TWO APPROACHES

There are a number of differences between the I-O model and the hospital's budget that might account for differences in cost forecasts. One is that some of the intermediate output measures are slightly different. General stores, admitting, and medical records are combined with the administration department in the hospital's budget, and different output measures are used for plant operation, plant maintenance, and nursing office departments. All changes in output measures made in the I-O model resulted in higher correlations between past measures of resource utilization and output.

The two systems also assume different patterns of services among the intermediate departments. The I-O model places no restrictions on service relationships among intermediate departments, whereas the step-down method assumes that the order of cost allocation among intermediate departments is crucial. Costs of departments that service the greatest number of other departments are the first to be allocated. No transfers of cost are then permitted back to those departments even though other departments may have rendered service to them. In most, if not all, hospitals the step-down assumption is not valid.

Another major difference between the two systems is the method of estimating external input coefficients. In the hospital's budget, cost forecasts were made by individual departments and were later negotiated and integrated by the hospital's director of financial services. The estimates developed for the I-O budget were statistical extrapolations using past data. The advantages and disadvantages of centralized versus decentralized budgeting in terms of accuracy and motivation have been discussed extensively [8]. At a minimum, it should be feasible to use statistically extrapolated estimates as an initial input into the budget negotiation process.

The use of price level-adjusted depreciation in one of the I-O cost projections constitutes another difference between the two systems. For hospitals with relatively old fixed assets, differences may be crucial in terms of estimating future capital needs.

Finally, the two systems make different assumptions about cost variability. The hospital's budget does not separate costs into variable and fixed components for individual departments, as does the I-O budget. A surrogate for variable or marginal cost often used in these circumstances is department direct cost per unit of output. The projected variable cost in the I-O budget may differ for two reasons. First, not all direct costs of a department may be considered variable in the I-O budget. To the extent that a large element of fixed cost is present, the projected variable cost in the I-O budget may be lower than direct cost per unit. Second, some elements of indirect cost transferred from the intermediate departments may be considered variable in the I-O budget. For example, if the production of a final product or service requires marginal products or services from intermediate departments that have variable costs, these costs will be defined as variable in the I-O budget.

IMPACT ON PRICING DECISIONS

There is no real consensus concerning how hospital price decisions are made. This failure can be attributed to the absence of an empirically tested economic theory for not-for-profit hospitals. In a recent article, Davis [9] attempted to test five alternative theories: cost recovery, output maximization, output and quality maximization, utility maximization, and cash flow maximization. Although her conclusions were quite tentative, the data provided some general support for the cash flow maximization hypothesis; the first three hypotheses were disproved in many instances. The utility maximization theory could not be tested because actual objective functions could not be specified.

Kaitz, in a case study of six Massachusetts hospitals, also identified a number of variables involved in hospital pricing decisions [10]. The study was more detailed in that pricing decisions were classified by service (routine, ancillary, and ambulatory). Kaitz identified three major factors of importance in hospital pricing: the total financial requirements of the hospital, the costs of individual services, and the prices of comparable services in competing hospitals. Kaitz found that the major objective of hospital administrators was to establish a set of rates that would generate sufficient funds to meet anticipated operating requirements. Prices for routine services were set approximately at computed cost. Ancillary services exhibited a greater degree of variance; it was presumed that this variance was largely because of price competition. No general pattern was noted for pricing ambulatory services.

Discussions with the administrative staff of the study hospital identified the importance of cost in the standard method of establishing hospital rates. In general, the overall hospital profit objective was 2.5 percent of budgeted hospital costs. This appears to be borne out by the hospital's budget, since budgeted profit was 2.8 percent of budgeted costs. Furthermore, the administrative staff stated that 2.5 percent was the profit target for each product line, although modifications were made to adjust for unusual circumstances. Specifically, the hospital administration expected losses in several established departments (for example, nursery, delivery, and outpatient) and initial losses in several of the new departments (isotope, pulmonary function, and health screening). Rates were also modified by existing past rates because the hospital administration was reluctant to raise rates excessively in some areas on the sole basis of abnormal cost increases. Competitive pressure was indicated in several areas, primarily in the laboratory, where strong commercial competition was just beginning to develop. Posted daily room rates were mentioned as being highly visible to patients and physicians. Discussions with the administrative staff pinpointed the fear that Blue Cross was becoming less willing to reimburse hospitals on the basis of posted charges. (Blue Cross of Northern California reimburses hospitals on the basis of negotiated charges. At the time of the study, the study hospital had succeeded in having posted charges accepted as negotiated charges and Blue Cross was still paying all posted charges, but external pressure on Blue Cross to assume a more active role in hospital cost containment was becoming more intense.)

In summary, all three views on how to make hospital pricing decisions stress the importance of cost information. To the extent that this observation is valid, differences in budgeted cost information generated under alternative budget systems may be expected to produce differences in posted hospital prices.

Analysis of the results in Tables 20.2 and 20.3 supports the pricing policies stated informally by the administrative staff of the study hospital. Nursery, delivery, and outpatient departments are budgeted to incur losses, as indicated by charge/full cost ratios of less than one. Also, two of the three new departments, pulmonary function and health screening, are budgeted for initial losses. Except for the nursery, the routine service departments show moderate profit ratios in a fairly narrow band (1.042 to 1.105). The role of cost in price setting appears critical here. The ancillary services exhibit a wider range of profit ratios, from 0.487 to 1.297. When new departments are removed from the ancillary services area, the profit ratios on average (1.086) exceed those in the routine services

TABLE 20.2
Projected Dollar Cost per Unit

Department	Hospital Budget			I-O Budget			1970 Budgeted Charges per Unit
	Full Cost	Direct Cost	Full Cost	Variable Cost	Full Cost (replacement)		
Routine services							
Medical/surgical	69.10	38.56	65.88	37.67	67.10		72.00
Obstetrics	60.16	31.64	62.23	40.59	67.51		66.50
Intensive care	112.03	73.15	109.38	104.30	113.49		118.00
Nursery	41.62	24.76	48.61	23.56	49.65		35.00
Elderly	65.03	38.37	60.59	20.55	61.83		69.00
Ancillary services							
Surgery	104.28	76.22	118.45	78.13	120.93		107.00
Delivery	132.49	91.29	110.63	60.04	112.25		95.00
Radiology	5.55	3.45	6.35	4.18	6.41		5.90
Radiation therapy	16.10	13.26	17.56	14.22	17.80		18.25
Laboratory	2.18	1.49	2.30	1.46	2.32		2.44
EKG	14.21	10.02	15.15	11.22	15.21		17.30
Isotope	67.43	38.62	61.66	41.81	61.96		80.00
Physical therapy	6.10	3.52	5.90	2.70	5.96		6.80
EEG, EMG	30.84	21.37	33.74	25.54	33.90		40.00
Pulmonary function	66.04	28.70	51.81	29.75	52.02		32.14
Other services							
Outpatient	28.01	16.50	26.60	8.27	27.45		13.35
Health screening	44.39	27.50	56.90	43.21	57.06		35.00

TABLE 20.3

Charge/Cost Ratios for Selected Departments

Department	Charges/Budgeted Full Cost	Charges/I-O Full Cost	Charges/I-O Replacement Cost	Charges/Budgeted Direct Cost	Charges/I-O Marginal Cost
All departments	0.984	0.965	0.948	1.551	1.640
Routine services					
All routine services	1.020	1.020	0.984	1.677	1.905
Medical/surgical	1.042	1.093	1.073	1.867	1.911
Obstetrics	1.105	1.069	0.985	2.102	1.638
Intensive care	1.053	1.079	1.040	1.613	1.131
Nursery	0.841	0.720	0.705	1.007	1.486
Elderly	1.061	1.139	1.116	1.798	3.358
Ancillary services					
All ancillary services	1.036	1.019	1.010	1.589	1.594
Ancillary services excluding new departments*					
Surgery	1.086	1.034	1.023	1.588	1.618
Delivery	1.026	0.903	0.885	1.404	1.370
Radiology	0.717	0.859	0.846	1.041	1.582
Radiation therapy	1.062	0.929	0.920	1.710	1.412
Laboratory	1.134	1.039	1.025	1.376	1.283
EKG	1.120	1.061	1.052	1.638	1.671
Isotope	1.217	1.142	1.137	1.727	1.542
Physical therapy	1.186	1.297	1.291	2.071	1.913
EEG, EMG	1.115	1.153	1.141	1.932	2.519
Pulmonary function	1.297	1.186	1.180	1.872	1.566
Other services	0.487	0.620	0.618	1.120	1.080
Outpatient	0.477	0.502	0.486	0.809	1.614
Health screening	0.788	0.615	0.613	1.273	0.810

*Isotope, pulmonary function.

area (1.020). In short, the pricing and profit structure of the study hospital does not appear to be radically different from that of similar short-term general care community hospitals [10-12], which indicates that the results from this hospital may be widely applicable.

Comparisons of projected costs for individual departments under the two budget systems are presented in Tables 20.2 and 20.4. Differences between the two systems appear substantial. The average absolute differences for full cost and marginal cost were 0.103 and 0.214, respectively. The importance of these differences in pricing decisions cannot be tested empirically. For that portion of hospital revenue generated under cost reimbursement, charges would be adjusted automatically provided the same magnitude of cost differences was observed on an ex-post basis. In this vein, it is interesting to note that costs for the elderly department, which is largely a Medicare nursing center, are 6.8 percent greater in the hospital budget than in the I-O forecast.

Examination of Table 20.3 reveals several significant differences between the hospital's budgeted charge/cost figures and those determined by the I-O budget. The obstetrics department, which has a charge/cost ratio of 1.105 on a budgeted full cost basis, shows a loss when replacement cost is used in the I-O full cost projection (0.985). Such a large reduction in projected departmental profit would very likely produce a price increase. The obstetrics department is located in an older wing of the hospital, which accounts for the unrealistically low depreciation charge allocated to this department compared to other departments. Surgery and radiology turn out to be loss areas under the I-O full cost and replacement cost projections. The results of these calculations were quite surprising since these two departments had been viewed as profit areas.

IMPACT ON OUTPUT DECISIONS

In attempts to determine the impact of I-O cost estimates on hospital output decisions, several tentative decision models have been posited. Some researchers have argued that staff physicians rather than hospital administrators control hospital output [13]. The real issue, however, is the extent to which the hospital administrator can influence the physician and can shape the relevant objectives of the hospital.

In the analysis that follows, a short-run profit maximization model is posited. Under this assumption, if the same output decisions are made regardless of the budgetary system used, there would be little reason to expect any major changes when alternative objectives were applied that placed less emphasis on profit and cost factors.

TABLE 20.4

Differences between Hospital Budget and I-O Budget in Cost per Unit

Department	Full Cost[a]	Marginal Cost[b]	Full Cost Replacement[c]
All departments			
Average deviation	0.023	0.022	0.010
Absolute average deviation	0.103	0.214	0.010
Routine services			
Average deviation	0.013	0.034	0.036
Absolute average deviation	0.068	0.248	0.036
Medical/surgical	−0.046	−0.023	0.018
Obstetrics	0.034	0.282	0.084
Intensive care	−0.023	0.425	0.037
Nursery	0.167	−0.048	0.021
Elderly	−0.068	−0.464	0.020
Ancillary services			
Average deviation	0.009	0.015	0.006
Absolute average deviation	0.108	0.133	0.006
Surgery	0.135	0.025	0.020
Delivery	−0.164	−0.342	0.014
Radiology	0.144	0.211	0.009
Radiation therapy	0.090	0.072	0.013
Laboratory	0.055	−0.020	0.008
EKG	0.066	0.119	0.003
Isotope	−0.085	0.082	0.004
Physical therapy	−0.032	−0.232	0.010
EEG, EMG	0.094	0.195	0.004
Pulmonary function	−0.215	0.036	0.004
Other services			
Outpatient	−0.050	−0.498	0.031
Health screening	0.281	0.571	0.002

[a] (I-O full cost − budgeted full cost)/ budgeted full cost.
[b] (I-O marginal cost − budgeted direct cost)/budgeted direct cost.
[c] (I-O replacement full cost − I-O full cost)/I-O full cost.

If the hospital made its output decisions in a linear programming context [14], the choice variables would be the individual department output levels and the coefficients would be marginal profit, that is, price minus marginal cost. Specification of constraints is beyond the scope of this paper. Operating within this restriction, a possible decision rule might be to expand or attempt to expand output in departments with relatively high charge/marginal cost ratios. Recent trends toward expansion of ancillary services provided per patient day are consistent with this decision rule in view of their traditionally higher charge/direct cost ratios [11].

Comparison of the ratio of charges to budgeted direct cost (assumed to be the hospital's method of estimating marginal cost) and the ratio of charges to I-O marginal cost (see Table 20.3) reveals a striking similarity between the results of the two approaches. Using a Spearman's rank correlation coefficient, the two sets of ratios are positively correlated (the correlations are significant at the 0.05 confidence level). Such a positive association indicates that output decisions reached under the two budget systems would probably be very similar.

Examination of the results with respect to individual departments, however, reveals some important individual differences between the two budget systems. The outpatient department, viewed as a loss area using the hospital's regular budget (ratio of charge to budgeted direct cost = 0.809), is regarded as a profit area using the I-O budget (ratio of charges to marginal cost = 1.614). The delivery department, which ranks fifteenth in ratio of charges to budgeted direct cost under the regular system, ranks eighth in ratio of charges to I-O marginal cost. On the other hand, the health screening department is judged to be a loss area when I-O marginal cost data are used (the hospital's budget approach indicates that the department makes a small profit on its services). The more accurate I-O estimate should be useful in making decisions concerning prices and continuance of this new department.

If charges are not viewed as fixed, another guideline for output expansion might be to expand output in departments with relatively low ratios of marginal cost to full cost. This course of action would be especially relevant for hospitals with large percentages of cost reimbursement. Since the effective price to the hospital would be full cost, the difference between full cost and marginal cost would be marginal profit to the hospital.

The rankings of the two sets of ratios in this instance are not nearly as isomorphic as the rankings of the ratios of charges to marginal cost or of charges to direct cost. Using a Spearman's rank correlation coefficient, the null hypothesis of independence is not rejected at the 0.05 level of significance. Departments whose relative rankings shift by six positions or more are: obstetrics, intensive care, delivery, isotope, pulmonary function, and health screening.

IMPACT ON PLANNING DECISIONS

The general budgeting objectives in hospitals are not unlike budgeting objectives in other industries; according to the AHA's <u>Budgeting Procedures for Hospitals</u> [1], hospital budgets should facilitate short-term planning and management control of operations—objectives that could come from any standard accounting or finance text. Budgets based on departmental expenses, such as the two budgets compared in this article, are the most common.

Budgets may be either fixed or flexible. A fixed budget contains expense estimates only for a single level of activity. Flexible budgeting, however, is based on the assumption that certain costs will vary with the level of activity and may be stated either as a series of budgets for alternative levels of activity or as a mathematical formula that allows restatement to any specified level of activity, for example, cost = \$5000 + \$150 × units of output. According to the AHA, flexible budgeting is the most effective tool management has to control costs [1], but flexible budgeting is not yet used extensively because many hospitals are still in a rudimentary stage of budget development.

The study hospital's budget and the I-O model may both be described as flexible. The I-O model recognizes that a certain component of labor cost may be fixed, whereas the hospital's budget assumes all labor costs are totally variable. To a certain extent this is an oversimplification of the hospital's knowledge of cost behavior in that the administrative staff, while recognizing the existence of fixed costs, does not believe the effort involved in estimating the separable fixed and variable coefficients plus the more extensive processing requirements is justified.

In this section the accuracy of the labor budgets of the two budget systems is compared for the last 13 two-week periods of 1970. Only budgets for final product centers are discussed because the two systems specify intermediate outputs in different units. Radiation therapy was not included because data for the last half of 1970 were unavailable. Two measures of accuracy are used: percent error over the entire budget period and number of individual periods during which one system is more accurate (as measured by percent error) than the other.

The two systems are compared in Table 20.5. Both accuracy measures indicate that the I-O labor budget was more accurate than the hospital's budget. For the entire 26-week period, the hospital's budget underestimated labor hours by 11.2 percent whereas the I-O

TABLE 20.5

Comparison of Labor Budget Accuracy

Department	Percent Error Over 26-Week Period		No. of 2-Week Periods in Which I-O Budget Was More Accurate
	Hospital's Budget	I-O Budget	
All departments	-11.2	1.3	9.375
Routine services			
Medical/surgical	-9.7	-1.9	13
Obstetrics	-11.7	-9.7	11
Intensive care	0.0	3.2	4
Nursery	-5.5	1.1	10
Elderly	-4.8	8.5	6
Ancillary services			
Surgery	-0.6	4.5	8
Delivery	-5.6	-3.9	9
Radiology	-40.1	-2.3	13
Laboratory	-12.4	-7.4	12
EKG	1.4	42.2	2
Isotope	-1.7	-9.4	8
Physical therapy	3.0	1.2	12
EEG, EMG	-11.4	-5.9	10
Pulmonary function	-19.1	6.0	11
Other services			
Outpatient	5.8	-3.5	8
Health screening	-67.1	-2.1	13

labor budget overestimated labor hours by 1.3 percent. The I-O labor budget also showed a smaller percent error in 150 of the 208 observations (16 departments, 13 two-week periods). Using a sign test this is significant at a 0.000001 level of confidence. Budget accuracy could have been greatly improved if the I-O statistical methodology had been used instead of the existing negotiated labor budget.

IMPACT ON COST CONTROL DECISIONS

Effective cost control requires a detailed cost accounting system that will report when and where costs were incurred and a budgeted or standard cost for each defined department or cost control center. Differences between actual and budgeted costs may then be analyzed to determine whether the variance should be subjected to further investigation.

Decision rules for determining when to investigate a given variance may be based on the absolute size of the variance, the size of the variance relative to the size of the standard cost, or the probability that the observed variance is caused by random, noncontrollable factors. Since these measures are related, there is no logical reason for selecting one over the others. The probability that the variance is due to random, noncontrollable factors (q) is some decreasing function of the size of the variance.

The current policy of the study hospital is to investigate variances when they seem to be too large. No differentiation is made between favorable and unfavorable variances. The hospital administration views consistent favorable variances as indications of either outdated budgets or changes in operating technology (which may or may not be desirable). The I-O budget, on the other hand, supplies an objective measure of q for each variance. It is not possible to determine from the data here which approach is more valid. However, an analysis of the rank orderings of the absolute sizes of the variances is possible for the two systems. A significant positive association between the two budget systems might imply that "investigate" decisions generated by the two sets of variances would differ only slightly. This assumes that the absolute size of the variance is the only variable determining the decision to investigate. Obviously other factors may be of importance, for example, past record of favorable and unfavorable variances, output level, and operating conditions.

A measure of the association between the two sets of variances for 16 departments in the study hospital is presented in Table 20.6. Using Spearman's rank correlation coefficient, eight of the departments have positive measures of association significant at the 0.05 level; five of these eight are significant at the 0.01 level. On this

TABLE 20.6

Association of Labor Budget Variances

Department	Spearman Rank Correlation Coefficient
Routine services	
Medical/surgical	0.467
Obstetrics	0.901[a]
Intensive care	0.780[a]
Nursery	−0.148
Elderly	−0.269
Ancillary services	
Surgery	0.577[b]
Delivery	0.714[a]
Radiology	0.231
Laboratory	0.912[a]
EKG	0.082
Isotope	0.242
Physical therapy	0.626[b]
EEG, EMG	0.742[a]
Pulmonary function	−0.060
Other services	
Outpatient	−0.210
Health screening	0.511[b]

[a]Significant at 0.01 confidence level.
[b]Significant at 0.05 confidence level.

basis, it appears likely that different "investigate" decisions would have been made under the two systems for at least half of the 16 departments. The actual efficacy of the two cost-control systems cannot be measured since the randomness of the variances cannot be assessed from the available data, nor can management decision rules be specified for either of the two information sets.

SUMMARY AND CONCLUSIONS

From a retrospective point of view it is difficult to determine the impact of two alternative information systems on management decision making, especially when the decisions do not lend themselves to the specification of well-defined rules. Such is the case encountered in this study, in which an attempt was made to determine the impact of two alternative budget systems on four broad areas of management decision problems: pricing, output, planning, and cost control.

It appears that the I-O budget would have produced substantial changes in posted hospital rates for individual revenue centers. This conclusion is based on fairly significant differences in projected full cost for individual hospital final product centers between the two budget systems (average absolute error was 10 percent). If full cost is a critical variable in hospital rate setting, which many have hypothesized (including the sample hospital's administrative staff), important differences in prices might have occurred.

The potential impact of the two approaches on hospital output determination is much harder to assess. This is due in part to the absence of an empirically validated theory of hospital objectives, but also to the inconclusiveness of hospital administrator control in this decision area. Aside from these two factors the two budgets did not generate significantly different information signals for the hypothesized decision model. There is then less reason to believe that decisions generated under each of the two budget systems would differ significantly.

Using labor budget accuracy as the principal criterion in determining the relative usefulness of the two systems for planning purposes, it was observed that the I-O model was consistently superior to the existing hospital budget.

Cost control decisions were hypothesized to be a function of the absolute size of the budget variance. From a rank order comparison of the absolute size of the variances reported under the two systems for 13 reporting periods in each of the sample departments, it was concluded that the I-O model might significantly change management cost control decisions, for example, the decision to investigate a given budget variance.

REFERENCES

1. American Hospital Association, Budgeting Procedures for Hospitals. Chicago: American Hospital Association, 1971.

2. N. Churchill, "Linear Algebra and Cost Allocation: Some Examples," Accounting Rev. 39 (October 1964):894.

3. G. Feltham, "Some Quantitative Approaches to Planning for Multi-product Production Systems," Accounting Rev. 45 (January 1970):11.

4. S. Livingstone, "Input-Output Analysis for Cost Accounting, Planning and Control," Accounting Rev. 44 (January 1969):48.

5. R. Minch and E. Petri, "Matrix Models of Reciprocal Service Cost Allocation," Accounting Rev. 47 (July 1972):576.

6. A. McCosh, "Computerized Cost Finding Systems," Hosp. Financial Mgmt. 23 (November 1969):18.

7. American Hospital Association, Statement on the Financial Requirements of Heath Care Institutions and Services. Chicago: American Hospital Association, 1969.

8. W. J. Bruns and D. T. DeCoster, Accounting and Its Behavioral Implications. New York: McGraw-Hill, 1969.

9. K. Davis, "Economic Theories of Behavior in Nonprofit, Private Hospitals," Econ. & Bus. Bull. 24 (Winter 1972):2.

10. E. Kaitz, Pricing Policy and Cost Behavior in the Hospital Industry. Lexington, Mass.: D. C. Heath, 1968.

11. K. Davis and R. Foster, Community Hospitals: Inflation in the Pre-Medicare Period. Research Report No. 41, Social Security Administration. DHEW Pub. No. (SSA) 72-11803. Washington, D.C.: U.S. Government Printing Office, 1972. P. 46.

12. K. Davis, "Hospital Costs and the Medicare Program," Soc. Security Bull. 36 (August 1973):18.

13. M. Pauly and M. Redisch, "The Not-for-profit Hospital as a Physicians' Cooperative," Am. Econ. Rev. 63 (March 1973):87.

14. H. H. Baligh and D. J. Laughhunn, "An Economic and Linear Model of the Hospital," Health Serv. Res. 4 (Winter 1969):293.

21

TIME SERIES ANALYSIS

INTRODUCTION

This paper describes five computerized time-series models that forecast patient tray demand in a hospital food service. In a large hospital, forecasting the demand for special diet meals is often a very complicated problem. The authors examine five forecasting models, programmed in Fortran IV, and compare the results with the traditional intuitive forecasts made by the food service supervisor of the hospital. The adaptive exponential smoothing model appears to be the best model for forecasting patient tray demand.

Introduction to Technique

A time series is a set of ordered observations of a quantitative variable taken at successive points in time. Time-series analysis is a technique used for developing a model for forecasting demands. The model consists of a description and measurements of the various changes or fluctuations as they appear in the series during a period of time. The analysis normally begins by decomposing the time series into components that account for the fluctuations—trend (T), seasonal (S), cyclical (C), and erratic (E) components. The time series is then constructed by any one of the following models:

1. Additive model: the four components are added together to give the series,

$$Y = T + S + C + E$$

2. Multiplicative model: the actual value of the time series is obtained by multiplying the four components,

$$Y = T \times S \times C \times E$$

where S, C, and E are usually expressed as percentages.

3. Hybrid model: the value of the series is obtained by a combination of multiplication and addition of the components, such as in

$$Y = T \times S \times C + E$$

Moving average, linear trend, semi-average method, least square method, and nonlinear trend are some of the methods used for measuring the trend component. The exponential smoothing model used in the paper is a special type of weighted moving average method for measuring the trend component.

REFERENCES

Arkin, Herbert, and Raymond Colton, Statistical Methods. New York: Barnes and Noble, 1970.

Clark, Frederick, and Lawrence Schkade, Statistical Methods for Business Decisions. Cincinnati, Ohio: Southwestern, 1969.

Griffith, John R., Quantitative Techniques for Hospital Planning and Control. Lexington, Mass.: D. C. Heath, 1972.

McClain, John O., "Exponential Smoothing: Appropriate and Inappropriate Application," Health Services Research 6 (Fall 1971): 256-59.

Pegels, C. C., "Exponential Forecasting: Some New Variations," Management Science 15 (January 1969):311-15.

Phillip, Joseph P., "On Exponential Smoothing: An Extension," Health Services Research 5 (Winter 1970):370-77.

Sposato, Donald, and A. H. Spinner, "Forecasting by a Modified Exponential Smoothing Method," Health Services Research 5 (Summer 1970):414-47.

Swartzman, Gordon, "The Patients Arrival Process in Hospitals: Statistical Analysis," Health Services Research 5 (Winter 1970): 320-29.

FORECASTING PATIENT TRAY CENSUS
FOR HOSPITAL FOOD SERVICE

Ronald J. Harris
and
Everett E. Adam, Jr.

Five computerized forecasting models were tested with data on daily patient tray demand in a large medical center food service, and results were compared with intuitive forecasts made by the food service supervisor. All five models gave more accurate results than the intuitive procedure; an adaptive exponential-smoothing model was most accurate. The effects of model complexity and data storage requirements are discussed, and simple exponential smoothing is suggested for forecasting patient tray demand in this setting.

Forecasting demand for individual items is a problem approached by managers either intuitively or statistically, or with some combination of both modes. In a medical environment the most common approach to the forecasting problem on the department level seems to be intuitive, and often this intuitive forecast of demand for supplies or services becomes the basic input for computerized statistical planning and control procedures in the medical complex. Statistical forecasting can provide more accurate estimates of demand, improving input for larger-scale planning and control.

The primary goal of the dietetic department in a hospital is to provide meals that meet the individual physiological needs of the various patients and personnel. Achieving this goal requires nutritional and managerial expertise to establish standards and procedures for planning and producing meals and to coordinate food, labor, facilities, equipment, and money within the limitations of the hospital's budget. The immediate need for forecasting is associated with production demand, but the problem is multi-echelon in that one must

Reprinted with permission from Health Services Research 10, No. 4 (Winter 1975). Copyright 1975 by the Hospital Research and Educational Trust, 840 North Lakeshore Drive, Chicago, Ill. 60611.

first forecast patients (or patient trays), then forecast the distribution of special diets ordered by physicians, and finally forecast individual servings of various foods. In a large hospital on any one day there may be four or five hundred patients, a dozen diets (liquid, sodium restricted, etc.), and hundreds of different food items. This is an enormous problem for "intuitive" forecasting, and certainly a situation in which operations research techniques should be able to free substantial managerial labor and improve decision making. The purpose of this article is to examine the problem, to evaluate existing models, and to recommend an item-forecasting model for daily patient tray demand.

A number of studies have focused on evaluation of item-forecasting models [1-6], but most of these have used hypothetical data, and the range of experimental designs makes it difficult to judge the suitability of models for application to other settings than that of the particular study. Other factors in addition to forecast accuracy need to be considered: model complexity, amount of historical data that must be maintained, and lead time (that is, how far in advance the forecasts are made). Box-Jenkins models [7], for example, give usefully accurate results but tend to be too complex for easy use by untrained personnel. (Groff [8] compared Box-Jenkins models with exponential-smoothing models and found that the latter performed as well or better with the time series he examined; the authors are aware of a similar unpublished comparison study in a food service environment.)

Konnersman [9] discussed the time requirement for food preparation as one of the determinants of the need for forecasting in hospital dietetic departments, but the ten-week weighted moving-average model he suggested would seem to require considerable data storage, and he reported no application of that model to actual demand data. Uhrich and Noort [10] identified three time horizons over which forecasts may be needed: short-term forecasting for food purchasing, labor utilization, and production; medium-term forecasting for annual budgeting and planning functions; and long-term forecasting for guiding future growth of the facility. Uhrich and Noort collected demand data and analyzed them to assist a manual (intuitive) short-term forecasting procedure, but they did not compare that procedure with other techniques such as exponential smoothing or moving average.

An unpublished study by Dougherty [11] reported a model she developed for the department of nutrition and dietetics at the University of Missouri Medical Center at Columbia, the site of the present study. Dougherty's model derives forecasts from regression of a modified moving average over historical census data. She applied the model to daily tray demand data covering 91 weeks and found that the forecasts were within ±5 percent of the actual values 64 percent of the time and within ±10 percent 90 percent of the time. Dougherty's model has never been implemented in this institution, perhaps partly because of the complexity and the data requirements of her model and partly because she did not compare her model's results with the intuitive forecasts that were used by the food service supervisor. A part of the present study makes use of Dougherty's 91-week time series; her model is described among the others tested in the present study.

MODELS TESTED

Among the criteria considered most important in selecting models to be evaluated were high ranking in previous evaluations of forecasting accuracy, simplicity of computation, and amount of historical data required. The models chosen for testing were simple (first-order) exponential smoothing, double exponential smoothing, adaptive exponential smoothing, simple moving average, and Dougherty's method [11], moving-average regression. These models were compared with the manual forecasting procedure that was in use at the dietetic department where the data originated.

The first two models, first-order and double exponential smoothing, have been discussed by Brown [12]. The first-order model is expressed by the following equation:

$$S'_{t+1} = \alpha S_t + (1 - \alpha)S'_t \tag{1}$$

where S'_{t+1} = forecast demand for period $t + 1$

S_t = observed demand for period t (the current period)

S'_t = forecast demand for period t (forecast period $t - 1$)

α = a constant smoothing coefficient ($0 \leq \alpha \leq 1$)

The doubly-smoothed model applied the smoothing constant to the forecast derived from Eq. 1 to produce a modified forecast, S'', for that period:

$$S''_{t+1} = \alpha S'_{t+1} + (1 - \alpha)S''_t \tag{2}$$

where S'_{t+1} = the forecast for period $t + 1$ from Eq. 1

S''_t = the doubly-smoothed forecast for period t

Adaptive exponential smoothing has been described by Trigg and Leach [13]. It is adaptive in that the smoothing coefficient ("tracking signal") is not a constant, but instead varies as a function of the estimated absolute error. Given a previous forecast for period t, the forecast error (E) for period t is the difference between the observed demand for the period (S_t) and the forecast demand (S'_t). From E_t, the next period's forecast error is estimated by exponential smoothing:

$$E'_{t+1} = (1 - \gamma)E_t + \gamma E'_t \tag{3}$$

where γ = a smoothing constant ($0 \geq \gamma \geq 1$)
E'_t = the error forecast (in period t - 1) for period t

The absolute error, $|E_{t+1}|'$, is obtained by substituting the absolute value of E_t in Eq. 3. The estimated absolute error is not necessarily equal to the absolute value of the estimated error; that is, in the notation used here, $|E_{t+1}|' \neq |E'_{t+1}|$. The smoothing coefficient, β, to be used in the demand forecast for period t + 1 is simply the absolute value of the ratio of the two values forecast by the two applications of Eq. 3:

$$\beta = \left| \frac{E'_{t+1}}{|E_{t+1}|'} \right| \tag{4}$$

The procedure, then, is to calculate E_t for each period, update the two exponentially smoothed estimates for forecast error, and then compute β by Eq. 4; β may then be used in an equation similar to Eq. 1 to provide a demand forecast that reflects changes in the demand pattern. In the present work the procedure described by Trigg and Leach was modified in that the value of β used in forecasting for period t + 1 was not adjusted from the previous value unless the calculated value of β changed by at least 0.05 between periods t - 1 and t.

The fourth model, the simple moving average, requires determining the average demand for N periods prior to the forecast period. The forecast for period t + 1 is calculated as follows:

$$S'_{t+1} = 1/N \sum_{t-(N-1)}^{t} S_i \quad [i = t - (N - 1), t - (N - 2), \ldots, t] \tag{5}$$

where S'_{t+1} = forecast for period t + 1
S_i = observed demand for period i
N = number of periods over which the moving average is found

The moving-average regression model developed by Dougherty [11] involves a simple linear regression of the form

$$Y = mX + b \qquad (6)$$

where Y = the predicted patient tray census for a given day
       m = the slope coefficient
       b = the Y intercept

The independent variable, X, is a function of two moving averages and one observed census:

$$X = A(B/C) \qquad (7)$$

where A = nine-week moving average of demand for the given day (that is, given Friday as the forecast day, A is the average demand for nine previous Fridays)
       B = observed demand for the fourth weekday prior to the forecast day (that is, the previous Monday's demand, if Friday is being forecast)
       C = nine-week moving average of demand for the fourth weekday prior to the forecast day (for example, for nine previous Mondays)

If a weekend day is to be forecast by Eq. 6, the values used for B and C are averages over the nine previous Saturdays or Sundays instead of nine occurrences of the fourth prior day.

EXPERIMENTAL DESIGN AND DATA

The objective was to select the model that gave the least overall forecast error. Numerous measures are available for the error; the measures chosen were the mean absolute deviation (M), the bias (B), and the U coefficient developed by Thiel [14]. These error measures are specified as follows:

$$M = 1/N \sum_{1}^{N} |S_t - S'_t| \qquad (t = 1, \ldots, N)$$

$$B = 1/N \sum_{1}^{N} (S_t - S'_t) \qquad (t = 1, \ldots, N)$$

$$U = \left(\frac{\sum_{1}^{N} (S_t - S'_t)}{\sum_{1}^{N} (S_t - S_{t-1})^2} \right)^{\frac{1}{2}} \qquad (t = 1, \ldots, N)$$

where S indicates an observed value, S' a forecast, and N the number of periods observed. (The unit of demand throughout this study was one patient tray daily, regardless of the number of meals the patient had.)

The evaluation was conducted in three phases. In phase I the model parameters were set, using results of a systematic search over Dougherty's 91 weeks of historical data to select seven smoothing coefficients—one coefficient for each day of the week—for the exponential models. The 91 weeks of historical data were also used to determine the most efficient value for the parameter N (the number of weeks over which the average is taken) for the simple moving-average model. This was done by varying N over 1, 3, 5, and 7 weeks and selecting the value that yielded the lowest U coefficient.

Phase II involved comparing error measures of forecasts by all five computerized models on the basis of 31 days' demand data collected by Dougherty at the University of Missouri Medical Center. In phase III forecasts from four of the models (excluding Dougherty's) were compared with the department supervisor's intuitive estimates, using new data collected by the authors over 61 days at the medical center. The demand data for phases II and III are shown in Tables 21.1 and 21.2 respectively.

Procedure

The models were programmed in FORTRAN IV and run on an IBM 360-65 computer. Programs were verified by hand calculations on the intermediate and final output of test runs of each model, and the outputs were checked for reasonableness by the programmers and by dietary department personnel.

The exponential models were structured to forecast Monday to Monday, Tuesday to Tuesday, etc.; that is, there were seven separate averages and subsequent forecasts, each with a seven-day lead time. The manual technique and the moving-average regression used a four-day lead time (reflected in variables B and C in Eq. 7). After phase I was completed (setting parameters, validating the models, and verifying the program), the simulation was conducted over the

TABLE 21.1

Daily Patient Tray Census, March 1971

Week	Mon	Tues	Wed	Thur	Fri	Sat	Sun
1	375	391	402	396	369	304	315
2	380	384	387	362	369	286	301
3	376	388	368	366	341	285	294
4	341	370	378	384	349	295	295
5	355	360	356	—	—	—	—

TABLE 21.2

Daily Patient Tray Census, June 12, 1972 to August 13, 1972

Week	Mon	Tues	Wed	Thur	Fri	Sat	Sun
1	273	282	287	273	305	190	163
2	291	283	289	266	283	204	219
3	301	230	272	264	277	162	153
4	193	170	310	264	294	206	195
5	266	294	300	272	283	189	203
6	254	232	277	267	290	231	228
7	279	290	292	274	292	211	201
8	254	308	275	297	278	189	215
9	258	246	286	316	264	208	189

new data covering a 31-day period for phase II (Table 21.1) and a 61-day period for phase III (Table 21.2).

RESULTS

Phase I. The grid search for exponential-smoothing coefficients yielded coefficients with values of either 0.1 or 0.3, depending on the day of the week, as shown in Table 21.3. For the moving-average forecast, N, the optimal number of weeks over which each weekday's demand should be averaged, was either one week or three weeks (Table 21.3). A smoothing coefficient as low as 0.1-0.3 should correspond to a high N for the moving-average forecast, but this did not occur here: the U coefficient of the moving average was rather insensitive over the values N = 1, 3, 5, and 7. Had mean absolute deviation or bias been used as the critical error measure, there would have been more correlation between the smoothing coefficient and N.

Phase II. Table 21.4 shows the error measures for all five computer models, calculated on forecasts over a test period of 31 days (Table 21.1 data). There seems to be very little difference in model performance, depending on the error measure used; one-period simple moving average seems to have a slight advantage, being best on two of the three error measures. Figure 21.1 shows the actual daily demand in March 1971, together with forecasts made with the adaptive exponential-smoothing model and Dougherty's moving-average regression model.

Phase III. Table 21.5 shows error measures for the three exponential-smoothing models, the simple moving-average model, and the manual procedure. Because the moving-average regression model requires substantially more data storage, it is not included in the comparison with the manual procedure: the data storage requirement made this model impractical for use in the dietetic department. All four computer models outperformed the manual procedure, with the adaptive exponential-smoothing model showing the lowest mean absolute deviation and bias and a reasonably low U coefficient. Forecasts from the adaptive exponential-smoothing model and the manual procedure are plotted in Fig. 21.2 with the observed patient tray demand over 61 days.

DISCUSSION

Personnel in the food service department had hoped for a forecasting procedure that was always within ±5 percent of actual demand.

TABLE 21.3

Error Measure Values Resulting from Selected Model Parameters

Parameters and Measures	Time Series						
	Mon	Tues	Wed	Thur	Fri	Sat	Sun
	Exponential Smoothing						
Smoothing coefficient	0.3	0.1	0.1	0.3	0.3	0.3	0.1
Mean absolute deviation	17.69	18.40	18.71	22.3	22.11	20.66	17.70
Bias	0.98	1.85	2.07	−0.58	−0.96	−1.34	−0.88
U coefficient	0.87	0.90	0.90	0.87	0.85	0.87	0.85
	Moving Average						
Number of weeks, N	3	1	1	1	3	1	3
Mean absolute deviation	19.6	18.3	20.7	21.6	19.2	18.2	18.2
Bias	−0.2	−0.5	−0.3	−0.2	−0.6	−0.1	−0.5
U coefficient	0.988	1.000	1.000	1.000	0.992	1.000	0.965

TABLE 21.4

Error Measure Values over 31 Daily Forecasts by Five Computer Models

Model	Error measure		
	Mean absolute deviation	Bias	U coefficient
Exponential smoothing	38.0	−2.1	0.92
Double exponential smoothing	38.7	−2.6	0.92
Adaptive exponential smoothing	39.9	−1.4	0.98
Simple moving average			
($N=1$ week)	26.2	0.6	1.00
($N=3$ weeks)	41.3	2.6	1.27
Moving-average regression	10.0	−2.0	1.04

TABLE 21.5

Error Measure Values over 61 Daily Forecasts by Four Computer Models and the Manual Estimate

Model	Error measure		
	Mean absolute deviation	Bias	U coefficient
Exponential smoothing	32.2	−3.1	1.07
Double exponential smoothing	30.7	−5.9	1.08
Adaptive exponential smoothing	28.3	0.3	1.06
Simple moving average			
($N=1$ week)	39.3	1.4	1.00
($N=3$ weeks)	43.9	2.5	1.04
Manual estimate	104.0	104.0	3.33

FIGURE 21.1

Observed Daily Patient Tray Count (▲), Adaptive Exponential-Smoothing Forecast (●), and Moving-Average Regression Forecast (■): 31 Days

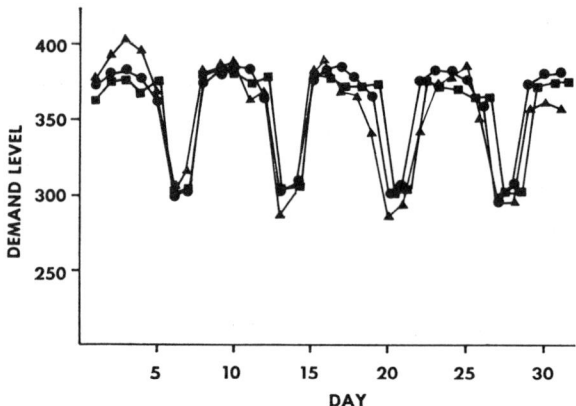

FIGURE 21.2

Observed Daily Patient Tray Count (▲), Adaptive Exponential-Smoothing Forecast (●), and "Manual" Intuitive Forecast (■): 61 Days

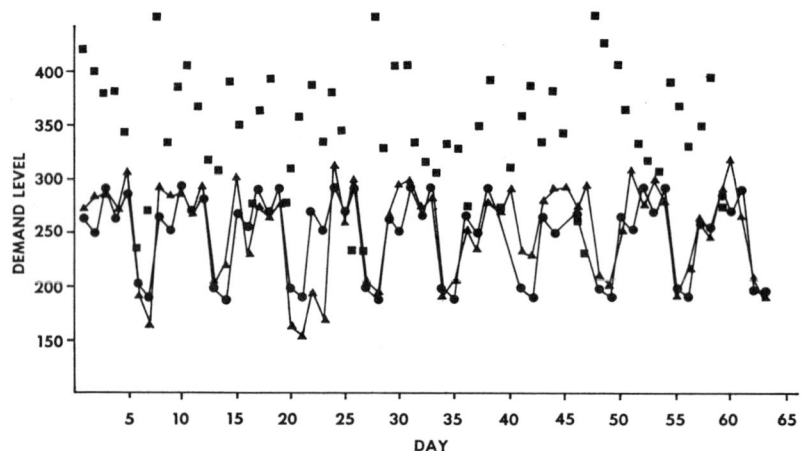

In 61 days, however, the exponential-smoothing model was over this limit 13 times and under 18, the double-smoothing model was over 15 times and under 20, the adaptive exponential-smoothing model was over 16 times and under 16, the one-week simple moving average was over 24 times and under 27, and the three-week simple moving average was over the 5-percent limit 24 times and under 28 times.

Although this performance was disappointing to the food service personnel, it contrasted sharply with that of the manual procedure, which exceeded the limit each day. Bias was a major factor, since the manual procedure is deliberately conservative, seeking to minimize the risk of patient tray stockouts.

The model that appears best for forecasting patient tray demand in this hospital setting is adaptive exponential smoothing, but the simplicity of first-order exponential smoothing and simple moving average (and their success relative to that of the manual forecast) recommend these, too, for consideration. The moving average is easy to understand, and was readily accepted by dietary department personnel, but it can require substantially more data in storage as N increases. It appeared that the initial reaction of department personnel to first-order smoothing was negative because of "model complexity." However, initial uncertainties were overcome by going over examples on a calculator until department personnel understood the model. Model complexity increases with double smoothing, adaptive smoothing with a tracking signal, moving-average regression, and the Box-Jenkins models. There is a real question as to whether increased model complexity will retard usage of item-forecasting models in dietary applications. Considering accuracy, model complexity, and data storage requirements, simple exponential smoothing was suggested for this application.

A further step in this research is to look at the multi-echelon forecasting problem of patient tray demand, menu-item demand, and serving demand. Costs should be incorporated into the evaluation, in addition to mean absolute deviation, bias, and other such measures. The cost of forecast error (above a small bias introduced as a safety margin) in a hospital should take the form of some penalty function. Another consideration is that some facilities have dining rooms where overproduction is "dumped" at a less than total loss: there are operations research techniques that can incorporate such savings into analysis. We would not suggest that the costs of underproduction are such that a hospital can operate without some bias, but we question the necessity for the magnitude of bias shown in Fig. 21.2.

REFERENCES

1. E. E. Adam, Jr., "Individual Item Forecasting Model Evaluation," Decis. Sci. 4 (October 1973):458.

2. E. E. Adam, Jr., J. M. Berthot, and H. E. Riley, Jr., "Individual Item Forecasting Models: A Comparative Evaluation Based on Demand for Supplies in a Medical Complex," in Proceedings of the 14th International American Production and Inventory Control Conference. Washington, D.C.: American Production and Inventory Control Society, 1971. Pp. 82-90.

3. E. E. Adam, Jr., W. L. Berry, and D. C. Whybark, "Forecasting Demand for Medical Supply Items Using Exponential and Adaptive Smoothing Models," in Annual Proceedings of the American Institute for Decision Sciences. Atlanta, Ga.: The Institute, 1972. Pp. 469-76.

4. R. M. Kirby, "A Comparison of Short and Medium Range Statistical Forecasting Methods," Manage. Sci. 13 (December 1966): B202.

5. J. E. Raine, "Self-Adaptive Forecasting Reconsidered," Decis. Sci. 2 (April 1970):181.

6. G. P. Torfin and T. R. Hoffmann, "Simulation Tests of Some Forecasting Techniques," Prod. Inventory Manage. 9 (1968):71.

7. G. E. P. Box and G. M. Jenkins, Time Series Analysis: Forecasting Control. San Francisco: Holden-Day, 1970.

8. G. K. Groff, "Empirical Comparison of Models for Short Range Forecasting," Manage. Sci. 20 (September 1973):22.

9. P. M. Konnersman, "Forecasting Production Demand in the Dietary Department," Hospitals 43 (September 1969):102.

10. R. V. Uhrich and J. J. Noort, "Production Demand Forecasting," Hospitals 45 (February 1, 1971):106.

11. D. A. Dougherty, "Development of a Computer-Assisted Forecasting Model for Patient Census." Unpublished technical paper, Department of Nutrition and Dietetics, Medical Center, University of Missouri-Columbia, 1971.

12. R. G. Brown, Smoothing, Forecasting, and Prediction of Discrete Time Series. Englewood Cliffs, N.J.: Prentice-Hall, 1963.

13. D. W. Trigg and A. G. Leach, "Exponential Smoothing with an Adaptive Response Rate," Oper. Res. Q. 18 (January 1967): 53.

14. H. Theil, Economic Forecasts and Policy. Amsterdam: North Holland, 1965.

APPENDIX
Health Care Journals

Journal	Published By	Main Target Audiences	Contents
Aging	Government Printing Office	Policymakers, and general public	Description of government programs and policy in long-term care.
Allied Health Trend	American Society of Allied Health	Allied health professionals	Policy-oriented, and takes the form of a newsletter.
American Journal of Law & Medicine	American Society of Law & Medicine	Health care professionals and insurance companies	Descriptive materials dealing with problems concerning the legislature and other legal aspects of medicine.
American Journal of Public Health	American Public Health Association	Graduates of public health programs	Descriptive materials dealing with environmental and occupations health preventive and public health programs.
American Medical News	AMA	Physicians	Newsletter-like policy-oriented materials.
Aviation, Space and Environmental Medicine	Aerospace Medical Association	Environmentalists and aviation-related personnel	Deals with studies pertaining to health issues involving the environment and aviation.
Canadian Journal of Public Health	Canadian Public Health Association	Health professionals in administrative level in Canada	Similar to the American Journal of Public Health with the focus on Canadian issues.

Journal	Published By	Main Target Audiences	Contents
Community Health	Royal Institute of Public Health and Hygiene	Canadian general public and health policy-makers	Qualitative report on a wide range of topics in community health.
Journal of Academy of Arts and Sciences (DAEDALUS)	American Academy of Arts	General public	Deals with health care problems in a nontechnical way.
Family Health	Family Media Corporation	General public and M.D.s	Descriptive and very nontechnical treatment to problems of family health maintenance.
Health/PAC Bulletin	Health Policy Advisory Center	Health policy-makers and hospital administrators	Provides views on health political problems.
Health Services Research	Hospital Research and Educational Trust	Hospital administrators, system analyst, and health care management researchers	Highly technical treatment of health care systems management and planning. Utilizes different statistical and operation research techniques to solve health care problems.
Hospitals	American Hospital Association (AHA)	Hospital administrators	Serves as reference for basic hospital information and major source of statistics on hospital systems and performance.
Hospital and Health Services Administration	American College of Hospital Administration	Hospital administrators	More technical than "Hospitals." It deals with organization of hospital systems, and policy-related questions

Journal	Published By	Main Target Audiences	Contents
Hospital Financial Management	Hospital Financial Management Association	Hospital administrators	Deals with issues in financial management such as planning, cost analysis, etc.
Hospital Progress	Catholic Hospital Association	Catholic hospital administrators	Very nontechnical description on policy-related matters.
Inquiry	Blue Cross	Health-related administrators and researchers	Deals with both policy-related as well as quantitative economic issues of health delivery.
International Journal of Health Services	Baywood Publishing Company, Inc.	Students, policymakers and researchers	Deals with local and international issues of health care. Many studies were done in foreign countries. Contains articles that are both technical and descriptive.
Journal of American Society for Information Systems	American Society for Information Science	Computer programmers, students, and hospital administrators	Attention is directed on computer application in health care areas.
Journal of American Medical Association (JAMA)	AMA	Physicians, health systems analysts	A directory which contains the geographical distribution of physicians in this country.
Medical Care	American Health Association: Division of Medical Care	Health system analysts	Technical treatment of the economics of medical care delivery.

Journal	Published By	Main Target Audiences	Contents
Milbank Memorial Fund Quarterly	Milbank Memorial Fund	Health system analysts and administrators	Contains both policy-related and quantitative studies on health care systems management.
Modern Hospital	McGraw-Hill Inc.	Hospital administrators	Innovations in hospital management.
Nursing Home	Cogswell House Inc.	Nursing home administrators	Descriptive studies of long-term care.
Nursing Research	American Journal of Nursing Company	Nurses, administrators	Contains research done in area of management that could improve the methods of nursing practice.
Journal of Nursing Administration	Journal of Nursing Administration Inc.	Nurses, and hospital administrators	Deals with nursing research and management problems.

BIBLIOGRAPHY OF ARTICLES

Ball, M., and G. Hammon. "Overview of Computer Applications in a Variety of Health Care Areas." CRC Critical Reviews in Bioengineering 2 (January 1975):183-208.

Cleverley, W. O. "Input-Output Analysis and the Hospital Budgeting Process." Health Services Research 10 (Spring 1975):36-50.

Dowling, W. L. "The Application of Linear Programming to Decision Making in Hospitals." Hospital Administration 16 (Summer 1971): 66-75.

Frankfurter, G. M., K. E. Kendall, and C. C. Pegels. "Management Control of Blood Through a Short-Term Supply-Demand Forecast System." Management Science 21 (December 1974): 444-52.

Garland, H. R. "Hospital Utilization by Characteristic of Industry in Southwestern Ohio." Inquiry 6 (March 1969):60-71.

Grimes, R. M., C. L. Allen, T. R. Sparling, and G. Weiss. "Use of Decision Theory in Regional Planning." Health Services Research 9 (Spring 1974):73-78.

Gupta, I., J. Zoreda, and N. Kramer. "Hospital Manpower Planning by Use of Queueing Theory." Health Services Research 6 (Spring 1971):76-82.

Gustafson, D. H., and D. C. Holloway. "A Decision Theory Approach to Measuring Severity in Illness." Health Services Research 10 (Spring 1975):97-106.

Harris, R. J., and E. E. Adam, Jr. "Forecasting Patient Tray Census for Hospital Food Service." Health Services Research 10 (Winter 1975):384-93.

Hopkins, C. E., R. W. Hetherington, and E. M. Parsons. "Quality of Medical Care: A Factor Analysis Approach Using Medical Records." Health Services Research 10 (Summer 1975):199-208.

Lave, J. R., and L. B. Lave. "The Extent of Role Differentiation Among Hospitals." Health Services Research 6 (Spring 1971): 15-38.

Lyons, J. P., and J. P. Young. "A Staff Allocation Model for Mental Health Facilities." Health Services Research 11 (Spring 1976): 53-68.

Mahajan, V., and M. Schoeman. "A Discriminant Analysis of Users and Nonusers of Computers in the Hospital Industry." Working Paper, School of Management, State University of New York at Buffalo, Buffalo, N. Y.

Meade, J. "A Mathematical Model for Deriving Hospital Service Areas." International Journal of Health Services Research 4 (Spring 1974):353-64.

Morrill, R. L., and R. Earickson. "Locational Efficiency of Chicago Hospitals: An Experimental Model." Health Services Research 4 (Summer 1969):128-41.

Pegels, C. C., and A. E. Jelmert. "A Comparison of Two Blood Bank Crossmatch Policies." AIIE Transactions 3 (March 1971): 69-75.

Phillip, P. J., and S. Gibson. "Simple, Multiple and Canonical Correlations." Inquiry 7 (June 1970):55-59.

Phillip, P. J., and R. N. Iyer. "Classification of Community Hospitals." Health Services Research 10 (Winter 1975):349-68.

Schweitzer, S. O. "Cost Effectiveness of Early Detection of Disease." Health Services Research 9 (Spring 1974):22-32.

Starkweather, D. B., L. Gelwicks, and R. Newcomer. "Delphi Forecasting of Health Care Organization." Inquiry 12 (March 1975): 37-46.

Steiner, K. C., and H. Smith. "Application of Cost Benefit Analysis to a PKU Screening Program." Inquiry 10 (December 1973):34-40.

Wan, T. T. H., and A. S. Yates. "Prediction of Dental Service Utilization: A Multivariate Approach." Inquiry 12 (June 1975): 143-56.

Wind, Y., and L. K. Spitz. "Analytical Approach to Marketing Decisions in Health Care Organizations." Operations Research 24 (September-October 1976):973-90.

ABOUT THE AUTHORS

VIJAY MAHAJAN is Assistant Professor of Marketing in the College of Administrative Sciences at Ohio State University. His teaching and research interests include health care systems analysis, health care marketing, and the management of innovations.

Professor Mahajan received his M.S. and Ph.D. degrees from the University of Texas at Austin in 1972 and 1975, respectively. He is the author of over 30 articles on marketing models and innovation diffusion in such professional journals as <u>Journal of Marketing Research</u>, <u>Decision Sciences</u>, <u>IEEE Transactions on Engineering Management</u>, <u>Socio-economic Planning Sciences</u>, <u>Technological Forecasting and Social Change</u>, <u>Interfaces</u>, <u>Journal of Consumer Research</u>, and <u>Management Science</u>.

C. CARL PEGELS, Associate Professor of Management Systems in the School of Management at the State University of New York at Buffalo, is an expert on health care systems analysis, health care financing, health maintenance organizations, and the management of regional blood banking.

Between 1968 and 1974 he did extensive federally funded contract and grant research in the management of regional blood banking. Since 1974 he has been involved in feasibility and planning of the marketing and financial aspects of health maintenance organizations.

Professor Pegels received his M.S. and Ph.D. degrees from Purdue University in 1963 and 1966, respectively. He is the author of two textbooks and over 40 articles on systems analysis and related topics in such professional journals as <u>Medical Care</u>, <u>Socio-economic Planning Sciences</u>, <u>Decision Sciences</u>, <u>Management Science</u>, <u>Transfusion</u>, and <u>AIIE Transactions</u>.

RELATED TITLES

Published by Praeger Special Studies

HEALTH SERVICES: The Local Perspective
    edited by Arthur Levin, M.D.

THE MANAGERIAL PROCESS IN HUMAN SERVICE AGENCIES
    David W. Young

ORGANIZATION DESIGN FOR PRIMARY HEALTH CARE: The Case of the Dr. Martin Luther King, Jr. Health Center
    Noel M. Tichy